Cardiac Rehabilitation Manual

Josef Niebauer

Editor

Cardiac Rehabilitation Manual

Second Edition

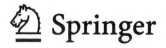 Springer

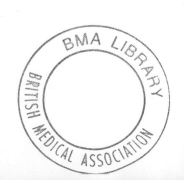

Editor
Josef Niebauer
University Institute of Sports Medicine
Prevention and Rehabilitation
Paracelsus Medical University
Institute of Sports Medicine
of the State of Salzburg
Salzburg
Austria

ISBN 978-3-319-47737-4 ISBN 978-3-319-47738-1 (eBook)
DOI 10.1007/978-3-319-47738-1

Library of Congress Control Number: 2017930674

Printed on acid-free paper

This Springer imprint is published by Springer Nature
The registered company is Springer International Publishing AG
The registered company address is: Gewerbestrasse 11, 6330 Cham, Switzerland

Preface

Secondary Prevention: A Second Chance to Make Inevitable Lifestyle Changes

Cardiac diseases are not only the leading causes of death in industrialized countries but also on the rise in many emerging countries worldwide. They also induce considerable harm to survivors and often lead to severe and irreversible physical and neurological disabilities. Despite the fact that there is no cure, a lot can be done to prevent coronary artery disease, i.e., primary prevention, or to slow the progression of the disease, i.e., secondary prevention. Both can be achieved by tackling the panoply of modifiable risk factors, which have been identified to be amenable to lifestyle changes.

As a matter of fact, according to current guidelines, a long list of risk factors ought to be treated first by lifestyle changes before medical therapy is considered or initiated. These risk factors include:

- Physical inactivity
- Smoking
- Hypercholesterolemia
- Hypertriglyceridemia
- Low HDL cholesterol
- Arterial hypertension
- Hyperglycemia

As an example, physical inactivity has been recognized to be among the strongest predictors of morbidity and mortality for both otherwise healthy persons and already affected patients. Often, however, medical therapy has to be initiated concomitantly to avoid further vascular damage and thus to halt or slow the progression of atherosclerosis. All doctors have received excellent training in choosing the right medication for their patients. We even have sales representatives from companies approach us on a regular basis who further try to provide us with up-to-date – albeit not always unbiased – information. The only effective treatment that no one is offering us or our patients is exercise training. Neither do we receive information on dieting. We, thus, have to set out to try and find current and reliable information ourselves: an obvious deficit that this book is trying to reduce.

At the time that we start medical therapy, we also tell our patients to change their lifestyle.

But what exactly does this mean?

What are the lifestyle changes that they are now being expected to make?

And above all, can we provide our patients with an infrastructure that really helps them to deviate from current unhealthy behavior?

Now it not only becomes very demanding for our patients but also for us, which is why many doctors, as shown in the EUROASPIRE trials, do not even recommend lifestyle changes; many because they lack detailed knowledge on how to implement it. Such training however is a prerequisite in order to convince a patient to say goodbye to many of his or her unhealthy habits. Indeed, the vast majority has been leading an unhealthy lifestyle all their lives and may not wish to change this. Usually, there is a narrow window right after a cardiac event during which patients are amenable to our advice. This is the time to initiate changes that nobody can afford to miss. At the same time, these changes have to be agreed on with a patient who we see as partner on a lifelong journey of lifestyle changes, since otherwise patients may not necessarily stick to their good intentions in the long run. They need encouragement but also an infrastructure that ought to be available to them to actually modify their lifestyle. Indeed, all our countries lack out-patient cardiac rehabilitation facilities that would provide a convenient and adequate infrastructure for our patients to not only initiate but also to provide a base for lifelong compliance with current guidelines. Such facilities have to be close to home, since otherwise it is not possible to attend exercise, nutritional, psychological, and other classes several times a week for an extended period of time. Only then, however, can long-lasting lifestyle changes be introduced into our patients' daily lives. Such facilities are especially warranted for those who want to return to work and wish to be on sick leave for as little as possible.

The network of institutions of ambulatory cardiac rehabilitation facilities has to increase, but also general hospitals have to start to establish ambulatory rehabilitation programs, so that patients get a fair chance to actually change their lifestyle. It is not enough if hospitals only concentrate on revascularizing patients, but do little or nothing to ensure optimal reduction in morbidity and mortality thereafter.

If we fail to do this, then we are in a situation that can be compared to prescribing drugs in a place where there are no drug stores.

But even if we were to get better infrastructure, even then we doctors have to improve our skills. Unfortunately, too few physicians have experience in cardiac rehabilitation, which comes as no surprise as it has never been taught in medical school, internist, or subspecialty training. It is only those of us who have chosen to work in cardiac rehabilitation centers or hospitals who know what to recommend and how to prescribe exercise training and other healthy treatment choices. I am no exception to this rule and had to learn the hard way by initiating training groups in various medical centers, what is best for our patients. Also several of the coauthors not only pursued a career in cardiac rehabilitation but got to where they are by trial and error. It is with this background and understanding that we hope to provide knowledge and advice to those who would like to learn more about cardiac rehabilitation.

After all, it becomes obvious that cardiac rehabilitation has not only come to stay but will become increasingly important, since it is a cost-effective treatment option. As a matter of fact, the number and quality of cardiac rehabilitation programs have to increase, which in turn will require an increasing number of skilled staff. More doctors have to be trained adequately to receive the skills that are required to effectively recommend appropriate measures to patients, let alone to actually guide or accompany them on this lifelong journey. It is thus the aim of this book to provide doctors with in-depth but still hands-on information to quickly grasp the leading problems of our patients and to design or recommend appropriate programs.

In this book, we have refrained from presenting exciting and exotic cases, but rather concentrate on the vast majority of our everyday patients in ambulatory or in-hospital cardiac rehabilitation.

All authors were or still are members of the nucleus of the working group on cardiac prevention and rehabilitation of the European Society of Cardiology. Their expertise not only spans the whole spectrum of cardiac diseases but also contributes various aspects of challenges in cardiac rehabilitation from centers throughout Europe. It is our wish to make a little but significant contribution to further excel the knowledge of our readers by writing this book which at first addresses general issues of cardiac rehabilitation, until it then teaches how to treat patients by focusing on individual patients with specific but very common cardiac conditions.

At first, this book will cover general principals of exercise testing and training as well as nutritional and psychological support. After these fundamentals of cardiac rehabilitation have been laid out in appropriate depths, chapters follow on the most common cardiac diseases. Cases include symptomatic coronary artery disease with or without diabetes, myocardial infarction or revascularization, and cases of heart failure in rather stable conditions, with or without cardiac devices. Our book will then be wrapped up with cardiac rehabilitation in patients with congenital cardiovascular diseases, valvular surgery, and peripheral arterial disease with claudication.

Contents is not presented in textbook style, but rather taught on representative clinical cases. Each chapter focuses on a particular patient and discusses pros and cons of the most appropriate diagnostic tools and treatment options. It is thus designed to be a practical guide for doctors and geared to help them guide their patients. Medical therapy, which most doctors will be very familiar with, has been addressed from the perspective of primary or secondary prevention and is of course in line with current guidelines of our national and international medical societies and associations. A therapeutic option that has long and that still is terribly neglected will receive the attention that it deserves – physical exercise training. Data on reduction of morbidity and mortality but also on improvement in quality of life are so striking that neither we nor our patients can afford to not use this poly-pill. Most of the modifiable risk factors of cardiovascular diseases can be treated by these lifestyle changes. Nevertheless, in the real world, treatment strategies concentrate almost solely on pharmaceutical interventions, neglecting the beneficial effects of heart-healthy diets and exercise training programs. For managing both long- and short-term risk, lifestyle changes are the first-line interventions to reduce the metabolic risk factors. Indeed, the importance of physical activity and heart healthy nutrition cannot be overestimated. This will be highlighted in several chapters. Primary and secondary prevention of cardiovascular diseases need to focus on all modifiable risk factors and implement pharmaceutical therapy wherever appropriate.

Exercise training has to become an integral part of it. It is inacceptable that it is only integrated into the daily routine by a minority of patients. Further cardiac rehabilitation programs have to be installed and doctors need to be trained to be able to refer and treat patients at this stage in their disease history appropriately. We strongly believe that this book will add to the knowledge of our readers and that it will enable them to better guide their patients on a lifelong journey of primary and secondary prevention.

Salzburg, Austria   Josef Niebauer MD, PhD, MBA
January 2017

Contents

Contributors

Paul Bennett, PhD Department of Psychology, University of Swansea, Swansea, UK

Werner Benzer, MD, FESC Outpatient Cardiac Rehabilitation Centre, Cardiac Disease Management Centre, Feldkirch, Austria

J. Berger Rehabilitation and Health Centre, Jesse Hospital, Hasselt, Belgium

Birna Bjarnason-Wehrens Institute for Cardiology and Sports Medicine, German Sportuniversity Cologne, Cologne, Austria

Konrad Brockmeier Department of Peadiatric Cardiology, University of Cologne, Salzburg, Germany

V. Cornelissen Department of Rehabilitation Sciences, Biomedical Sciences, KU Leuven, Leuven, Belgium

Paul Dendale Faculty of Medicine and Life Sciences, Hasselt University, Hasselt, Belgium Department of Cardiology, Jessa Hospital, Hasselt, Belgium Rehabilitation and Health Centre, Jesse Hospital, Hasselt, Belgium

Gernot Diem, MD Clinical Center Bad Hall for Cardiac and Neurological Rehabilitation, Bad Hall, Austria

Sigrid Dordel Institute for Cardiology and Sports Medicine, German Sportuniversity Colgene, Cologne, Germany

Ines Frederix Faculty of Medicine and Life Sciences, Hasselt University, Hasselt, Belgium Department of Cardiology, Jessa Hospital, Hasselt, Belgium Faculty of Medicine and Health Sciences, Antwerp University, Antwerp, Belgium

Helmut Gohlke, FACC, FESC Department of Cardiology II, Herzzentrum Bad Krozingen, Ballrechten-Dottingen, Germany Deutsche Herzstiftung, e.V. Frankfurt, Germany

Gabriel Guşetu, MD, PhD University of Medicine and Pharmacy "Iuliu Haţieganu" Rehabilitation Hospital, Cluj-Napoca, Romania

Martin Halle Department for Prevention, Rehabilitation and Sports Medicine, Munich, Germany

Miguel Mendes Hospital de Santa Cruz/Centro Hospitalar de Lisboa Ocidental, Carnaxide/Lisboa, Portugal

Josef Niebauer, MD, PhD, MBA Institute of Sports Medicine, Prevention and Rehabilitation, Paracelsus Medical University, Institute of Sports Medicine of the State of Salzburg, Sports Medicine of the Olympic, Salzburg, Austria

David Niederseer, MD, PhD, BSc Department of Cardiology, University Heart Center, University Hospital Zurich, Zurich, Switzerland Institute of Sports Medicine, Prevention and Rehabilitation, Paracelsus Medical University, Institute of Sports Medicine of the State of Salzburg, Sports Medicine of the Olympic, Salzburg, Austria

Massimo F. Piepoli Heart Failure Unit, Cardiology, Guglielmo da Saliceto Hospital, Piacenza, Italy

Dana Pop University of Medicine and Pharmacy "Iuliu Haţieganu" Rehabilitation Hospital, Cluj-Napoca, Romania

Sabine Schickendantz Department of Peadiatric Cardiology, University of Cologne, Salzburg, Germany

Jean-Paul Schmid Department of Cardiology, Tiefenau Hospital, Bern, Switzerland

Narayanswami Sreeram Department of Peadiatric Cardiology, University of Cologne, Salzburg, Germany

F. Vandereyt Rehabilitation and Health Centre, Jesse Hospital, Hasselt, Belgium

L. Vanhees Department of Rehabilitation Sciences, Biomedical Sciences, KU Leuven, Leuven, Belgium

Dumitru Zdrenghea University of Medicine and Pharmacy "Iuliu Haţieganu" Rehabilitation Hospital, Cluj-Napoca, Romania

Part I

Introduction to Cardiac Rehabilitation

General Principles of Exercise Testing in Cardiac Rehabilitation

1

Miguel Mendes

1.1 Introduction

Before the admission into a cardiac rehabilitation program (CRP), every patient is submitted to a clinical assessment which must include a medical consultation, an evaluation of LV function (usually by echocardiography), a maximal exercise test (ET) limited by symptoms, and blood tests to evaluate the CVD risk factor profile. In special cases, after the clinical assessment, the patients need further diagnostic tests like a 24 h Holter monitoring, an imaging technique to study perfusion or coronary anatomy or bypass grafting [1–5].

The ET is a very important part of this clinical assessment performed before admission and repeated at the end of the CRP phase, because it gives indispensable data regarding functional capacity and information regarding the hemodynamic adaptation to maximal and submaximal levels of exercise (HR and BP), residual myocardial ischemia, and cardiac arrhythmias induced or worsened by exercise and permits the identification of the training heart rate (THR) for the aerobic training [2–4].

Besides the objective parameters mentioned above, the ET is very important from the psychological point of view for many patients and partners, because they realize that the patient usually has a better functional capacity than they could predict. In the follow-up period, the ET is very useful to detect or confirm eventual clinical status changes which occurred during the program, update exercise prescription intensity, measure the gains obtained after the CRP, and perform global prognostic assessment.

M. Mendes
Hospital de Santa Cruz/Centro Hospitalar de Lisboa Ocidental, Carnaxide/Lisboa, Portugal
e-mail: miguel.mendes.md@gmail.com

© Springer International Publishing AG 2017
J. Niebauer (ed.), *Cardiac Rehabilitation Manual*,
DOI 10.1007/978-3-319-47738-1_1

1.2   What Kind of Exercise Test

Cardiopulmonary exercise test (CPX) is the ideal ET to be used in all kinds of patients in the setting of a CRP [6]. Although it is almost mandatory to use it in heart failure patients [3], due to its higher cost, more complicate delivery, and interpretation, it is usually replaced in many CR centers, mainly in CAD patients with normal or near-normal LV function, by the standard ET which is more widely available and familiar to most cardiologists.

During the CPX, peak VO_2, ventilatory thresholds, VE/VCO_2 slope, and O_2 kinetics are measured beyond all the parameters recorded in the standard ET, like maximal load reached, HR and BP changes from rest to maximal exercise, and, during recovery, the eventual arousal of symptoms like angina pectoris or ECG abnormalities (ST changes or arrhythmias) [7].

Considering the parameters obtained from the CPX, peak VO_2 is the most important because it is the gold standard for functional capacity and it was identified as the strongest prognostic parameter in CVD [8–13]. Peak VO_2 is also very important to prescribe exercise intensity since continuous moderate aerobic training, the classical modality, is performed at a percentage of peak VO_2 ranging from 50 to 70 % [16].

The first and second ventilatory thresholds (VT1 and VT2), which are expected to occur at submaximal level during the CPX, are independent of motivation, contrary to peak VO_2. Due to this fact, they are considered good indicators of the training effect of the program, if they occur at a higher percentage of VO_2 max. The determination of the ventilatory thresholds is also useful to calculate the training intensity for moderate continuous aerobic training, which must start at the HR attained at the level of VT1 and increased to HR reached at the VT2 moment [14, 15].

1.3   How to Perform an ET in the Setting of a CRP

A fully equipped exercise lab test, including at least one ergometer (bike or treadmill), an ECG system with several exercise protocol options, and an emergency cart, together with a well-trained and experienced staff (cardiologist and technician), must be available to perform the exercise tests in the setting of a CRP [7, 17, 18].

After the team welcome of the patient immediately before the ET, he must be asked about his usual exercise tolerance, in order to estimate his maximal functional capacity and to choose the test protocol. The test must be programmed in a way that the patient's physical exhaustion or high-grade fatigue will be attained around 10±2 min of exercise [19]. In case of test interruption before 8 min, a less intense protocol must be used and a steeper one in the reverse situation to evaluate correctly functional capacity.

It's important to rule out a possible recent worsening of clinical status, which may oblige to postpone the test and the interruption of the regular cardiovascular medication before the test. The exercise tests integrated in a CRP must be performed under the patient's usual medication, and one must try to schedule the test for a moment of the day similar to the foreseen moment of the CRP sessions.

The respect of these two issues, medication and moment of the day, will prevent that the drug effect and consequently the patient's protection will be different during

ET and the exercise sessions of the CRP. This is very important, for example, in patients under beta-blockers which are usually taken in the morning and whose effect can decrease during the day, namely, in the afternoon. If the THR was calculated after a test performed at a certain time of the day, it may happen that it will be difficult to reach if the test was performed late in the day and the session is in early morning, where the beta-blocker effect is more intense or will be easily surpassed in late-afternoon exercise sessions if the ET took place in the morning.

The decision to stop exercise during the ET is crucial to quantify exercise tolerance accurately. If no medical contraindications to continue the effort are present, like major ST changes, serious arrhythmias, blood pressure (BP) drop, or hypertensive response, and if the patient seems to be relatively comfortable, the exercise period must be interrupted only upon patient request, based on the perception that he reached his maximal exercise capacity or feels a major discomfort, like claudication, eventually related to peripheral arteriopathy or orthopedic disease [17, 18].

The exercise period must never be stopped based on the attainment of any level of predicted maximal HR, due to the large variability of peak HR among subjects. This procedure, followed in some centers, prevents an accurate quantification of exercise tolerance and maximal HR. When THR is calculated based on the chronotropic reserve, it is crucial to not stop the test without reaching maximal HR because the peak HR may not be the maximal attainable HR during the ET.

After confirming that the patient is in the desired situation in terms of clinical status and medication, it's time to choose the ergometer and the protocol to be used.

If both of the usual possibilities are available (bicycle or treadmill), the choice must be made or performed taking into consideration which ergometer will be more used for aerobic training, the patient's preference, and the clinical staff familiarity.

Regarding the protocol choice, two issues must be considered:

1. The patient's predicted exercise tolerance
2. Type of protocol (ramp type or with small or large increments between stages)

Considering the type of increments of the ET protocol, there is a preference for ramp or short increment (around 1 MET) protocols [20, 21], because the error of the functional capacity estimation will be lower, in the case that respiratory gas analysis will not be performed. The ergometer must also be taken into consideration because the load is more accurately determined on a bike than with the treadmill, since the treadmill calibration is more difficult and especially if the patient grasps the handrails during effort, diminishing the oxygen demand needed to perform the test (Tables 1.1 and 1.2) [7, 17, 18].

Table 1.1 Stationary bike most used protocols [22, 23]

Designation	Load (watts)			Duration (min)		Peak estimated METs
	Start	Increase	Peak	Stage	Total	
Balke (men)	50	25	175	2	12	9.5
Balke (women)	25	25	150	2	12	8.3
Astrand	25	25	150	3	18	8.3

Table 1.2 Treadmill most used protocols [24–26]

Designation	Estimated METs		
	At 8 min	At 9 min	At 12 min
Naughton	4	NA	6
Balke-Ware[a]	5	NA	8
Modified Bruce	NA	7	10
Bruce	NA	10	13

NA not applicable

[a]Usually not acceptable for old people and frail patients, because it has a constant speed (5.47 km/h), which is not tolerated by most patients

1.4   When to Do It

The ET must be performed at the admission of the CRP in the majority of program participants, sometimes in the middle of a phase when it seems that the patient's clinical status changed or THR is inadequate due to the acquisition of a better exercise tolerance as a consequence of exercise training and at the end of each phase to measure the final functional capacity [2, 4, 16].

Patients recently submitted to cardiac surgery are usually admitted in the CRP, without performing an ET, because they may face physical limitations that advise to postpone the test for 2–4 weeks. During these early weeks, the patients are involved in respiratory and global physiotherapy and may even start exercising in a stationary bike or on the treadmill, below a THR of 100 or 120, respectively, if they are or not under β-blocker medication, till they reach a satisfactory exercise tolerance that enables them to be submitted to the ET, after what an individualized THR will be calculated [2].

1.5   How to Report the ET in the Setting of a CRP

A standard ET must be reported not only in terms of the presence or absence of myocardial ischemia but also about enlightening the global prognosis, as it is shown in the Table 1.3.

The test must be reported not only in terms of myocardial ischemia but also on functional capacity, chronotropic index, HR recovery, BP, and ventricular or supraventricular arrhythmias.

Despite having informed the patient at the beginning of the ET about the need to spontaneously report the occurrence of any unexpected symptom, namely, angina or a disproportionate grade of dyspnea or fatigue, it's also advised to ask periodically, for example, at the end of each stage and at the moment of ST depression occurrence, if the patient is experiencing angina and what is his perception of exercise intensity (Borg scale). During the exercise period, it is also recommended to record every minute a full ECG in order to define accurately the eventual moment after which ST segment depression reaches 1 mm and 60 or 80 ms after the J point, the so-called ischemic threshold.

Table 1.3 Parameters to describe in the ET report in the CR setting [18, 27]

1. *Exercise capacity*
   (a) Test duration and reason to stop the exercise
   (b) In a classical ET, estimate exercise tolerance, as ratio between the achieved and the predicted METs, calculated by the following equations:
      (i) Men: Predicted METs = $14.7 - 0.11 \times$ age
      (ii) Women: Predicted METs = $14.7 - 0.13 \times$ age
   (c) In a CPX, measure exercise tolerance and use Weber classification and percentage of predicted VO_2 max
   Classify functional capacity below normal if lower than 85 % of the predicted value

2. *Heart rate*
   HR at rest, at the end of each stage, at the moment of the ischemic threshold, ventricular or supraventricular arrhythmias starting, abnormal BP (drop or hypertensive response) at peak exercise and in recovery at 1, 3, and 6 min
   Classify chronotropic evolution during exercise as:
      Normal, if peak HR value is above 85 % of the predicted value (220 bpm minus age), for individuals not under β-blocker or above 62 % under β-blocker
      Abnormal, if below the mentioned values
   Classify chronotropic evolution during recovery as
      Normal, if HR difference between peak exercise and min 1 > 12 on protocols where there is an active recovery (slow walking or pedaling) or >18 bpm, if exercise is immediately stopped at peak effort
      Abnormal, if below the mentioned values

3. *Blood pressure*
   Classify blood pressure evolution as
      Normal, if SBP increases ~10 mmHg per MET and there is no change or a small drop is found in DBP. It's acceptable to find a drop <15 mmHg at peak exercise
      Hypertensive, if SBP reaches values >250 or >DBP 120 mmHg
      Insufficient, if SBP increases <30 mmHg

4. *Ischemia*
   Classify the test as *negative, positive, equivocal,* or *inconclusive* for myocardial ischemia, taking into consideration the presence or absence of angina or ST depression/elevation induced during the test, in the exercise or the recovery period, according to the criteria defined in the guidelines
   Use the ST/HR index, the ST rate-recovery loops, and/or the ST/HR slope to increase the accuracy of the diagnosis of ischemia
   Grade ischemia as severe, moderate, or low level, taking into consideration the precocity of appearance, magnitude of ST changes, time until normalization in the recovery period, association with limiting angina, BP fall, chronotropic deficit, or ventricular arrhythmias
   Identify clearly the HR of the ischemic threshold, because the THR to be observed during the exercise sessions must be 10 bpm below this value for safety reasons

5. *Prognosis*
   Assess globally the prognosis, considering functional capacity, ST/HR index, chronotropic response, HR recovery, ventricular ectopy during recovery, and ST/HR slope, which are implicated in global and cardiovascular mortality and events

6. *Aerobic training intensity*
   Classically, THR is calculated as the HR at (50), 60–70 % of HR reserve or (50), or the HR reached at 60–70 % of VO_2 reserve or at HR of the VAT level, respectively, if the patient was submitted to a standard ET or to a CPX [16]

(continued)

Table 1.3 (continued)

More recently, important changes in terms of determination of THR occurred, due to the adoption of new modalities of exercise training like high-intensity exercise training (HIIT) and to the change of concept of the submaximal exercise thresholds. Today, the concept of only one threshold, previously called ventilatory anaerobic threshold (VAT), was abandoned, and it was adopted the concept of two submaximal thresholds, the first and the second ventilatory thresholds identified, respectively, by the nadir of the curves of the O_2 and VCO_2 equivalents [14, 15]

In the case of continuous moderate aerobic training, exercise training must start at the level of HR attained by the subject at the level of the first ventilatory threshold (LVT1) and move till the HR attained at the level of the second ventilatory (LVT2)

After the seminal paper of Wisloff [28] and coworkers, a new paradigm emerged: HIIT. In this case, exercise intensity is prescribed at up to 95 % of HR attained during the ET for periods of 4 min, intercalated by 3 min periods of not so intense training at 50–75 % of peak exercise

Ischemia is diagnosed by the occurrence of angina and/or definitive ST changes on the exercise or in the recovery period. In order to increase the diagnostic accuracy of the ET, ST changes must be interpreted considering ST/HR index, which must be superior to 1.6 µV/bpm, and rate-recovery loops that are suggestive of myocardial ischemia if there is a counterclockwise rate-recovery loop.

Functional capacity is probably the most important finding after an ET as it is the best parameter to predict all-cause mortality. When peak VO_2 is not measured, it can be estimated by the ratio between the estimated METs achieved at the last stage of the ET and the predicted value given by the following formula: Predicted METs = 14.7–0.11 × age or 14.7–0.13 × age, respectively, for men and women. To allocate the estimated METs of a stage, the patients must exercise at least 1 min at that stage. If he was not able to do it, his maximal METs attained will be the ones estimated for the previous completed stage.

The Duke score tries to put together the presence/absence of ischemia and functional capacity and classifies the patients in low, intermediate, and high categories of risk, according to the value of the score.

Chronotropic index, HR recovery, and ventricular arrhythmias predict increased/decreased risk of death if they are negative or positive.

1.6 How to Assess Exercise Training with a Standard ET or a CPX

At the end of a CRP phase, the ET or the CPX must be repeated to be compared with the test performed at the phase start, in order to document eventual gains provided by the program.

These gains must be observed in terms of maximal and submaximal functional capacity, ischemic threshold, exercise-induced or exercise-worsened arrhythmias, heart rate, and blood pressure evolution during the exercise and the recovery periods [2, 6, 16].

To make a correct comparison between both tests, they must be performed under the same medication, at the same time of the day, and using the same ergometer and protocol. If any revascularization procedure, like a PCI, is performed, the medication is changed between the tests, or if the ergometer or the protocols are also different, a direct comparison of both tests is impossible.

1.6.1 Standard ET

If exercise training is successful, the standard ET will usually show in the second test:

(a) Higher duration/load attained
(b) Lower levels of HR and BP at each stage and an early normalization of HR during recovery
(c) Starting of ischemia later during the test, although at the same or higher double product
(d) Lower frequency and complexity of ventricular arrhythmias, in the exercise or recovery periods

Functional capacity can be estimated for each patient in terms of METs (metabolic units of oxygen consumption: 1 MET = 3.5 ml/kg/min) considering the oxygen consumption previously known to be inherent to the highest stage attained at peak exercise, if the patient was able to keep this stage more than 1 min. If the test was stopped before staying 1 min or more in the last stage, the attributed estimated METS must be those predicted for the previous completed, since usually it takes, at least, 1 min to stabilize oxygen consumption in each exercise protocol stage.

Functional capacity must also be classified regarding the predicted values for the same age, gender, and physical activity status, provided by several equations.

The maximal load reached by the patients can also be considered as a measure of functional capacity, especially when a stationary bike is used. In a treadmill, due to the body weight dislocation effect and the walking, the peak load values are less accurate.

The estimation of aerobic capacity by the standard ET is not very accurate, since it usually overestimates the load, namely, in the case of patients and old people and when treadmill protocols with high increment protocols are used, like the Bruce protocol.

1.6.2 Cardiopulmonary Exercise Test

The CPX allows the best identification of maximal aerobic capacity because peak VO_2, the gold standard for exercise capacity, is directly measured "breath by breath" during the entire test. Due to some variability, the values should be determined by calculating the rolling average of each period of 20–30 s [29].

Peak VO_2 is the most used parameter to evaluate the CRP benefit. In case of doubt that the CPX is a maximal test, one must specially look at VO_2, HR, and

Table 1.4 How to assess the training effect with an exercise test [7, 17, 18]

Standard ET	Cardiopulmonary exercise test
Test duration, maximal load, and estimated METs	The same parameters as in standard ET, plus:
Presence or absence of ischemia	Peak VO_2
HR at rest, at each stage, at peak exercise, and on recovery	VO2 and HR at VAT
Blood pressure at rest, at each stage, at peak exercise, and on recovery	O_2 kinetics in the recovery period
Ischemic threshold: HR, double product, and load	Peak RER
Grade of myocardial ischemia, in terms of ST normalization, ST depression morphology	VE and breathing reserve
Ventricular arrhythmias	VE/VCO_2 slope

respiratory exchange ratio (RER) and RPE at peak exercise level. VO_2 and/or HR must fail to increase significantly despite load further increments; RER and RPE must be, respectively, equal or over 1.10 and 8/10 at peak [30].

Recently, the terminology of the events observed at submaximal level during a CPX was changed. Now, two thresholds are recognized instead of the only one, the formerly designed ventilatory anaerobic threshold (VAT), presently called the first VT (VT1). Also, the formerly designated respiratory compensation point is called now the second ventilatory threshold. These thresholds are defined, respectively, as the nadir points of the curves of the O_2 and CO_2 equivalents, which have a U shape form during the exercise period. These equivalents are, respectively, the ratios of O_2 and CO_2/ventilation [14, 15].

VT1, formerly designated by VAT, can also be calculated by the V slope method and defines the end of the period where exercise intensity is not perceived by the individual as difficult to be performed. Between VT1 and VT2, exercise intensity is perceived as moderate and after surpassing VT2 as very intense and difficult to maintain for a few minutes.

To overcome the limitations of peak VO_2, the VO_2 attained at the VT1 can be used to evaluate the training effect, because it is independent of patient motivation and expresses better the patient capacity to perform daily life activities.

In cardiac patients, peak VO_2 and VO_2 at the VT1 increase between 7 and 54 % after a period of some weeks of exercise training, although the average increase is usually around 20–30 % [31–33].

VE/VCO_2 slope, which evaluates ventilatory efficiency, one of the most important parameters for prognosis assessment in CHF, is also expected to decrease as a demonstration of a favorable exercise training period (Table 1.4) [34, 36].

Compare pre- and post-exercise tests, performed at the same time of the day, under the same medication and protocol.

1.7   Clinical Cases

Case #1

Male, 41 years old

Apparently healthy till 20th of April 2009 when he suffered an anterior myocardial infarction. Tobacco smoking, obesity, and psychological stress were identified as risk factors for CVD in this case: he smoked one pack a day during 25 years and has a BMI of 30.6 (99 kg of weight and 180 cm height). His BP, blood cholesterol, and glucose levels were normal.

He was submitted to primary PCI of LAD (middle portion) that was totally occluded by a thrombus. The PCI was performed within 2 h of symptoms and was very successful, with the exception of the occurrence of a right thigh hematoma related to the femoral puncture, which obliged him to rest in bed for a week. No other lesions were found in the coronary arteries, and LV function was near normal.

He was discharged from the hospital on the fifth day after ACS under ASA, clopidogrel, ramipril (2.5 mg, od), bisoprolol (2.5 mg, od), and pravastatin (40 mg, od).

When he started to go out of bed and to move around 1 week after hospital discharge, he felt dizziness, nausea, and a thoracic discomfort, different from the one that arose during the ACS, which stopped immediately when he lay down. No pericardial effusion was found on echocardiography. After this he took the initiative to contact our CRP 3 weeks after the ACS.

After a medical consultation and physical examination, where everything seemed to be OK, he was submitted to an ET (Table 1.5; Fig. 1.1).

Table 1.5 Exercise test parameters (case #1)

Stage	Speed km/h	Grade %	METs	HR bpm	SBP mmHg	DBP mmHg	Symptoms	ECG
Rest	0	0	1	75	130	80	No	T wave inversion V1-V4
I	2.7	10	4.6	98	150	80	No	Almost normal
II	4.0	12	7.0	117	175	90	Mild fatigue	Normal
III	5.4	14	10.0	138	200	100	Moderate fatigue	Normal
IV	6.7	16	12.5	150	210	100	Severe fatigue	Normal
Exercise duration: 10 min 20 s								
Rec. 1'	1.5	0		132	200	90	No	Normal
Rec. 3'	0	0		104	190	90	No	Normal
Rec. 6'	0	0		95	170	85	No	Normal

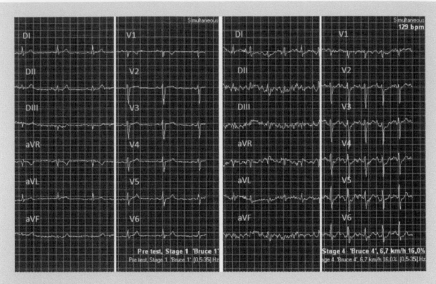

Fig. 1.1 Rest and peak exercise 12-lead ECG (case #1)

Comments ET#1

Confronting the findings of this ET with what is supposed to be found in a normal ET, this patient shows:

1. Good exercise tolerance: 10–20 min exercise duration on the Bruce protocol ~12.5 METs (122 % of the predicted).
2. Normal evolution of HR: from 75 to 150 bpm at peak effort and a drop of 18 bpm on the first minute of an active recovery.
3. Normal increase of SBP: from 130/80 at rest to 210/100 at peak exercise.
4. Hypertensive pattern on DBP: increase from 80 to 100 mmHg
5. No arrhythmias, ST changes, and angina were found.
6. The normalization during the exercise period of the T wave previously present in the rest ECG suggests the presence of stunned myocardium.

Comments

This is a typical case of a low-risk patient for CR, with normal LV ejection fraction, no residual ischemia, no arrhythmias, good exercise tolerance, and a normal adaptation of hemodynamic parameters to maximal exercise.

He was admitted to a formal CRP under medical supervision during some weeks, since he was wishing to start an exercise program and he didn't had any previous physical activity habits.

A THR of 120 bpm was calculated using the Karvonen formula, adding 60 % of his HR reserve [(150 − 75)*0.60 = 45 bpm] to his rest HR (75 bpm): 45 + 75 = 120 bpm [31–34].

Case #2

Male, 54 years old

CVD risk factors: Type 2 diabetes and hypertension.

Assessment performed before admission to CRP on the 4th of October 2004, following a noncomplicated CABG on the 11th of July 2004 and a previous inferior myocardial infarction in an indeterminate date.

He was submitted to complete revascularization, by a triple CABG with LIMA to LAD and single saphenous grafts to the second diagonal and posterior descendent arteries. Three months after surgery, a nuclear perfusion scan requested for routine clinical assessment and identified residual silent ischemia in the inferior wall (Fig. 1.2).

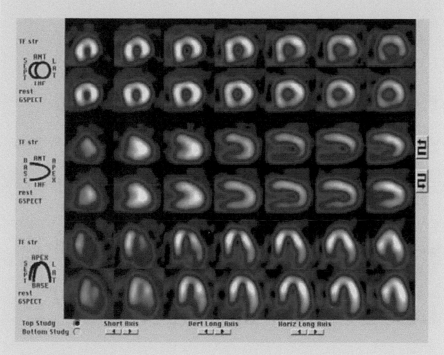

Fig. 1.2 Myocardial nuclear perfusion scan (case #2)

After this test, he was re-submitted to coronary angiography, and it was found that the graft to the posterior descendent artery was occluded and the artery was not amenable to PCI. He had good collateral circulation from the left coronary artery, and the other bypasses were patent, with normal flow. His attending cardiologist decided to keep him on medical therapy and send him to CR.

Before the CRP, he was submitted to an ET, under his usual medication: bisoprolol (5 mg, od), IMN (50 mg, od), losartan (50 mg, od), enalapril (20 mg, od), HCTZ

Table 1.6 Admission exercise test (case #2)

Stage	Speed Km/h	Grade %	METs	HR bpm	SBP mmHg	DBP mmHg	Symptoms	ECG
Rest	0	0	1	59	130	80	No	Q waves on DII, DIII, and aVF
I	2.7	10	4.6	113	150	80	No	No change
II	4.0	12	7.0	131	170	80	Intense fatigue	ST downslope of 1 mm in V5-V6
Exercise duration, 6 min 00 sec; onset of ischemia, at 4 min 00 s with 123 bpm								
Rec. 1'	1.5	0	1	112	140	80	No	ST downslope of 1 mm in V5-V6
Rec. 3'	0	0	1	90	130	80	No	ST downslope of 1 mm in V5-V6
Rec. 6'	0	0	1	82	120	75	No	ST downslope of 1 mm in V5-V6
Rec. 9'	0	0	1	79	120	80	No	Equal to rest ECG

Table 1.7 End of CRP exercise test (case #2)

Stage	Speed Km/h	Grade %	METs	HR bpm	SBP mmHg	DBP mmHg	Symptoms	ECG
Rest	0	0	1	68	120	90	No	Inferior Q waves
I	2.7	10	4.6	91	160	80	No	No change
II	4.0	12	7.0	103	170	80	No	No change
III	5.4	14	10.0	125	190	80	Mild fatigue	ST downslope of 1 mm in V5-V6
IV	6.7	16	12.5	142	190	80	Intense fatigue	ST downslope of 1 mm in V5-V6
Exercise duration, 10 min 00 s; onset of ischemia, at 10 min 00 s of exercise with 123 bpm								
Rec. 1'	1.5	0	1	123	190	80	No	ST downslope of 1 mm in V5-V6
Rec. 3'	0	0	1	95	180	80	No	ST downslope of 1 mm in V5-V6
Rec. 6'	0	0	1	88	130	80	No	ST downslope of 1 mm in V5-V6
Rec. 9'	0	0	1	80	120	75	No	Equal to the rest ECG

(12.5 mg, od), simvastatin (20 mg, od), ASA (100 mg, od), and two oral antidiabetic drugs (Table 1.6).

After 12 weeks of CRP, he was reassessed by a new ET, under the same protocol (Bruce) and medication (Table 1.7).

Comments

First test:

The patient had residual ischemia with a moderate compromise of functional capacity (7 estimated METs). He was admitted to the CRP, with a THR of 100 bpm, calculated with the Karvonen formula, adding 60 % of his HRR to the rest HR: $[(131–59) \times 0.60] = (43+59) = 102 \sim 100$ bpm. If the calculated value for THR would be superior or equal to the HR of the ischemia threshold, the THR would be assigned to a HR 10 bpm lower than the HR of the ischemic threshold that would be around 110–115 bpm.

He didn't complain about any symptom during the program and he progressed very well.

Second test:

The second test was performed immediately at the end of the program. It shows a very good evolution [35]:

1. Better functional capacity (12.5 vs 7.0 estimated METs).
2. Lower values of HR at each stage of the protocol, with silent ischemia appearing almost at the same HR value, although much later in the ET. Although some references show that ischemic threshold can appear at a higher HR and double product after exercise training, in this case, like in the majority of the published articles, only a delayed appearance of the threshold was found.
3. Higher HR and BP values at peak exercise.

Case #3

Male, 64 years old, asymptomatic, submitted to ET on the 3rd of December 2009, 5 days after inferior STEMI

Risk factors: dyslipidemia, hypertension, smoking, and family history of CVD below 60 years.

Medication: aspirin, clopidogrel, ß-blocker, ACE inhibitor, and statin.

Baseline ECG: sinus rhythm and Q waves on inferior leads.

Coronary angiography: LM lesion <50 %. RCA occlusion at the middle segment with retrograde filling from the left coronary. No significant lesions were found on LAD and circumflex arteries (Table 1.8; Figs. 1.3 and 1.4).

Table 1.8 Admission exercise test (case #3)

Exercise data								
Stage	Speed Km/h	Grade %	METs	HR bpm	SBP mmHg	DBP mmHg	Symptoms	ST-T changes
Rest	0	0	1	75	120	60	None	
I	2.7	10	4.6	111	150	80	Fatigue	ST depression: 1.0 mm
II	4	12	7	113	150	80	Fatigue, not-limiting angina	ST depression: 1.5 mm

Test stopped at 3 min and 33 s of Bruce protocol due to fatigue:				
Stage	HR bpm	SBP mmHg	DBP mmHg	Symptoms	ST-T changes
Rec. 1'	102	150	80	None	ST depression: 1.5 mm
Rec. 3'	90	140	80	None	ST depression: 1.5 mm
Rec. 6'	78	120	70	None	ST depression: 1 mm
Rec. 9'	81	120	70	None	Absent

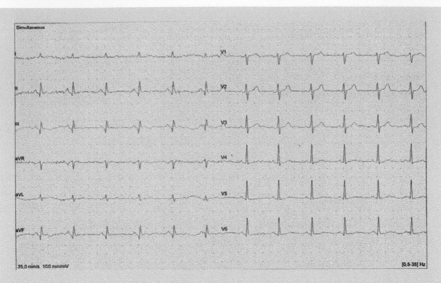

Fig. 1.3 Rest 12-lead ECG (case #3)

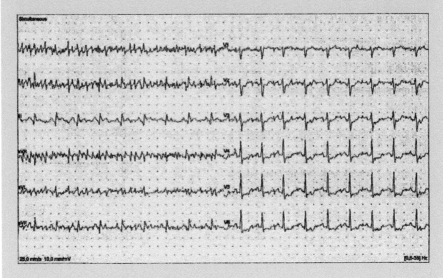

Fig. 1.4 Peak exercise 12-lead ECG (case #3)

1.8   Summary

METS = 4.6 (59 % of the predicted)
  Peak HR: 113 ppm = 72 % predicted HR
  % HR reserve use: 72.4 % (abnormal if ≤62 %)
  HR decay in the first minute of recovery: 11 bpm (abnormal ≤12 ppm)
  Peak double product = 16,950
  ST changes: Horizontal downslope ST segment depression starting at 3 min of
the exercise, with maximal amplitude of 1.5 mm in V4, V5, and V6. ST depression
normalized at 9 min of recovery, after sublingual TNG at 6 min
  Arrhythmias: absent

Conclusions
  1. Moderate exercise tolerance limitation (<5 METs)
  2. Myocardial ischemia starting at low exercise level (Table 1.9)

Table 1.9   Risk classification grades of exercise training for cardiovascular patients

Risk	Low stable conditions	Moderate	High unstable conditions
Decision regarding patient admission in the CRP	Accept	Decide case by case	Consider to reject or return to referral MD for stabilization
Type of CRP team	Basic experience	Advanced experience	
Individualized exercise prescription	Yes	Yes	Exercise training recommended only in few specific situations
Session supervision	Nonmedical personnel with advanced cardiac life support	Medical and nonmedical with advanced cardiac life support, until safety apparently guaranteed	As in moderate-risk patients
ECG and BP monitoring	6–12 sessions	≥12 sessions	≥12 sessions
NYHA	I or II	III	IV
Exercise capacity	≥7 METs	<5 METs	<5 METs
Myocardial ischemia	Absent or ≥7 METs	<7 METs	<5 METs
Ejection fraction	≥50 %	40–49 %	<40 %
Rise of BP and HR	Appropriate	Appropriate	Fall or non-increase of SBP or HR during exercise
VT at rest or during exercise	Absent		Complex arrhythmias
Self-monitoring	Able	Some difficulties	Unable

Adapted from Refs. [2, 14]

Fig. 1.5 Left main IVUS
(case #3)

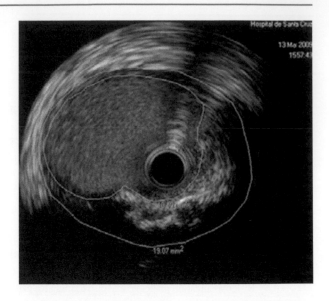

Comments

The patient was not accepted in the CRP, since he had myocardial ischemia starting below 5 METs, a contraindication for CRP admission.

This patient's myocardial ischemia must be considered serious, since it starts at low level of exercise, is associated with angina (although non-limiting), and is normalized only at 9 min in the recovery period after a sublingual TNG.

He was submitted to a new coronary angiography where IVUS was performed. The LM lesion, with an area of 10.4 mm^2 and a plaque burden of 47 % on IVUS, was considered as nonsignificant (Fig. 1.5), but a lesion of 70 % of the first marginal obtuse was defined as the lesion responsible for the ischemia. This lesion was submitted successfully to PCI with DES implantation.

He was reevaluated and admitted in the CRP 1 week later, after being submitted to a new ET that showed good exercise tolerance (9 min on Bruce protocol) and no residual ischemia.

Case #4

Male, 64 years old

Patient with an ischemic cardiomyopathy (ejection fraction of 28 %) in NYHA class III, after an anterior STEMI occurred 6 years before the clinical assessment for the CRP in February 2016.

He was submitted to primary PCI on his proximal LAD. No residual ischemia was diagnosed in a myocardial perfusion scan although several lesions on the right coronary artery were found. Moderate pulmonary hypertension and mitral and tricuspid regurgitation were present. An ICD was implanted 3 years before based on a primary prevention strategy. Cardiovascular risk factors: type 1 diabetes mellitus, former heavy smoker (quit smoking 30 years ago).

Current medication: bisoprolol, ivabradine, lisinopril, furosemide, simvastatin, ezetimibe, insulin, metformin, sitagliptin, and clopidogrel.

The ECG showed sinus rhythm and slow progression of R waves from V1 to V5.

Before admission he was submitted to a treadmill CPX under a ramp protocol (speed, from 2 to 5 km/h; grade, from 0 to 20 %; increments every 15 s; ECG recording and BP measurement every 2 min during exercise and on min 1 and 3 of the recovery period (Table 1.10).

Table 1.10 CPX parameters of case #4

	Rest	VT1	VT2	End of exercise
Time (min)	01:52	4:20	6:40	9:03
Ex Time (min)	00:00	02:20	4:40	7:03
Vt BTPS (L)	0.86	0.93	1.23	1.62
RR (br/min)	24.5	27.9	27.6	35.7
VE BTPS (L/min)	21.0	26.0	34.0	58.0
VO_2 (mL/kg/min)	7.1	8.7	10.4	11.7
VO_2 (mL/min)	524	641	773	864
VCO_2 (mL/min)	420	541	752	1073
RER	0.80	0.85	0.97	1.24
HR (BPM)	70	79	86	93
VO_2/HR (mL/beat)	7.5	8.1	9.0	9.3
VE/VO_2	34.0	35.4	40.4	62.9
VE/VCO_2	42.4	41.9	41.4	50.6
$P_{ET}CO_2$ (kPa)	4.11	4.17	4.04	3.33

Stage	HR	SBP	DBP	Borg scale	ST-T changes
Rest	70	85	60	6	Q waves V1 to V5
Min 2	84	90	60	10	
Min 4	84	90	60	14	
Min 6	91	130	80	16	
Min 7:09	90	135	90	18	No ST changes
Exercise duration: 7:09 min					
Rec. 1 min	71	70	40	16	
Rec. 3 min	68	80	55	12	

Exercise duration: 7:03 min	*Stop exercise due to:* exhaustion
Peak HR: 91 bpm (58 % of predicted maximal HR)	*HR decay peak – recovery min 1:* 22 bpm
Chronotropism: limited even for a patient under β-blocker	
Delta SBP = 15 mmHg	*Double product* = 9100
ST-T changes: none	*Arrhythmias*: none

Comments

The patient demonstrated a severe compromise of exercise tolerance: peak VO_2 is 11.7 ml/kg/min (41 % of the predicted value) being classified as Weber class C

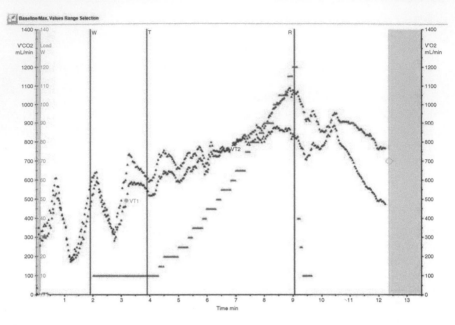

Fig. 1.6 VO$_2$ uptake and VCO$_2$ output (case #4)

(>10<16 ml/kg/min). The VO$_2$ at VT1 is 8.7 ml/kg/min, which is 30 % of the predicted VO$_2$ maximum and 74 % of the reached peak VO$_2$, confirming a severe exercise limitation.

Although his VO$_2$ max is still over 10 ml/kg/min, all the other three bad prognosis criteria mentioned by Guazzi and coworkers [13] are found: a VE/VCO$_2$ slope of 46, exercise oscillatory ventilation, and P$_{ET}$CO$_2$ non-increase.

The patient was considered to be in the gray zone for heart transplantation, and it was decided to enroll him into CR in order to find if it is possible to improve his condition with the exercise program, the drug therapy optimization, and the adoption of a healthy lifestyle.

It was discussed to prescribe him a high-intensity interval training similar to the one of Wisloff and coworkers [29], alternating 4 min bouts of high-intensity exercise at 90–95 % of peak heart rate with 3 min active pauses at 50–75 % of peak HR or to a moderate continuous aerobic program starting at the HR met at VT1 (79 bpm) and moving to the HR found at VT2 (86 bpm) with the progression of the training effect.

Due to the superior results found with the U. Wisloff method and to the clinical situation of the patient, it was decided to submit him to this kind of training program (Figs. 1.6, 1.7, and 1.8).

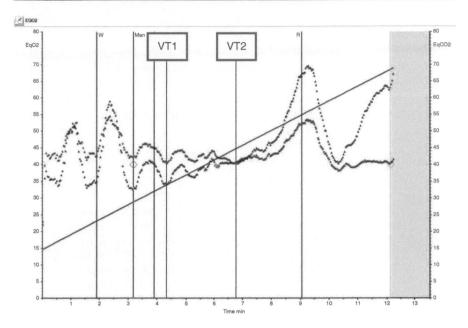

Fig. 1.7   Ventilatory thresholds: VT1 and VT2 (case #4)

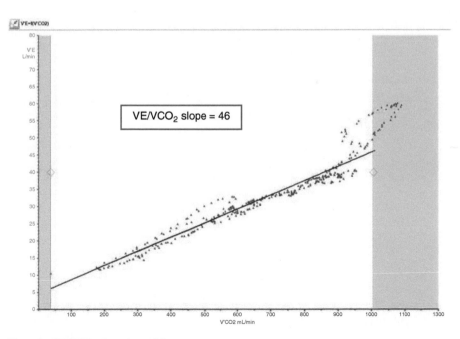

Fig. 1.8   VE/VCO$_2$ slope (case #4)

Case #5

Male, 53 years old, submitted to CPX in June 2007, after heart transplant performed in July 2006. No symptoms under tacrolimus, MMF, pravastatin, and amiodarone.

Despite being asymptomatic, he contacted the rehab center to increase his physical fitness, because he wished to compete in the World Games for transplanted people (Tables 1.11 and 1.12; Figs. 1.9, 1.10, 1.11 and 1.12).

Table 1.11 Admission CPX parameters (case #4)

Treadmill CPX under a modified Bruce protocol:

Stage	HR	SBP	DBP	Borg scale	ST-T changes
Rest	107	130	90	6	No ST-T changes
I	108	130	90	8	No ST-T changes
II	114	155	80	10	No ST-T changes
III	127	155	80	12	No ST-T changes
IV	138	170	70	13	No ST-T changes
V	151	180	70	15	No ST-T changes
VI	158	180	70	17	No ST-T changes
Rec. 1'	157	170	60	14	No ST-T changes
Rec. 3'	150	150	70	10	No ST-T changes

Exercise duration: 17:34 min	*Stop exercise due to*: exhaustion
Peak HR: 159 bpm = 96 % predicted maximal HR	*HR decay: peak – recovery min 1*: 1 bpm
Chronotropism: typical of heart transplant	
Peak BP: 180 mmHg/70 mmHg	*Double product* = 28,620
Delta SBP = 50 mmHg	
ST-T changes: no changes	*Arrhythmias*: None

Table 1.12 CPX parameters (case #5)

	Rest	VT1	Peak VO_2	Pred
Time (min)	02:01	11:38	18:37	
Ex Time (min)	00:00	09:35	16:34	
Vt BTPS (L)	0.62	1.77	2.1	
RR (br/min)	19	31	39	
VE BTPS (L/min)	11.9	54.6	80.9	134
VO_2 (mL/kg/min)	5.2	25.4	30.5	34.5
VO_2 (mL/min)	351	1731	2131	2344
VCO_2 (mL/min)	276	1699	2277	2836
RER	0.79	0.98	1.11	
METS	1.5	7.3	9.0	9.9
HR (BPM)	102	129	156	167
VO_2/HR (mL/beat)	3	13	14	14
VE/VO_2	34	32	37	40
VE/VCO_2	43	32	35	33

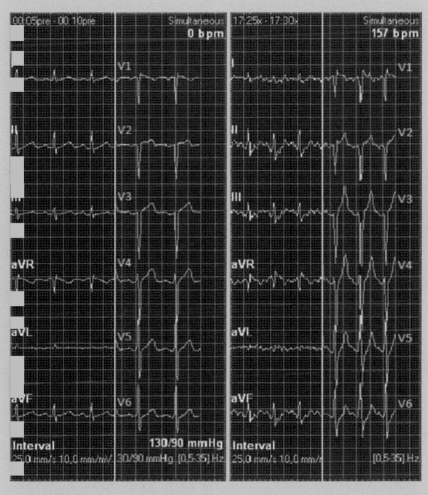

Fig. 1.9 Comparison of rest and peak exercise ECG of case #5

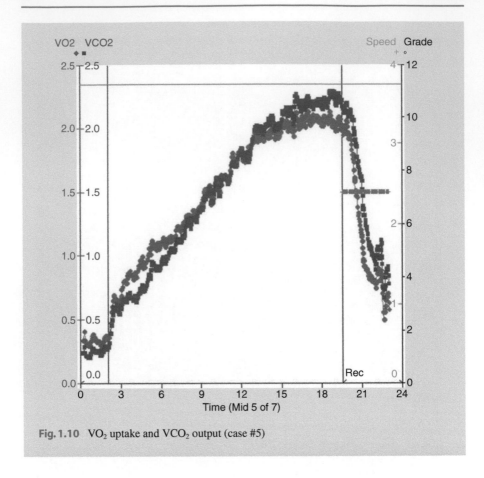

Fig. 1.10 VO$_2$ uptake and VCO$_2$ output (case #5)

Comments

This patient has a good exercise tolerance, confirmed by a near normal peak VO$_2$ (88 % of the predicted value), although he has an abnormal evolution of the HR during the exercise and recovery period. His HR curve is typical of a transplanted heart, with a high HR at rest and a slower and lower increase during effort than what is found in normal individuals.

In the transplanted heart, the linear relationship of VO$_2$ and HR is lost. In this case exercise intensity can't be prescribed by the usual Karvonen formula or the VO$_2$ reserve, and it will be prescribed by the rate of perceived exertion (RPE).

Considering the grades of RPE described by the patient during the CPX exercise period, the load which provoked a RPE of 12 must be selected for the training intensity at the beginning of the program and will be periodically increased till a RPE of 14.

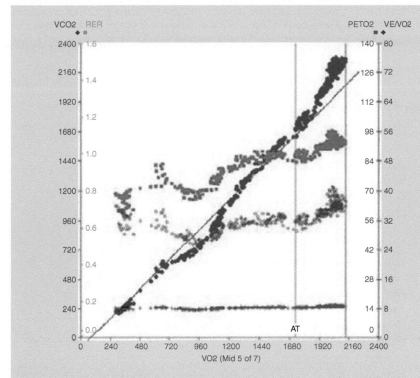

Fig. 1.11   First threshold/VT1 – V slope method (case #5)

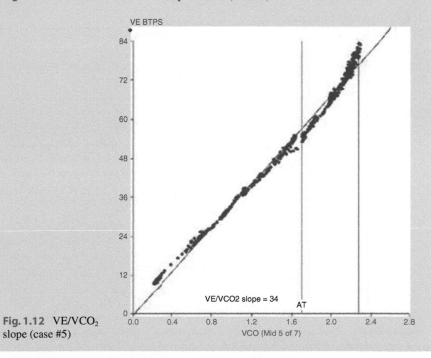

Fig. 1.12   VE/VCO$_2$ slope (case #5)

Acknowledgments I express my gratitude to my colleagues from Instituto do Coração and Hospital de Santa Cruz (Carnaxide/Portugal), António Ventosa and Frederik AA de Jonge, for allowing the publication of the nuclear scintigraphy image of case #2 and to Luís Raposo for the IVUS image on case #3.

Glossary

BMS	Bare metal stent
BP	Blood pressure
bpm	Beats per minute
CAD	Coronary artery disease
CHF	Congestive heart failure
CPX	Cardiopulmonary exercise test
CR	Cardiac rehabilitation
CRP	Cardiac rehabilitation program
CVD	Cardiovascular disease
ECG	Electrocardiogram
ET	Exercise test
HR	Heart rate
HRR	Heart rate reserve
LV	Left ventricle
MET	Metabolic unit
RPE	Rate of perceived exertion
THR	Training heart rate
VAT	Ventilatory anaerobic threshold
VT1	First ventilatory threshold
VT2	Second ventilatory threshold

References

1. Giannuzzi P, Mezzani A, Saner H, Björnstad H, Fioretti P, Mendes M, Cohen-Solal A, Dugmore L, Hambrecht R, Hellemans I, McGee H, Perk J, Vanhees L, Veress G, Working Group on Cardiac Rehabilitation and Exercise Physiology European Society of Cardiology. Physical activity for primary and secondary prevention. Position paper of the Working Group on Cardiac Rehabilitation and Exercise Physiology of the European Society of Cardiology. Eur J Cardiovasc Prev Rehabil. 2003;10:319–27.
2. American Association for Cardiovascular and Pulmonary Rehabilitation. Guidelines for cardiac rehabilitation and secondary prevention programs. 4th ed. Champaign: Human Kinetics Publishers; 2004.
3. Corrà U, Giannuzzi P, Adamopoulos S, Bjornstad H, Bjarnason-Weherns B, Cohen-Solal A, Dugmore D, Fioretti P, Gaita D, Hambrecht R, Hellermans I, McGee H, Mendes M, Perk J, Saner H, Vanhees L; Working Group on Cardiac Rehabilitation and Exercise Physiology of the European Society of Cardiology. Executive summary of the position paper of the Working Group on Cardiac Rehabilitation and Exercise Physiology of the European Society of Cardiology (ESC): core components of cardiac rehabilitation in chronic heart failure. Eur J Cardiovasc Prev Rehabil 2005;12:321–325.

4. Balady GJ, Williams MA, Ades PA, Bittner V, Comoss P, Foody JM, Franklin B, Sanderson B, Southard D. Core components of cardiac rehabilitation/secondary prevention programs: 2007 update: a scientific statement from the American Heart Association Exercise, Cardiac Rehabilitation, and Prevention Committee, the Council on Clinical Cardiology; the Councils on Cardiovascular Nursing, Epidemiology and Prevention, and Nutrition, Physical Activity, and Metabolism; and the American Association of Cardiovascular and Pulmonary Rehabilitation. Circulation. 2007;115:2675–82.
5. Wenger NK. Current status of cardiac rehabilitation. J Am Coll Cardiol. 2008;51:1619–31.
6. Mezzani A, Agostoni P, Cohen-Solal A, Corra U, Jegier A, Kouidi E, Mazic S, Meurin P, Piepoli M, Simon A, Laethem V, Christophe, Vanhees L. Standards for the use of cardiopulmonary exercise testing for the functional evaluation of cardiac patients: a report from the Exercise Physiology Section of the European Association of Cardiovascular Prevention and Rehabilitation. Eur J Cardiovasc Prev Rehabil. 2009;16:249–67.
7. Myers J, Arena R, Franklin B, Pina I, Kraus WE, McInnis K, Balady GJ, on behalf of the American Heart Association Committee on Exercise, Cardiac Rehabilitation and Prevention of the Council on Clinical Cardiology, the Council on Nutrition, Physical Activity and Metabolism, and the Council on Cardiovascular Nursing. Recommendations for Clinical Exercise Laboratories: A Scientific Statement from the American Heart Association. Circulation. 2009;119:3144–61.
8. Prakash M, Myers J, Froelicher VF, Marcus R, Do D, Kalisetti D, Atwood JE. Clinical and exercise test predictors of all-cause mortality: results from > 6,000 consecutive referred male patients. Chest. 2001;120:1003–13.
9. Myers J, Prakash M, Froelicher V, Do D, Partington S, Atwood JE. Exercise capacity and mortality among men referred for exercise testing. N Engl J Med. 2002;346:793–801.
10. Ghayoumi A, Raxwal V, Cho S, Myers J, Chun S, Froelicher VF. Prognostic value of exercise tests in male veterans with chronic coronary artery disease. J Cardpulm Rehabil. 2002;22: 399–407.
11. Kokkinos P, Myers J, Kokkinos JP, Pittaras A, Narayan P, Manolis A, Karasik P, Greenberg M, Papademetriou V, Singh S. Exercise capacity and mortality in black and white men. Circulation. 2008;117:614–22.
12. Kodama S, Saito K, Tanaka S, Maki M, Yachi Y, Asumi M, Sugawara A, Totsuka K, Shimano H, Ohashi Y, Yamada N, Sone H. Cardiorespiratory fitness as a quantitative predictor of all-cause mortality and cardiovascular events in healthy men and women. A meta-analysis. JAMA. 2009;301:2024–35.
13. Guazzi M, Adams V, Conraads V, Halle M, Mezzani A, Vanhees L, Arena R, Fletcher GF, Forman DE, Kitzman DW, Lavie CJ, Myers J. EACPR/AHA Joint Scientific Statement. Clinical recommendations for cardiopulmonary exercise testing data assessment in specific patient populations. Eur Heart J. 2012;33:2917–27.
14. Carvalho VO, Mezzani A. Aerobic exercise training intensity in patients with chronic heart failure: principles of assessment and prescription. Eur J Cardiovasc Prev Rehabil. 2011;18:5–14.
15. Mezzani A, Hamm LF, Jones AM, McBride PE, Moholdt T, Stone JA, Urhausen A, Williams MA, European Association for Cardiovascular Prevention and Rehabilitation; American Association of Cardiovascular and Pulmonary Rehabilitation; Canadian Association of Cardiac Rehabilitation. Aerobic exercise intensity assessment and prescription in cardiac rehabilitation: a joint position statement of the European Association for Cardiovascular Prevention and Rehabilitation, the American Association of Cardiovascular and Pulmonary Rehabilitation and the Canadian Association of Cardiac Rehabilitation. Eur J Prev Cardiol. 2013;20:442–67.
16. Fletcher GF, Balady GJ, Amsterdam EA, Chaitman B, Eckel R, Fleg J, Froelicher VF, Leon AS, Piña IL, Rodney R, Simons-Morton DA, Williams MA, Bazzarre T. Exercise standards for testing and training: a statement for healthcare professionals from the American Heart Association. Circulation. 2001;104:1694–740.
17. Gibbons RJ, Balady GJ, Timothy BJ, Chaitman BR, Fletcher GF, Froelicher VF, Mark DB, McCallister BD, Mooss AN, O'Reilly MG, Winters WL, Gibbons RJ, Antman EM, Alpert

JS, Faxon DP, Fuster V, Gregoratos G, Hiratzka LF, Jacobs AK, Russell RO, SC S. ACC/ AHA 2002 guideline update for exercise testing: summary article: a report of the American College of Cardiology/American Heart Association Task Force on practice guidelines (committee to update the 1997 exercise testing guidelines). J Am Coll Cardiol. 2002;40:1531–40.

18. Smokler PE, MacAlpin RN, Alvaro A, Kattus AA. Reproducibility of a multi-stage near maximal treadmill test for exercise tolerance in angina pectoris. Circulation. 1973;48:346–51.

19. Kaminsky LA, Whaley MH. Evaluation of a new standardized ramp protocol: the BSU/Bruce Ramp protocol. J Cardpulm Rehabil. 1998;18:438–44.

20. Davis JA, Whipp BJ, Lamarra N, Huntsman DJ, Frank MH, Wasserman K. Effect of ramp slope on determination of aerobic parameters form the ramp exercise test. Med Sci Sports Exerc. 1982;14:339–43.

21. Balke B, Nagle F, Baptista G. Compatibiliy of progressive treadmill, bicycle and step test based on oxygen uptake responses. Med Sci Sports. 1971;3:149.

22. Astrand PO, Rodahl K. Textbook of work physiology. 2nd ed. New York: McGraw Hill; 1977.

23. Patterson JA, Naughton J, Pietras RJ, Gumar RN. Treadmill exercise in assessment of patients with cardiac disease. Am J Cardiol. 1972;30:757–62.

24. Balke B, Ware R. An experimental study of physical fitness of air force personnel. U S Armed Forces Med J. 1959;10:675–88.

25. Bruce RA. Exercise testing of patients with coronary heart disease. Ann Clin Res. 1971;3:323–30.

26. Kligfield P, MS L. Exercise electorcardiogram testing: beyond the ST segment. Circulation. 2006;114:2070–82.

27. Wisløff U, Støylen A, Loennechen JP, Bruvold M, Rognmo Ø, Haram PM, Tjønna AE, Helgerud J, Slørdahl SA, Lee SJ, Videm V, Bye A, Smith GL, Najjar SM, Ellingsen Ø, Skjaerpe T. Superior cardiovascular effect of aerobic interval training versus moderate continuous training in heart failure patients: a randomized study. Circulation. 2007;115: 3086–94.

28. Myers J, Walsh D, Sullivan M, Froelicher VF. Effect of sampling on variation and plateau in oxygen uptake. J Appl Physiol. 1990;68:404–10.

29. Howley ET, Basset Jr DR, Welch HG. Criteria for maximal oxygen uptake: review and commentary. Med Sci Sports Exerc. 1995;27:1292–301.

30. Thompson PD, Buchner D, Piña IL, Balady GJ, Williams MA, Marcus BH, Berra K, Blair SN, Costa F, Franklin B, Fletcher GF, Gordon NF, Pate RR, Rodriguez BL, Yancey AK, Wenger NK. Exercise and physical activity in the prevention and treatment of atherosclerotic cardiovascular disease: a statement from the Council on Clinical Cardiology (Subcommittee on Exercise, Rehabilitation, and Prevention) and the Council on Nutrition, Physical Activity, and Metabolism (Subcommittee on Physical Activity). Circulation. 2003;107:3109–16.

31. O'Connor CM, Whellan DJ, Lee KL, Keteyian SJ, Cooper LS, Ellis SJ, Leifer ES, Kraus WE, Kitzman DW, Blumenthal JA, Rendall DS, Miller NH, Fleg JL, Schulman KA, McKelvie RS, Zannad F, Piña IL, for the HF-ACTION Investigators. Efficacy and safety of exercise training in patients with chronic heart failure: HF-ACTION randomized controlled trial. JAMA. 2009;301:1439–14.

32. Myers J, Hadley D, Oswald U, Bruner K, Kottman W, Hsu L, Dubach P. Effects of exercise training on heart rate recovery in patients with chronic heart failure. Am Heart J. 2007;153:1056–63.

33. Arena R, Myers J, Abella J, Peberdy MA, Bensimhon D, Chase P, Guazzi M. Development of a ventilatory classification system in patients with heart failure. Circulation. 2007;115: 2410–7.

34. Franklin BA, Whaley MH, Howley ET. General principles of exercise prescription. In: Franklin BA, Whaley MH, Howley ET, editors. ACSM's guidelines for exercise testing and prescription. Philadelphia: Lippincott Williams & Wilkins; 2000. p. 137–64.

35. Meyer T, Gabriel HHW, Kindermann W. Is determination of exercise intensities as percentages of VO2max or HRmax adequate? Med Sci Sports Exerc. 1999;31:1342–5.
36. Jones AM, Carter H. The effects of endurance training on parameters of aerobic fitness. Sports Med. 2000;29:373–86.

General Principles of Nutrition Support in Cardiac Rehabilitation

2

Helmut Gohlke

This chapter will review epidemiologic studies, prospective observational cohort studies, and metabolic and clinical interventional studies that guide our recommendation for the best possible nutrition in patients at risk for or with established cardiovascular disease. This includes quantitative and qualitative aspects of nutrition as well as of drinks.

The type of nutrition is one of the important factors that contribute to the development of cardiovascular disease. The way we eat is part of our lifestyle and poor dietary habits and physical inactivity together contribute to 15 % of the causes of death in the general population [99, 103, 153], whereas a low-risk diet with low-risk lifestyle habits has a protective effect [2, 168].

A diet with a low proportion of fruits and vegetables contributes to more than a quarter of the population attributable fraction of coronary artery disease and strokes [39]. Accordingly dietary recommendations are a key element in the management of patients with cardiovascular disease. More and more studies indicate that certain dietary patterns can influence cardiovascular health by modifying risk factors such as obesity, dyslipidemia, and hypertension as well as factors involved in systemic inflammation, insulin sensitivity, oxidative stress, endothelial function, thrombosis, and cardiac rhythm. A diet favorable for cardiovascular prevention can also reduce the risk of cancer substantially. Although the interventional database for dietary endpoint studies in primary as well as in secondary prevention is far from satisfactory, it is highly plausible that the type of nutrition will maintain its importance after a cardiovascular event has occurred. This is supported by the large international

H. Gohlke, FACC, FESC
Department of Cardiology II, Herzzentrum Bad Krozingen, Neue Kirchstrasse 22, D-79282
Ballrechten-Dottingen, Germany
Board member, Deutsche Herzstiftung, e.V. Frankfurt, Germany
e-mail: h.gohlke@t-online.de

© Springer International Publishing AG 2017
J. Niebauer (ed.), *Cardiac Rehabilitation Manual*,
DOI 10.1007/978-3-319-47738-1_2

study performed in 41 countries, the "Organization to Assess Strategies in Acute Ischemic Syndromes 5" (OASIS 5) randomized clinical trial. Compliance after formal dietary counseling in this group of patients with acute ischemic syndrome was associated with an odds ratio for myocardial infarction, stroke, or death of 0.85 (95 % CI, 0.73–0.99; $P = 0.03$) although the details on the nature of the dietary advice or intensity of the program attended were not recorded. The compliance after exercise counseling resulted in a similar odds ratio. However patients who were adherent to both diet and exercise advice had an odds ratio of 0.52 (95 % CI, 0.38–0.57; $P < 0.0001$) indicating that behavioral modification should be given priority similar to other preventive medications immediately after acute coronary syndrome and that dietary counseling is an important component of it and apparently has a greater effect than in the general population [16].

2.1 Overweight and Obesity as Risk Factors for Heart Disease

The relationship between body size and body weight is expressed in the body mass index (BMI), calculated as weight in kilograms divided by the square of height in meters. A BMI of 18.5–25 kg/m^2 is regarded as normal weight, 25–29.9 kg/m^2 is generally referred to as "overweight," and a BMI of $\geq$ 30 kg/m^2 as "obesity." Only a third of the population in Europe or in the United States has a desirable BMI of less than 25 kg/m^2 [42, 44, 167].

Overweight and obesity have increased globally, with only some regions experiencing stabilization of the average body mass index (BMI) [42, 132]. In 2010, elevated BMI accounted for about 2.8 million deaths each year, and diet-related risk factors (e.g., low fruit consumption and high sodium intake) and physical inactivity accounted for 10 % of global disability-adjusted life years [89, 90]

There is a dichotomy of individual versus environmental drivers of obesity, and although people bear personal responsibility for their health, environmental factors can readily support or undermine the ability of people to act in their own self-interest [132]. Social networks play an important role, and the distribution of obesity in the society resembles the spread of an infection [17].

To evaluate the importance of overweight and obesity for life expectancy, more than one million adults in the United States were analyzed in a prospective study, with more than 200,000 deaths occurring during 14 years of follow-up. The relationship between BMI and the risk of death from all causes in four subgroups categorized according to smoking status and history of disease was examined. The most favorable BMI range in healthy male never-smokers with respect to prognosis was between 23.5 and 24.9 kg/m^2 and in females between 22.0 and 23.4 kg/m^2 [13]. A collaborative analysis of 57 prospective studies with 900,000 persons came to similar conclusions of an apparent optimum of the BMI between 22.5 and 25 kg/m^2 [167].

The database was used to assess the relative risk between BMI and mortality. To avoid confounding, Cox models were used for exact age at enrollment, level of education and physical activity, alcohol use, marital status, current use of aspirin, a crude index of fat consumption, vegetable consumption, and (in women) the use of estrogen replacement therapy.

Among subjects with the highest BMI (>40 kg/m^2), white men and women had a relative risk of death of 2.58 and 2.00, respectively, compared with those with a BMI of 23.5–24.9 kg/m^2. A high BMI was most predictive of death from CVD, especially in men. Heavier white men and women in all age groups had an increased risk of death. In black men and women, however, with the highest BMI, the risk of death was not significantly increased. A 35-year-old Caucasian man with a BMI of over 35 kg/m^2 has a loss of life expectancy of 10 years [44, 124]. Weight gain during adulthood is also a strong and independent risk factor for premature cardiovascular death [13]. There was also a significant increase in the risk of cancer with obesity in general and at multiple individual sites [14].

Obesity with a BMI of more than 30.0 kg/m^2 favors the early development of atherosclerosis, type 2 diabetes, hypertension, coronary artery disease, acute coronary syndromes, left atrial fibrosis with atrial fibrillation, and heart failure and shortens life expectancy [7, 95].

Reports on a so-called obesity paradox [87] that showed a lower mortality of overweight persons versus "normal weight" persons are largely due to the fact that the definition of "normal" weight extends at the lower end to a BMI of 18.5 kg/m^2. The mortality below a BMI of 21 kg/m^2 increases rather steeply. Because BMI is in itself a strong predictor of overall mortality both above and below the apparent optimum of about 22.5–25 kg/m^2 [167], it is debatable whether a lower limit of "normal weight" of 18.5 kg/m^2 or rather a lower limit of 21 kg/m^2 would be more appropriate.

A long-term goal-directed weight management in an atrial fibrillation (AF) cohort showed in a long-term follow-up study that sustained weight loss was associated with a significant reduction of AF burden and maintenance of sinus rhythm. Weight loss of >10 % resulted in a significant sixfold greater probability of arrhythmia-free survival compared with two other groups who achieved less or no significant weight loss. Weight fluctuation >5 % partially offset this benefit, with an increased risk of arrhythmia recurrence [123].

Long-standing obesity alters also myocardial structure and conduction properties not only in the left atrium but also in areas near the scar after myocardial infarction [128].

In patients with established coronary disease, obesity was associated with major adverse cardiovascular events (MACE) after adjusting for significant confounders in men but not in women. Further categorization of BMI showed a J-shaped association between BMI and MACE in men, and no association in women [13].

In a study examining obesity and age at a first non-ST-segment elevation myocardial infarction (NSTEMI) in more than 110,000 patients, there was a strong, inverse linear relationship between BMI and earlier age of first NSTEMI [94]. The mean patient ages (±SD) of first NSTEMI were 74.6 ± 14.3 years for the leanest (BMI < 18.5 kg/m^2) and 58.7 ± 12.5 years for the most obese (BMI > 40.0 kg/m^2) cohorts, respectively ($p < 0.0001$). In several studies, obese patients with acute coronary syndrome had a more favorable course after an event; however the event had occurred 7 years earlier compared to nonobese individuals [12]; in a patient group after STEMI, no significant advantage was seen for the obese, but again the event occurred at a 5-year younger age [3].

The progressive excess mortality above the BMI range of 22.5–25 kg/m² is mainly due to vascular disease and is probably largely causal. At 30–35 kg/m², median survival is reduced by 2–4 years; at 40–45 kg/m², it is reduced by 8–10 years. Body mass index at ages 30–49 years predicted mortality after ages 50–69 years [124].

The increased risk for CHD through excess body weight may be mediated in most population-based studies partly through its impact on individual risk factors such as hypertension, diabetes, and dyslipidemia [167]. Obesity however also results in reduced nitric oxide bioavailability, increased vascular tone, arterial stiffening, increased systolic and pulse pressures, and an overall atherogenic vascular phenotype.

Additional independent mechanisms may include chronic oxidative stress, local activation of the renin–angiotensin system, and a low-grade inflammatory state; the latter two may have their origin in the abdominal visceral fatty tissue [53].

2.1.1 Abdominal Obesity

An increased waist circumference has been recognized as an additional – possibly independent – risk factor for myocardial infarction and may be present despite a normal BMI.

In the European Prospective Investigation into Cancer and Nutrition (EPIC) study [129], waist circumference was measured either at the narrowest circumference of the torso or at the midpoint between the lower ribs and the iliac crest [160]. Hip circumference was measured horizontally at the level of the largest lateral extension of the hips or over the buttocks.

The association of body mass index (BMI), waist circumference, and waist-to-hip ratio with the risk of death was examined among more than 350,000 European subjects who had no major chronic diseases. General as well as abdominal adiposity were associated with the risk of death. The data support the use of waist circumference or waist-to-hip ratio in addition to BMI for assessment of the risk of death, particularly among persons with a lower BMI [129].

The risk for metabolic diseases is increased with a waist circumference of greater than 80 cm in women and 94 cm in men. Persons with abdominal obesity (the android pattern) are in a proinflammatory, prodiabetic, and prothrombogenic state. Visceral fatty tissue has been recognized as an active endocrine organ playing a central role in lipid and glucose metabolism. It produces a large number of hormones and cytokines involved in the development of metabolic syndrome, diabetes mellitus, and vascular diseases [53], whereas weight reduction and increasing physical activity improve the adipose tissue function.

2.1.2 Caloric Restriction

Increasing evidence from laboratory animals indicates that caloric restriction profoundly affects the physiological and pathophysiological alterations associated with aging and markedly increases life span in several species, including mammals. Although the ability of caloric restriction to prolong the life span in humans has not been demonstrated conclusively, it now seems plausible that caloric restriction may attenuate visceral fat accumulation and counteract the deleterious aspects of obesity. The cardioprotective effects of short-term caloric restriction are probably mediated by increased production of adiponectin and the associated activation of AMP-activated protein kinase [145].

Caloric restriction has also cardiac-specific effects that ameliorate aging-associated changes in diastolic cardiac function. These beneficial effects on cardiac function might be mediated by the effect of caloric restriction on blood pressure, systemic inflammation, and myocardial fibrosis.

Prolonged caloric restriction in obese type 2 diabetes patients decreases BMI and improves glucoregulation associated with decreased myocardial triglyceride content and improved diastolic heart function [54].

2.1.3 Weight Reduction

If weight reduction is intended, the daily caloric intake should be reduced by 500–800 Kcal, and physical activity should be increased [123]. Mediterranean and low-carbohydrate diets are effective alternatives to low-fat diets [141]. In a recent trial in moderately obese subjects, the low-carbohydrate diet had more favorable effects on lipids, and the Mediterranean diet leads to a better glycemic control which suggests that personal preferences and metabolic considerations allow individualized tailoring of dietary interventions. The mean weight loss over 2 years was between 3.3 and 5.5 kg with a plateau reached after 1 year suggesting that the lifestyle modification was difficult to maintain or intensify [136].

Diet-induced weight reduction over 2 years may reverse to some degree the atherosclerotic process; weight reduction was associated with a significant regression of measurable carotid vascular wall volume in a three-dimensional echo study. The effect was similar in low-fat, Mediterranean, or low-carbohydrate strategies and correlated with the weight loss-induced decline in blood pressure [142].

In an observational dietary study, increases in the consumption of potato chips, potatoes, sugar-sweetened beverages, unprocessed red meats, and processed meats were factors associated with weight gains. Associations with weight loss were seen for increased consumption of vegetables, whole grains, fruits, nuts, and yogurt. For each of these dietary factors, the weight change with increased consumption was the inverse of that with decreased consumption. Thus, less weight gain occurred with decreased consumption of potato chips, processed meats, sugar-sweetened beverages, potatoes, or trans fat, and more weight gain occurred with decreased consumption of vegetables, whole grains, fruits, nuts, or yogurt [108].

In an overweight cohort of patients with atrial fibrillation, a structured motivational and goal-directed program was able to achieve a more than 10 % weight reduction in more than a third of the participants. The program included dietary advice and a low to moderate exercise program using face-to-face counseling and repeated follow-up counseling depending on the progress of weight reduction. The program also achieved a reduction of the atrial fibrillation burden [123].

How the dietary modification and caloric restriction can be implemented in individual overweight or obese patients remains an unresolved problem, the discussion of which exceeds the scope of this chapter. A recent trial compared five ways of providing support for lifestyle modification. High-frequency telephone contact with a dietitian led to the same weight loss as a frequent personal contact and more weight loss than with low-frequency contact or e-mail contact or no contact at all [29].

The findings illustrate that a frequent contact is necessary to keep up the motivation for healthy lifestyle changes in patients trying to lose weight.

A comparison of weight loss diets with different compositions of fat, protein, and carbohydrates showed that the average weight loss over 2 years was similar (about 4 kg) in the low-fat average-protein group, in low-fat high-protein group, in high-fat average-protein group, and in the high-fat high-protein group and was altogether somewhat disappointing. Thus the composition of the diet was of less importance than the attendance of the participants in the weight counseling sessions. Behavioral factors and motivation for change appear to be of greater importance for weight loss than macronutrient composition of the diet [136].

It has been suggested that an individual approach to the societal problem of obesity is bound to fail, because obesity is favored by societal conditions [72, 133].

Network phenomena appear to be relevant to the biological and behavioral trait of obesity, and obesity appears to spread through social ties. The distribution of overweight in the community bears similarities to the spread of an infectious disease reflecting these social ties. These findings have implications for clinical and public health intervention [17].

The increasing prevalence of overweight in our communities is a threat particularly to the health of the children in our society. Communities have to get engaged to achieve a beneficial impact [83], and early results of such endeavors appear promising [129, 133].

A general lack of exercise is certainly one important component of this problem. The average American man is spending in his free time 3.05 h in front of the TV set and the average woman 2.61 h, i.e., [11]. Television viewing and low participation in vigorous recreation are independently associated with obesity and markers of cardiovascular disease risk [65], cardiovascular events, and all-cause mortality [150].

2.2   Individual Components of the Diet

Several individual components of the diet are of particular metabolic importance, although for the patient a dietary pattern (see below Sect. 2.3) rather than picking individual components should guide the eating habits.

2.2.1   Cardiovascular Risk Associated with Intake of Total Fats, Saturated and Unsaturated Fats

The consumption of fat as a risk-modifying factor has been debated since the early results of the Seven Countries Study. Probably the largest and most detailed analyses of the effects of fat consumption were performed in the Nurses' Health Study and the Health Professionals Follow-Up Study; in 2005 in an observational study of 14 years among more than 80,000 women in the Nurses' Health Study cohort [119], higher intakes of trans fat and, to a smaller extent, saturated fat were associated with increased risk, whereas higher intakes of non-hydrogenated polyunsaturated fatty acids (PUFAs) and monounsaturated fatty acids (MUFAs) and olive oil were associated with decreased risk. Probably because of opposing effects of different types of fat, total fat as percentage of energy was not appreciably associated with CHD risk [118]. Ten years later in a follow-up of the observational study of 83,349 women (Nurses' Health Study, 1980–2012), and of 42,884 men (Health Professionals Follow-Up Study, 1986–2012), an update on the ingestion of saturated and unsaturated fats and the use of whole grain and refined carbohydrates on CV risk were reported [166]. Replacing 5 % of energy intake from saturated fats with equivalent energy intake from PUFA and MUFA was associated with a 27 % (HR, 0.73; 95 % CI, 0.70–0.77) and 13 % (HR, 0.87; 95 % CI, 0.82–0.93) lower risk respectively $p < 0.001$; intake of ω-6 PUFA, especially linoleic acid, was inversely associated with mortality owing to most major causes, whereas marine ω-3 PUFA intake was associated with a modestly lower total mortality (HR comparing extreme quintiles, 0.96; 95 % CI, 0.93–1.00; $P = .002$ for trend). In an earlier study in this population [89], replacement with carbohydrates from whole grains was associated with a 9 % lower risk of CHD (HR, 0.91; 95 % CI, 0.85–0.98; $p = 0.01$), whereas replacing saturated fats with carbohydrates from refined starches/added sugars was not significantly associated with CHD risk reduction ($p > 0.10$). Fat and carbohydrate consumption has therefore to be looked at in a more differentiated manner.

From the preventive aspect, saturated fatty acids and trans-fatty acids should be reduced and replaced by PUFAs, MUFAs, or carbohydrates from whole grains.

Trans-fatty acids are of greater importance in the United States and are associated with a markedly increased risk for CHD [155].

In the Nurses' Health Study, the quartile of women with the highest erythrocyte trans fat content – as a validated indicator of trans fat consumption – had a relative risk of 3.3 for CHD after adjustment for the usual risk factors [119]. As compared with the consumption of an equivalent amount of calories from saturated or cis-unsaturated fats, the consumption of trans-fatty acids raises levels of low-density lipoprotein (LDL) cholesterol, reduces levels of high-density lipoprotein (HDL) cholesterol, and increases the ratio of total cholesterol to HDL cholesterol, a powerful predictor of the risk of CHD. Trans fats also increase the blood levels of triglycerides as compared with the intake of other fats, increase levels of Lp(a) lipoprotein, and reduce the particle size of LDL cholesterol, all of which are considered unfavorable for the CHD risk [105].

Industrial trans-fatty acids are considered as so important in the United States that the FDA has required that nutrition labels for all conventional foods and supplements must indicate the content of trans-fatty acids, and their use was prohibited in the state of New York in 2007 [120]. Also in Denmark the content of trans fats in foods has to be below 2 %.

The consumption of saturated fatty acids decreases the anti-inflammatory activity of HDL and inhibits endothelial function, whereas the consumption of polyunsaturated fatty acids improves the anti-inflammatory activity of HDL and endothelial function [116].

In the observational LURIC study of patients undergoing coronary angiography in Germany, the level of the naturally occurring trans-fatty acid (TFA C16:1n-7t) in dairy products was associated with reduced risk, whereas no increased risk was found for the low levels of industrially produced trans-fatty acids observed in this patient group [76]. Dairy products are listed on the protective side in a review on components of a cardioprotective diet [107]; this would support the idea that the differentiation between naturally occurring and industrially produced trans-fatty acids is of importance.

A breakfast rich in saturated fats increases the cardiovascular reaction in response to psychological stress in healthy young adults, whereas the addition of walnuts to a fat-rich meal improves acutely the flow-dependent endothelial dilatation [66].

The predominant consumption of a Western diet characterized by frequent use of red and processed meat, fried foods, soft drinks, and refined cereal products and a low consumption of fruits, vegetables, fish, and whole grain products is associated with an increased rate of the metabolic syndrome, whereas dairy consumption provides some protection. Also the consumption of a Mediterranean diet enriched with 30 g mixed nuts per day has beneficial effects on several cardiovascular risk factors [37] and decreased the prevalence of a metabolic syndrome compared with a low-fat control diet [139]; in addition this diet reduced the risk for cardiovascular events [38].

2.2.1.1 Cholesterol and Eggs

Elevated serum LDL cholesterol levels are an established risk factor for cardiovascular disease, and lowering of serum LDL cholesterol levels decreases the risk of cardiovascular disease in persons at increased risk [15]. However the assessment whether consumption of food items with high cholesterol content has a significant impact on serum cholesterol levels has undergone major changes during recent years. The American Heart Association (AHA) recommended in 1961 that people reduce cholesterol consumption, and eventually the AHA suggested a limit of

300 mg of cholesterol consumption per day because it was assumed that the total amount of cholesterol ingested would increase the serum cholesterol levels [50]. Egg consumption is one of the main sources of dietary cholesterol. The yolk of a single egg contains about 200 mg of cholesterol. Accordingly the recommendation of the AHA was for decades that the consumption of eggs should be limited to ≤2 egg yolks per week [50].

In the Nurses' Health Study and in the Health Professionals Follow-Up Study, daily consumption of >1 egg per day was however associated only in diabetic persons with a 100 % increase of the coronary heart disease incidence in men and a 50 % increase of coronary heart disease incidence in women compared to those who ate less than 1 egg per week [62]. In the Physicians' Health Study I, egg consumption of ≥1 per day was associated with an increased risk of heart failure among US male physicians [33].

On the basis of two meta-analyses [18, 60], an increase of daily dietary cholesterol intake by 100 mg would increase plasma total cholesterol by 2.2–2.5 mg/dl, LDL cholesterol by 1.9 mg/dl, and HDL cholesterol by 0.4 mg/dl. In addition, some cholesterol feeding studies observed that dietary cholesterol intake had little effect on the change in the ratio of LDL to HDL cholesterol. Furthermore the association between dietary cholesterol intake and risk of CVD remains unclear.

A more recent meta-analysis for the risk of CVD with respect to egg consumption based on 345,000 male and female individuals with a wide age range (20–90 years) and an average of 11.3 years of follow-up came to the conclusion that those who ate 1 egg per day or more compared with those who ate less than one egg per week were 42 % more likely to develop type 2 diabetes mellitus. Among diabetic patients, frequent egg consumers were 69 % more likely to suffer a CVD comorbidity [144]. There appears to be heterogeneity of risk in different regions of the world [34, 164]. When stratified by geographic area, there was a 39 % higher risk of diabetes (95 % CI, 21 %, 60 %) comparing the highest with the lowest egg consumption in US studies and no elevated risk of DM with egg intake in non-US studies from Europe and Japan ($P < 0.001$ when comparing US with non-US studies). The explanation for this heterogeneity is not obvious, but frequent consumption of eggs with processed meats and/or bacon that has been shown to be associated with a higher risk of diabetes could provide an alternative explanation for observed elevated risk of DM with >3 eggs/week in the United States [34]. In a smaller cross-sectional study of more than 1200 consecutive patients in Canada (mean age 61.5 years, 47 % women, 13 % with diabetes) who were referred to vascular prevention clinics, patients who ate <2 eggs/week had significantly less carotid plaque than those who ate three or more eggs per week [148].

Considering the above-cited meta-analysis of observational studies or cross-sectional studies, the 2014 AHA/ACC guideline on lifestyle management [36] concluded (correctly) that there is insufficient evidence to determine whether lowering dietary cholesterol consumption reduces LDL cholesterol in the blood and influences prognosis – a major change of the position the AHA had held for the last 50 years; the US Department of Health and Human Services stated in the Scientific Report of the 2015 Dietary Guidelines – consistent with the conclusions of the AHA/ACC report [36] – that "cholesterol is not a nutrient of concern for overconsumption" [161]. The lack of evidence from randomized controlled interventional trials [55] for the recommendations in the previous dietary fat guidelines introduced in 1977 and 1983, by the US and UK governments, respectively, was probably the reason for giving up this recommendation and possibly opening the way for new studies. (Of course it is worth to remember that the absence of proof is not the proof of absence). The AHA guidelines emphasize instead to reduce the consumption of saturated fats and of trans fats in the diet which is more effective in lowering of cholesterol levels compared to lowering cholesterol intake [36].

What conclusions can be drawn from these conflicting data and statements for patients with coronary disease? Diabetics are considered to be at a high risk for cardiovascular events [63, 122, 127, 140], and from the meta-analysis of observational studies, we can assume that diabetics with higher egg consumption are at a higher risk for CVD than diabetics who consume less eggs [144] at least in the United States [34]; therefore in the absence of randomized interventional studies, it appears reasonable that diabetics should limit their egg consumption. Patients with established cardiovascular disease are considered as very high risk for future cardiovascular events – higher than diabetics without cardiovascular disease. Therefore it appears – again despite the absence of randomized studies – in view of the recent large meta-analysis with long follow-up of observational studies [144] also reasonable that patients with cardiovascular disease should, like diabetic patients, limit the consumption of eggs and cholesterol in their diet. But the observational database with respect to egg consumption is heterogeneous and leaves room for individual decisions in Europe as well as in the United States.

2.2.1.2 Rapeseed Oil and Olive Oil

Rapeseed oil (canola oil) has been used in the Lyon Diet Heart Study which resulted in a reduction of cardiovascular events in patients after myocardial infarction [26].

Olive oil has been associated with longevity and good cardiovascular health since the Seven Countries Study and is an essential part of the Mediterranean diet. Olive oil also contains aside from monounsaturated oleic acid micronutrients like phenolic components, which have antioxidative, anti-inflammatory, and antithrombotic properties. The long-term consumption of olive oil improves endothelial function in persons with hypercholesterolemia, decreases oxidability of LDL cholesterol in vitro, and increases the antioxidative capacity of human plasma [37]. The latter can be shown after only short-term intake of olive oil; the higher the polyphenol content of the olive oil, the stronger the increase in HDL, the decrease of the total cholesterol/HDL cholesterol ratio, and the decrease of the oxidative stress indicators [22]. The ratio of monounsaturated to saturated fatty acids in the diet is of prognostic importance. The German, the European, and the US American cardiac societies consider olive oil as a favorable component of the diet. The PREDIMED study showed in a randomized trial that among persons at high cardiovascular risk, a Mediterranean diet supplemented with extra-virgin olive oil or nuts reduced the incidence of major cardiovascular events [38].

2.2.1.3 Omega-6 [n-6] Fatty Acids

Dietary recommendations for omega-6 polyunsaturated fatty acids (PUFAs) traditionally focused on the prevention of essential fatty acid deficiency [56]. Linoleic acid is the predominant n-6 PUFA in the Western diet and primarily from vegetable oils (e.g., sunflower, safflower, soya, rapeseed, and corn) and nuts. Temporarily n-6 PUFAs were also seen as competitors for n-3 PUFAs whose benefit in reducing CV disease appeared well established. In a review of prospective observational studies on the effects of dietary linoleic acid on the risk of coronary heart disease, a 5 % increment of energy in linoleic acid intake replacing energy from saturated fat intake was associated with a significant 9 % lower risk of CHD events and a 13 % lower risk of CHD deaths [40].

Dietary linoleic acid intake was inversely associated with CHD risk in a dose–response manner. These data provide support for the recommendations to replace saturated fat with polyunsaturated fat for primary prevention of CHD [40].

2.2.1.4 Omega-3 [n-3] Fatty Acids

Large long-term observational studies in women in the Nurses' Health Study [119] and in men in the Physicians' Health Study and the Zutphen Study [154], in randomized clinical trials after myocardial infarction [51], and experimental studies have evaluated the effects of fish and n-3 fatty acid consumption on fatal CHD and sudden cardiac death (SCD).

These different studies provide strong concordant evidence that modest consumption of fish or fish oil significantly reduces risk of coronary death and total mortality and may favorably affect other clinical outcomes. Intake of 250 mg/day of EPA and DHA appears sufficient for primary prevention with little additional benefit with higher intakes. An omega-3 index has been proposed which describes the percentage of EPA + DHA of total fatty acids measured in red blood cells. An omega-3 index of >8 % is associated with 90 % less risk for sudden cardiac death, as compared to an omega-3 index of <4 %; the index could be used as a benchmark for supplementation of omega-3 fatty acids [79, 165]. However interventional studies are necessary to confirm this percentage as a treatment goal.

The concordance of findings from different studies also suggests that effects of fish or fish oil on CHD death and SCD do not vary depending on presence or absence of established CHD. The evidence appears strong and consistent, and the magnitude of this effect is considerable. Because more than one-half of all CHD deaths and two-thirds of SCD occur among individuals without recognized heart disease, modest consumption of fish or fish oil, together with smoking cessation and regular moderate physical activity, should be among the first-line lifestyle modifications for prevention of CHD death and SCD. A review of the potential benefits of omega-3 fatty acids was given in 2009 [86].

In the Health Professionals Follow-Up Study, the associations between different patterns of intake of seafood and plant PUFAs and incident CHD among 45,722 men were investigated over the course of 14 years [104]. N-3 PUFAs from both seafood and plant sources may reduce CHD risk, with little apparent influence from

Table 2.1 Alpha-linolenic acid content in selected plant oils, nuts, and seeds

	A-LA-content; g/tablespoon
Flaxseed oil	8.5
Flaxseed	2.2
Walnut oil	1.4
Canola oil	1.3
Soja oil	0.9
Walnuts	0.7
Olive oil	0.1

Adapted from Ref. [81]
Estimated daily requirements 1.3–2.7 g

background n-6 PUFA intake. The alpha-linolenic acid content – an n-3 fatty acid – in selected plant oils, nuts, and seeds is shown in Table 2.1 [81].

Plant-based n-3 PUFAs may particularly reduce CHD risk when seafood-based n-3 PUFA intake is low, which has implications for populations with low consumption or availability of fatty fish [104]. However even in persons (without cardiovascular disease or malignancies) consuming adequate marine n-3 PUFAs, plant-based dietary n-3-PUFA alpha-linolenic acid (supplied mainly by walnuts and olive oil) was associated with an additional protective effect on all-cause mortality as could be shown in the PREDIMED study [138].

The mechanisms underlying the protective effects of omega-3 fatty acids are poorly understood. Telomere length is an emerging marker of biological age. Telomeres are tandem repeat DNA sequences (TTAGGG) that form a protective cap at the ends of eukaryotic chromosomes. Among patients with coronary artery disease, there was an inverse relationship between baseline blood levels of marine omega-3 fatty acids and the rate of telomere shortening over 5 years, suggesting that this could be one mechanism by which n-3 PUFAs might have a protective effect [41].

More recent studies however failed to demonstrate a benefit from use of omega-3 fatty acids in patients with multiple risk factors in a large general practice cohort who were treated according to the standard of care [131] or in patients early after acute myocardial infarction [130] who were treated according to current guidelines. The event rates in the control groups were lower than expected, and it is conceivable that the modern cardiovascular therapy (in patients recognized to be at increased risk) delivers already the effects formerly achieved by omega-3 fatty acids.

2.2.2   Fruits and Vegetables

The role of fruits and vegetables for the prevention of ischemic events has been examined in the Nurses' Health Study and the Health Professionals Follow-Up Study. 84,251 women 34–59 years of age who were followed for 14 years in the Nurses' Health Study and 42,148 men 40–75 years who were followed for 8 years in the Health Professionals Follow-Up Study were free of diagnosed cardiovascular disease, cancer, and diabetes at baseline. Participants in both studies completed mailed questionnaires about medical history, health behaviors, and occurrence of cardiovascular and other outcomes every 2 years.

After adjustment for standard cardiovascular risk factors, persons in the highest quintile of fruit and vegetable intake had a 31 % lower risk for ischemic stroke [70] and a 20 % lower relative risk for coronary heart disease [71] compared with those in the lowest quintile of intake. Green leafy vegetables and vitamin C-rich fruits and vegetables contributed most to the apparent protective effect of total fruit and vegetable intake. The optimal effect was reached with 5 servings per day, which is the current recommendation.

In the European Prospective Investigation into Cancer and Nutrition, a one portion (80 g) increment in fruit and vegetable intake was associated with a 4 % lower risk of fatal ischemic heart disease or ischemic stroke [23].

The results of the Cardiovascular Risk in Young Finns Study suggest that high consumption of fruits and vegetables during childhood and early adulthood is related to less arterial stiffness after 27 years of follow-up in young adulthood [1]. In the longitudinal CARDIA cohort study, higher intake of fruits and vegetable during young adulthood was associated with lower odds of prevalent coronary artery calcium after 20 years of follow-up [101].

A multicenter study from Europe [117] extends these findings to a diabetic population, where intake of vegetables, legumes, and fruits was associated with reduced risks of all-cause and CVD mortality. The findings support the current state of evidence from general population studies suggesting that the protective potential of vegetable and fruit intake is also seen in diabetic patients.

The results of these different studies reinforce the importance of establishing a high intake of fruits and vegetables as part of a healthy dietary pattern beginning early in life and continuing this pattern throughout late adulthood.

2.2.3   Whole grain Products

Although whole grain products are metabolically favorable, their prognostic implications have not been adequately examined. Whole grain products decrease total cholesterol and LDL cholesterol by about 18 %, decrease postprandial glucose levels, decrease the risk for type 2 diabetes mellitus, and improve insulin sensitivity in overweight and obese adults. Their influence on bodyweight however remains unresolved. There are no prospective studies evaluating the effect of whole grain products or diets on coronary death or on the occurrence of coronary artery disease. A retrospective analysis of ten US American and European studies found consumption of dietary fiber from cereals and fruits inversely associated with risk of coronary heart disease: for each 10 g cereal or fruit fiber intake, risk reductions of 10 and 16 % respectively for all coronary events were observed and 25 and 30 % risk reductions respectively for deaths; there were however no risk reductions for vegetable fiber intake. The results were similar for men and women [125].

Whole grain products for breakfast were associated with a lower occurrence of heart failure, as an observational sub-study on 21,000 physicians for more than 20 years of follow-up from the British Physician's Health Study suggested. It remains however unclear at present whether this benefit was achieved by prevention of hypertension and/or myocardial infarction [32]. In female type 2 diabetics, bran appears to be of prognostic benefit as shown in the Nurses' Health Study [57]. As mentioned above in the Nurses' Health Study and the Health Professionals Follow-Up Study replacement of 5 % of the total caloric content of saturated fats by a caloric equivalent of whole grain was associated with a 9 % reduction of the cardiovascular risk [89]. A recent meta-analysis of the association between whole grain intake and coronary heart disease risk indicated that whole grain intake has a protective effect against coronary heart disease in Europe as well as in the United States [156]. A more quantitative recent meta-analysis [169] based on 14 studies which included 786,076 participants, 97,867 total deaths, 23,957 CVD deaths, and 37,492 cancer deaths concluded that for each 16 g/day daily consumption increase in whole grain ($\approx$1 serving per day), relative risks of total mortality was 0.93 (95 % CI, 0.92–0.94; $P < 0.001$), the cardiovascular mortality was 0.91 (95 % CI, 0.90–0.93; $P < 0.001$), and the cancer mortality was 0.95 (95 % CI, 0.94–0.96; $P < 0.001$).

2.2.4 Meat

Lower consumption of red meats is part of the overall dietary recommendation for a Mediterranean-type diet, which is supported by the European Society of Cardiology [126] and also by the American Heart Association [109, 110]. Several constituents of red meats could potentially increase cardiometabolic risk, including saturated fatty acids, cholesterol, and heme iron; in processed meats, high levels of salt and other preservatives [107] are associated with higher incidence of CHD and diabetes mellitus [100]. Although not strictly related to cardiovascular disease but also of health concern for the CV patient is the recent statement of the International Agency for Research on Cancer that consumption of processed meats is "carcinogenic to humans" (Group 1) on the basis of sufficient evidence for colorectal cancer. Additionally, a positive association with the consumption of processed meat was found for stomach cancer. The Working Group classified consumption of red meat as "probably carcinogenic to humans" (Group 2A) [9]. Thus lower consumption of red meat, particularly of processed meat, should have a twofold favorable effect on health.

2.2.5 Snacks and Sweets

The diet of the coronary patient is characterized by quite a few restrictions and some degree of fat and cholesterol reduction. Therefore the addition of snacks to the diet is often more than welcome, particularly if these snacks have a beneficial effect on the course of the disease or at least modify risk factors in a favorable way or improve endothelial function.

2.2.5.1 Nuts and Almonds

Tree nuts, peanuts, and almonds have been thoroughly analyzed with respect to their effect on prognosis and lipid profile of persons with hypercholesterolemia.

Observations from the Adventist Health Study have shown that frequent consumption of nuts is associated with a substantial, independent reduction in the risk of myocardial infarction and death from ischemic heart disease [46]. In a small study on young healthy, normal-weight, nonsmoking males, replacement of 20 % of daily calories with walnuts decreased LDL cholesterol levels by 16.3 % and HDL cholesterol by 5 %, resulting in overall favorable changes of the lipid profile [135]. In two large, independent cohorts of nurses, in the Nurses' Health Study and of male health professionals in the Health Professionals Follow-Up Study, the frequency of nut consumption was inversely associated with total and cause-specific mortality, independently of other predictors of death [6]. This inverse association between nut consumption and CHD risk has also been found in the prospective Physicians' Health Study primarily due to a reduction in the risk of sudden cardiac death [4].

The average nut consumption in the Adventists' and the Nurses' Health Study was about 20 g/day – a handful. In a randomized nutritional study, larger but still moderate quantities of walnuts (84 g/day) within a cholesterol-lowering diet favorably modified the lipoprotein profile in normal men and decreased serum levels of LDL cholesterol by 16 % if the intake of total dietary fat and calories was maintained. The ratio of LDL cholesterol to HDL cholesterol was also lowered by the walnut diet and endothelial function was improved [134].

The beneficial effect of nuts on prognosis is plausible. Nuts are rich in monounsaturated and polyunsaturated fatty acids, which makes them a palatable choice of healthy fats. Monounsaturated fats may contribute to decreased CHD risk by amelioration of lipid profile, by reducing postprandial triglyceride concentrations, and by decreasing soluble inflammatory adhesion molecules in patients with hypercholesterolemia. Moreover, the relatively high arginine content of nuts has been suggested as one of the potential biological mechanisms for their cardioprotective effect, because consumption of arginine-rich foods is associated with lower CRP levels [82].

Also almonds used as supplements in the diet of hyperlipidemic subjects significantly reduce coronary heart disease risk factors: 73 g of almonds produced a significant 9.4 % reduction of LDL cholesterol, a 12 % reduction of the LDL-HDL ratio, a 7.8 % reduction of lipoprotein(a), and a reduction of oxidized LDL concentrations by 14.0 % – all significant and most likely beneficial for the course of the disease [82].

Also a macadamia nut-based diet high in monounsaturated fat has potentially beneficial effects on cholesterol and low-density lipoprotein cholesterol levels when compared with a typical American diet [24]. These changes are probably a result of the nonfat (protein and fiber) as well as the monounsaturated fatty acid components of the nut, but other additive effects of the numerous bioactive constituents may contribute to this effect.

A traditional Mediterranean diet enriched with nuts in a weight reduction program enhanced – as mentioned above in the PREDIMED study – the reversion of metabolic syndrome by 30 % compared with the control diet group [139].

In addition the consumption of peanuts and other nuts is significantly associated with a lower risk of gallstone disease – a welcomed side effect in persons with increased cholesterol levels. A review found the prognostic effects of nut and peanut studies somewhat greater than expected on the basis of the magnitude of the blood cholesterol lowering seen from the diet. Thus, in addition to a favorable fatty acid profile, nuts and peanuts may contain other bioactive compounds that could contribute to their multiple cardiovascular benefits. Other macronutrients include plant protein and fiber; micronutrients including potassium, calcium, magnesium, and tocopherols; and phytochemicals such as phytosterols, phenolic compounds, resveratrol, and arginine. Nuts and peanuts are food sources that are a composite of numerous cardioprotective nutrients, and if routinely incorporated in a healthy diet, the population risk of CHD would therefore be expected to decrease markedly [82].

The strongest argument for the beneficial prognostic effects however provides the already mentioned PREDIMED study, a randomized primary prevention trial involving persons at high cardiovascular risk: the study showed a significant reduction in major cardiovascular events among participants assigned to a Mediterranean diet – one component of which was supplementation with 30 g of walnuts, hazelnuts, or almonds per day – as compared with a control diet [38, 52].

2.2.5.2 Chocolate

In the sixteenth century, Aztec Emperor Montezuma was a keen admirer of cocoa, calling it a "divine drink, which builds up resistance and fights fatigue. A cup of this precious drink permits a man to walk for a whole day without food" was supposedly Hernán Cortés, the conquistador of the Aztecs convinced (cited in [20]). In the language of the Aztecs, this drink was called chocolatl. With the discovery of the New World, cocoa came to Europe in the sixteenth century. Also today the consumption of chocolate is often associated with or followed by an intense feeling of pleasure and gratification, where the desire of repetitive consumption is often difficult to resist (personal experience and unpublished observation). The total chocolate consumption in Germany is approximately 11.5 kg per person and year and even greater than the chocolate consumption of the Swiss of 11.1 kg per person and year (including the sales to tourists) (Fig. 2.1).

Because of its high caloric content (500–600 kcal/100 g), chocolate consumption may be an important aspect of overall energy balance in men as well as in women. It could contribute to 7–8 kg overweight/year in Germany if chocolate was used as an add-on to a normocaloric diet. The high fat and sugar content limit its use in a diet with the aim to minimize risk factors. Yet regular cocoa consumption – an essential ingredient for chocolate production – prevented high blood pressure in Kuna Indians of Panama [20]. Recent investigations have shown that flavanol-rich dark chocolate induces coronary vasodilation, improves coronary vascular function, and decreases platelet adhesion even in a short-term experiment 2 h after consumption. These immediate beneficial effects were

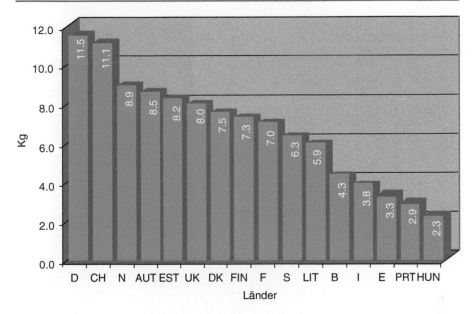

Fig. 2.1 Per capita annual chocolate consumption in kg in different European countries (Swiss 2015, other countries 2014); [61]

paralleled by a significant reduction of serum oxidative stress and were positively correlated with changes in serum epicatechin concentration [45]. The possible beneficial effects of cocoa on cardiovascular health by activation of nitric oxide (NO) and influencing antioxidant, anti-inflammatory, and antiplatelet effects, which in turn might improve endothelial function, lipid levels, blood pressure, insulin resistance, and eventually clinical outcome, have been reviewed [20]. Cocoa is contained in dark chocolate rather than in milk chocolate. The content of the bitter-tasting flavanols is responsible for the vasodilating and anti-oxidative effects of the chocolate, whereby epicatechin is probably the dominant if not the sole mediator. Interestingly the procyanidins, which are polymerized chains of epicatechin and catechin, and which represent the vast majority of the polyphenol content of cocoa, are also as flavanols present in red wine, apples, and tea [58] and presumably responsible for the beneficial vascular effects. Unfortunately – or rather on purpose – in the regular production process of the chocolate, the bitter-tasting flavanols are largely eliminated by a process called "dutching" [59]. Accordingly the liberal consumption of chocolate as a preventive measure is probably limited by the bitter taste. In the regular chocolate these prognostic beneficial ingredients have been partially eliminated to better please the taste of the majority of the consumers (Fig. 2.2).

Thus chocolate with high flavanol content has beneficial effects on endothelial function and can probably be enjoyed without untoward effects as a snack by persons who are fond of bitter chocolate. The bitter flavor will probably prevent any excessive caloric intake.

Fig. 2.2 A 70 %
chocolate which improves
endothelial function (www.
chocosuisse.ch accessed 22
February 2009)

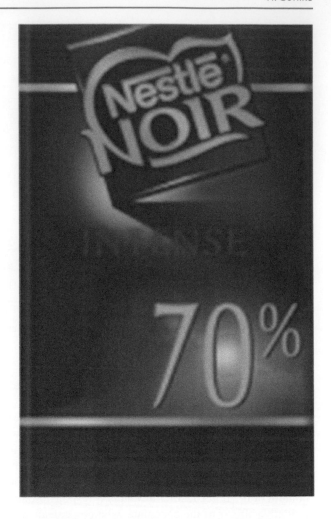

2.2.6   Non-pharmacological Decrease of the Postprandial Rise in Glucose

The postprandial rise in glucose appears to be of some importance for the development of diabetes and cardiovascular events; it also correlates with indicators of oxidative stress. A moderate (20 g of alcohol) "aperitif" results in a decrease of the postprandial rise in glucose; two tablespoons of vinegar, e.g., with salad before a meal with a high glycemic index, have a similar effect as well as almonds, walnuts, or peanuts (Figs. 2.3 and 2.4).

These components – which are part of the Mediterranean diet – can result in a noticeable decrease of postprandial lipid and glucose levels [118].

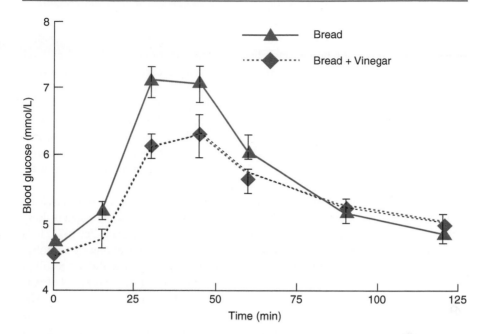

Fig. 2.3 Vinegar reduces postprandial glucose. The addition of two tablespoons of vinegar to two slices of white bread significantly reduced the postprandial glucose increase (Modified from O'Keefe et al. [118])

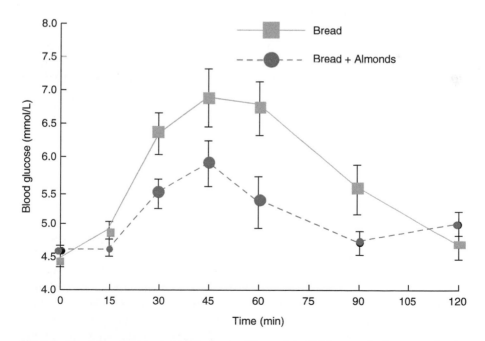

Fig. 2.4 Almonds reduce postprandial glucose. The postprandial increase in the area under the curve for glucose was reduced by 58 % when 90 g of almonds were added to a high glycemic index meal ($p < 0.01$) (Modified from O'Keefe et al. [118])

2.2.6.1 Glycemic Index

The glycemic index (GI) is an empiric measure describing the influence of carbohydrates on glucose-insulin homeostasis based on the extent to which they raise blood glucose levels 2 h after their consumption. Less refined carbohydrates with a high fiber content have a lower GI.

Food consumption with a low GI decreases postprandial glucose, insulin levels, and triglycerides, improves the total cholesterol/HDL cholesterol ratio, may support the decrease of body weight, and possibly has – via this pathway – a favorable effect on the development of diabetes and CHD. This concept may be particularly useful in type III hyperlipoproteinemia [118, 125]. However, whether these improvements translate into improved clinical outcomes is not known.

In randomized trials, reduced-glycemic-index diets have not resulted in increased weight loss beyond that explained by caloric restriction. In some aspects low-glycemic-index diets have features resembling the Mediterranean diet [97]. In a 5-week controlled feeding study, diets with low glycemic index of dietary carbohydrate, compared with high glycemic index of dietary carbohydrate, did not result in improvements of metabolic parameters or blood pressure if the baseline diet was structured as a DASH (Dietary Approaches to Stop Hypertension)-type diet. The DASH-type diet is rich in fruits, vegetables, and low-fat dairy and reduced in fats and cholesterol. Thus the negative prognostic importance of the glycemic index of single food items is diminished in persons consuming a "healthy" diet [137].

2.3   Dietary Patterns

Although scientific investigation of macro- and micronutrients remains essential to elucidate biological mechanisms, the concept of cardiovascular prevention by nutrition has moved from focusing on individual components of a diet to emphasizing a food pattern.

2.3.1   Mediterranean Diet

In general the type of diet is part of the lifestyle, and there may be some residual bias when correlating a diet with the occurrence of cardiovascular events. The Mediterranean lifestyle used to be more relaxed compared to the Central European or US American lifestyle.

The Mediterranean diet has been favored since the Seven Countries Study as promoting longevity and good cardiovascular health [73, 74].

In 1999 the Lyon Diet Heart Study had shown in a randomized interventional study that a strict Mediterranean diet in patients after myocardial infarction is associated with a 45 % reduction of the CV event rate [26]. The Mediterranean diet is a class 1 recommendation (Evidence Level B) in the European Society of Cardiology guidelines for CV prevention [127] and is also recommended by the AHA and ACC [36].

2.3.1.1 Mediterranean Diet Scores and Prognostic Implications (Observational Studies)

In the meantime however the components of the Mediterranean diet have been analyzed in many countries and have been correlated with events in more than half a million persons. The Mediterranean diet is characterized by a high proportion of vegetables, legumes, fruits, and cereals (primarily unprocessed), frequent fish consumption, less dairy products, rarely meat, a moderate consumption of alcoholic beverages mostly as wine and preferably with meals, and a small amount of saturated fatty acids, but a high proportion of unsaturated fatty acids, particularly olive oil.

In middle-aged persons, there was a significant inverse relation between the degree of compliance with the Mediterranean diet (as evaluated by a score) and mortality [147]. Because this score has been used extensively and repeatedly with only minor modifications in different studies [102, 159] and different countries, it will be outlined in some detail here; this score can also be used as a checklist in advising patients to change their diet into the direction of a Mediterranean diet. The traditional Mediterranean diet score includes nine components and results in values from 0 to 9 points reflecting minimal to maximal conformity with the score (Table 2.2).

One point each is given for intake at or above the gender-specific median intake for the six components considered to be healthy (fatty acid ratio, legumes, grains, fruits, vegetables [excluding potatoes], or fish), and one point if the consumption of the items considered to be less healthy (meat and dairy products) was below the gender-specific median. One point is given for alcohol consumption within a specified range (5–25 g/day for women; 10–50 g/day for men) (Fig. 2.5).

If participants met all the characteristics of the Mediterranean diet, their score was the highest (nine points), reflecting maximal conformance with a Mediterranean diet, and if they met none of the characteristics, the score was zero reflecting minimal or no conformity with a Mediterranean diet.

In two cohorts of elderly persons, the life-prolonging effects of the Mediterranean diet could be observed:

In the HALE Project among 2339 apparently healthy men and women, aged 70–90 years, adherence to a Mediterranean diet was associated with a 23 % lower rate of all-cause mortality [78].

Table 2.2 Components of the Mediterranean diet score: one point for above (high intake) or below (low intake) the age and gender adjusted consumption of the corresponding nutritional item	1. High ratio of monounsaturated: saturated fatty acids
	2. High intake of legumes
	3. High intake of grains
	4. High intake of fruit and nuts
	5. High intake of vegetables
	6. High intake of fish
	7. Low intake of meat and meat products
	8. Low intake of milk and dairy products
	9. Moderate consumption of alcohol (10–50 g/day for men, 5–25 g/day for women)

Fig. 2.5 The traditional and the alternative (marked with *yellow background*) Mediterranean diet score (*Trichopoulou et al. [159], **Fung et al. [47])

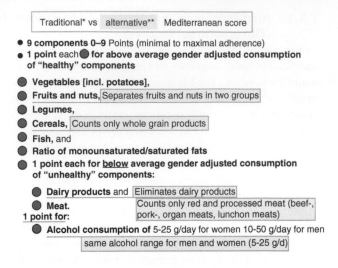

Traditional* vs alternative** Mediterranean score

● **9 components 0–9 Points** (minimal to maximal adherence)
● **1 point each● for above average gender adjusted consumption of "healthy" components**

● **Vegetables [incl. potatoes],**
● **Fruits and nuts,** Separates fruits and nuts in two groups
● **Legumes,**
● **Cereals,** Counts only whole grain products
● **Fish,** and
● **Ratio of monounsaturated/saturated fats**
● **1 point each for below average gender adjusted consumption of "unhealthy" components:**

  ● **Dairy products** and Eliminates dairy products
  ● **Meat.** Counts only red and processed meat (beef-, pork-, organ meats, lunchon meats)
  1 point for:
  ● **Alcohol consumption of** 5-25 g/day for women 10-50 g/day for men same alcohol range for men and women (5-25 g/d)

In the EPIC study of more than 74,000 above 60-year-old European persons without coronary heart disease, stroke, or cancer at enrolment, a two-unit increment in the modified Mediterranean diet score was associated with a statistically significant reduction of overall mortality of 8 % [160].

Also in a prospective observational study of more than 380,000 US Americans (age range 50–71 years), a 20 % reduced total mortality and CV mortality could be seen as well as a 12–17 % reduced cancer mortality in men and women who showed with 6–9 points a good conformity with a Mediterranean diet compared to persons with a score of 0–3. This relationship was seen in smokers and never-smokers alike [102]. A similar Mediterranean diet score was used for nutritional evaluation in the HALE Project [78] and the EPIC study [160]. Thus the database for the primary preventive effects of the Mediterranean diet has been greatly strengthened.

The beneficial effects of the Mediterranean diet were confirmed in the Nurses' Health Study in more than 74,500 women 38–63 years of age, without a history of cardiovascular disease and diabetes who were followed from 1984 to 2004.

The authors used the alternate Mediterranean diet score (Fig. 2.5) from self-reported dietary data collected through validated food frequency questionnaires administered six times between 1984 and 2002. During 20 years of follow-up, 2391 incident cases of CHD, 1763 incident cases of stroke, and 1077 cardiovascular disease deaths (fatal CHD and strokes combined) were ascertained. Women in the top alternate Mediterranean diet score quintile were at 29 % lower risk for CHD and 13 % lower risk for stroke compared with those in the bottom quintile. Cardiovascular disease mortality was 39 % lower among women in the top quintile of the alternate Mediterranean diet score ($p < 0.0001$) [49]. In a Danish cohort, the Mediterranean diet score was inversely associated with total mortality and with cardiovascular and MI incidence and mortality but not with stroke incidence or mortality [157].The concept of the Mediterranean diet was confirmed for high-risk patients with stable coronary heart disease where greater consumption of healthy foods appeared to be more important for secondary prevention of coronary artery disease than avoidance of less healthy foods typical of Western diets [154].

This inverse relationship between consumption of "healthy" foods in the sense of the Mediterranean-type diet and risk of myocardial infarction was also confirmed in the INTERHEART study where dietary patterns were analyzed in patients after MI and controls in 52 countries [64]. Three dietary patterns were identified and labeled as Oriental, Western, and prudent. The "Oriental" pattern had a high loading on tofu and soy and other sauces. The second dietary pattern was labeled "Western" because of its high loading on fried food, salty snacks, and meat intake. The third dietary pattern was labeled "prudent" because of its emphasis on fruit and vegetable intake.

The authors found significant, inverse, and graded associations between the intake of raw vegetables, green leafy vegetables, cooked vegetables, and fruits on the one hand and acute myocardial infarction on the other hand. Conversely, they observed a positive association between myocardial infarction and the intake of fried foods and salty snacks ($p < 0.001$) and a weaker association between quartiles of meat intake and AMI ($p = 0.08$) [64]. The typical US southern dietary pattern however characterized by added fats, fried food, eggs, organ and processed meats, and sugar-sweetened beverages was associated with greater hazard of CHD in a sample of 17,400 white and black adults in diverse regions of the United States with 5.8 years of follow-up [143]. In the 2013 AHA/ACC guideline on lifestyle management to reduce cardiovascular risk, dietary recommendations are given that are largely in agreement with the Mediterranean diet [36].

2.3.1.2 Effects of the Mediterranean Diet on Risk Indicators and Risk Factors

The exact mechanisms leading to decreased myocardial infarction, cardiovascular deaths, and all-cause deaths are not clear, but several indicators of risk such as indicators of inflammation and established CV risk factors are decreased by the Mediterranean diet.

Estruch et al. examined in the randomized controlled PREDIMED trial the effects of a Mediterranean diet supplemented with 1 l olive oil per week (for a family of four) or with 30 g of nuts/day in comparison to a low-fat diet in 772 asymptomatic persons 55–80 years of age at high cardiovascular risk.

Compared with a low-fat diet after 3 months, both Mediterranean diets lowered plasma glucose levels, systolic blood pressure, and the cholesterol-high-density lipoprotein cholesterol ratio. The Mediterranean diet supplemented by olive oil also reduced C-reactive protein levels compared with the low-fat diet [37].

In the same study the effects of the Mediterranean diet on in vivo lipoprotein oxidation were assessed. After the 3-month interventions, mean oxidized low-density lipoprotein (LDL) levels decreased in the traditional Mediterranean diet group supplemented by virgin olive oil significantly and to a lesser degree also in the group supplemented by nuts – without significant changes in the low-fat diet group. Change in oxidized LDL levels in the traditional Mediterranean diet virgin olive oil group reached significance vs. that of the low-fat group ($p = 0.02$) [37].

A Mediterranean diet supplemented with nuts (30 g/day) or olive oil (one liter per week for the family) resulted within 3 months in lower blood pressure, fasting blood sugar, and inflammatory markers as compared to a low-fat diet [43].

2.3.1.3 Mediterranean Diet and Inflammation

The inflammatory reaction of the body in relation to adherence to the Mediterranean diet was assessed in more than 300 middle-aged male twins using the mentioned diet score. A 1-unit absolute difference in the diet score was associated with a 9 % (95 % CI, 4.5–13.6) lower interleukin-6 level – an established marker of inflammation related to progression of atherosclerotic disease.

Thus reduced systemic inflammation appears to be an important mechanism linking Mediterranean diet to reduced cardiovascular risk [25, 47]. The hypothesis that inflammation impairs reverse cholesterol transport at numerous steps in the pathway from initial macrophage efflux to HDL acceptor function and the final step of cholesterol flux through the liver to bile and feces was confirmed for the first time in an in vivo study. The anti-inflammatory effect of the Mediterranean diet could to some degree contribute to its beneficial effects on cardiovascular but possibly also cancer incidence [98].

However it is not only the arterial system that benefits from a high intake of plant foods and fish and less red and processed meat: also the risk for venous thromboembolic events is reduced! In a prospective study as part of the Atherosclerosis Risk in Communities (ARIC) Study, almost 15,000 middle-aged adults were followed up over 12 years for incident venous thromboembolism. At baseline the average age of study participants was 54 years. A food frequency questionnaire assessed dietary intake at baseline and after 6 years. The risk of venous thromboembolism was assessed in quintiles of fruit and vegetable intake.

There was a significant risk reduction of venous thromboembolism incidence of 40–50 % in quintiles three to five compared with quintile one.

Eating fish one or more times per week was associated with 30–45 % lower incidence of venous thromboembolism for quintiles 2–5 compared with quintile 1, suggestive of a threshold effect. High intake of red and processed meat intake (quintile 5) doubled the risk (p trend = 0.02). Hazard ratios were attenuated only slightly after adjustment for factors VIIc and VIIIc and von Willebrand factor [151].

2.3.1.4 Mediterranean Diet and Diabetes

Considering the components of the Mediterranean diet, it may come as no surprise that the Mediterranean diet has a preventive effect for the development of diabetes. In a prospective cohort study from Spain, a relation between adherence to a Mediterranean diet and the incidence of diabetes among initially healthy participants (university graduates) could be shown [97] – after adjustment for covariables such as sex, age, years of university education, total energy intake, body mass index, physical activity, sedentary habits, smoking, family history of diabetes, and personal history of hypertension. Participants who adhered closely to a Mediterranean diet had a lower risk of diabetes. The incidence rate ratios in the fully adjusted analyses showed that a two-point increase in the score was associated with a 35 % relative reduction in the risk of diabetes with a significant inverse linear trend (p = 0.04) in the multivariate analysis. A high adherence (7–9 points) was associated with an 80 % reduced incidence rate of diabetes compared with a low score of 0–2 [97].Thus the traditional Mediterranean diet may have considerable protective effects against diabetes.

Similar results were obtained in patients after myocardial infarction [106]. In prospectively obtained data of 8291 Italian patients with a recent (<3 months) myocardial infarction, who were free of diabetes at baseline, the incidence of new-onset diabetes (new diabetes medication or fasting glucose ≥7 mmol/L) and impaired fasting glucose (fasting glucose ≥6.1 mmol/L and <7 mmol/L) were assessed up to 3.5 years. A Mediterranean diet score was assigned according to consumption of cooked and raw vegetables, fruit, fish, and olive oil. Associations of demographic, clinical, and lifestyle risk factors with incidence of diabetes and impaired fasting glucose were assessed with multivariable Cox proportional hazards regression analysis.

These patients had a 15-fold higher annual incidence rate of impaired fasting glucose and a more than twofold higher incidence rate of diabetes during a mean follow-up of 3.2 years (26,795 person-years) compared with population-based cohorts. Consumption of typical Mediterranean foods, smoking cessation, and prevention of weight gain were associated with a lower risk [106].

2.3.1.5 Meta-analysis of Mediterranean Diet Studies

The benefits of the Mediterranean diet pattern were evaluated in a meta-analysis of 514,816 subjects on the basis of 33,576 deaths occurring during the respective observation time. The overall mortality in relation to adherence to a Mediterranean diet showed that a two-point increase in the adherence score was significantly associated with a 9 % reduced risk of all-cause mortality and likewise a 9 % reduction on cardiovascular mortality as well as a 6 % lower incidence of or mortality from cancer. The message from these studies is that it is the completeness of adherence to the Mediterranean diet rather than the consumption of individual components, which is effective in improving the prognosis. Unexpectedly also the incidence of Parkinson's disease and Alzheimer's disease was significantly reduced by 13 % [147].

Thus a greater adherence to a Mediterranean diet is not only associated with a significant reduction in mortality from arterial cardiovascular diseases but also from a reduced incidence of venous thromboembolism. In addition other diseases that are a threat for the well-being and quality of life in the later years are decreased: cancer, Parkinson's disease, and Alzheimer's disease – diseases for which no specific strategies of prevention have been established. This makes it easy for the physician to recommend this type of diet to the cardiovascular patient after myocardial infarction: the side effects of this diet are most welcome [36, 127].

2.3.1.6 Mediterranean Diet in Primary Prevention: PREDIMED Study

The abovementioned randomized primary prevention PREDIMED study [37] in an older population at high cardiovascular risk (mean age 67 years, age range 55–80 years) which demonstrated in the early phase an improvement of several risk indicators showed after 4.8 years of follow-up that an energy-unrestricted Mediterranean diet supplemented with extra-virgin olive oil or nuts resulted in a substantial reduction in the risk of major cardiovascular events. The hazard ratios were 0.70 (95 % confidence interval [CI], 0.54–0.92) for the group assigned to a Mediterranean diet with extra-virgin olive oil and 0.72 (95 % CI, 0.54–0.96) for the group assigned to a Mediterranean diet with nuts, in comparison to the control group. The randomized study supported the results gained from observational studies and supports the benefits of the Mediterranean diet for the primary prevention of cardiovascular disease [38]. In a sub-study, the Mediterranean diet supplemented with olive oil or nuts was associated with improved cognitive function [162] and with a reduced incidence of invasive breast cancer in the participating women in the Mediterranean diet with extra-virgin olive oil group [158].

2.3.2 Other Dietary Patterns: Dietary Risk Score and Acute Myocardial Infarction (INTERHEART Study)

The authors from the INTERHEART study [64] computed from their data a dietary risk score (DRS) and observed a graded and positive association between this DRS and risk of AMI. Food items that were considered to be predictive (meat, salty snacks, and fried foods) or protective (fruits and green leafy vegetables, other cooked vegetables, and other raw vegetables) of CVD were used to generate a DRS. The authors used a point system. Compared with the lowest quartile, odds ratios (adjusted for age, sex, and region) varied from 1.29 in the second quartile of dietary risk score to 1.92 in the fourth quartile. The association of the score with AMI varied by region ($p < 0.0001$) but was directionally similar in all regions. The population attributable ratio for this score was 30 % (95 % CI, 0.26–0.35) in participants in the INTERHEART study (Fig. 2.6).

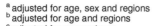

Population Attributable Fraction		Odds ratio for myocardial infarction Dietary Quartile 4 vs. Quartile 1
Overall[a]	0.30 (0.26-0.35)	
Male[b]	0.28 (0.23-0.33)	
Female[b]	0.39 (0.30-0.49)	
N. America, W.Europe and Australia[c]	0.30 (0.17-0.42)	
Central Europe[c]	0.31 (0.18-0.44)	
Middle East[c]	0.28 (0.17-0.40)	
Africa[c]	0.10 (-0.14-0.35)	
South Asia[c]	0.29 (0.18-0.40)	
China[c]	0.18 (0.07-0.29)	
Southeast Asia[c]	0.58 (0.45-0.71)	
S. America[c]	0.15 (-0.03-0.32)	

[a] adjusted for age, sex and regions
[b] adjusted for age and regions
[c] adjusted for age and sex

Odds ratio (95% CI)

Fig. 2.6 Population attributable risk and odds ratios for acute myocardial infarction associated with dietary risk score (Modified from Iqbal et al. [64])

Thus many observational and case–control studies have already suggested the prognostic importance of a healthy (prudent) or Mediterranean-type diet for a lower risk for myocardial infarction (and cancer), which was later verified by a randomized study [38].

However more randomized interventional studies are necessary to develop specific dietary recommendation for patients with CV disease and with different metabolic problems.

2.4 Drinks

The fluid requirements of the body vary depending on the environment and the physical activity. The type of fluid preferred to fulfill the requirements depend on tradition and environment.

2.4.1 Coffee or Tea Consumption and Cardiovascular Events

Coffee and tea and to a lesser degree chocolate have been the most widely used drinks during the course of the day for decades if not centuries but their relationship to the risk of coronary disease has been examined only in recent years.

2.4.1.1 Coffee

Coffee consumption has been associated with an increased risk in patients with coronary artery disease. The influence of coffee on cholesterol levels was already examined in 1989. After 9 weeks of coffee consumption, boiled coffee increased LDL cholesterol by 10 %, whereas filtered coffee showed no difference compared to a "no-coffee" group [5].

In the Health Professionals' Follow-Up Study, almost 42,000 male employees in the hospital (age range 40–75 years) were asked about their coffee consumption, lifestyle, and risk factors every 2 years for a total of 12 years. Similarly in the Nurses' Health Study, more than 84,000 nurses in the age range of 30–55 years were asked about their coffee consumption every 2 years for a total of 18 years. In both studies the prevalence of diabetes mellitus was examined: coffee consumption of 4–5 cups/day reduced the prevalence of diabetes mellitus by 29–30 % in males and females similarly after multivariate analysis. In males even a consumption of more than six cups of coffee per day reduced the risk of diabetes by 46 %, whereas in females there was no further decrease of the diabetes prevalence beyond the consumption of five cups of coffee [126].

In a systematic review habitual coffee consumption was associated with a substantial lower risk of type II diabetes which was also observed for decaffeinated coffee in postmenopausal women [126] as well as middle-aged and younger US women [163].Thus there may be ingredients in the coffee – other than caffeine – that protect from diabetes.

Coffee consumption in two observational studies showed no increased risk for the development of coronary artery disease. The consumption of up to five cups of coffee per day is without harm for the coronary patient and possibly beneficial by preventing or delaying the occurrence of diabetes – but beware of the sugar and cream!

Coffee consumption decreased the relative risks of stroke across categories of coffee consumption in the more than 83,000 women of the Nurses' Health Study [163]. After adjustment for high blood pressure, hypercholesterolemia, and type 2 diabetes, the relative risk reduction was 43 % among never and past smokers (RR for >4 cups a day versus <1 cup a month; $p < 0.001$), but not significant among current smokers. Similarly there was a protective effect among non-hypercholesteremics (HR 0.77, $p < 0.003$), nondiabetics (HR 0.79, $p = 0.009$), and non-hypertensives (HR 0.72; $p = 0.001$). However, no protective effect was seen in women with diabetes, hypertension, or hypercholesterolemia, suggesting that the moderate beneficial effects of coffee consumption cannot override the detrimental effects of these important risk factors. The authors also observed a slightly lower risk of stroke in women who drank moderate amounts of decaffeinated coffee (2–3 cups/day vs. <1 cup/month; HR 0.84; $p = 0.002$) suggesting that components in coffee other than caffeine may be responsible for the potential beneficial effect of coffee on stroke risk [91]. A similar effect was seen in a large Japanese population study (more than one million person-years with a follow-up time of 13 years) where 1–2 cups of coffee per day reduced the hazard ratio for stroke by 20 % compared to persons who seldom drank coffee, but there was no effect on coronary events [80]. In a large observational study of more than 208,000 American persons (74,890 women in the Nurses' Health Study, 93,054 women in the Nurses' Health Study II, and 40,557 men in the Health Professionals Follow-Up Study) and more than 4.6 million person-years of follow-up significant inverse associations were observed between coffee consumption and deaths attributed to cardiovascular disease, neurologic diseases, and suicide. No significant association between coffee consumption and total cancer mortality was found. Restricting the analysis to never-smokers, the lowest hazard ratio of 0.85 (0.79–0.92) was seen for 3.1–5.0 cups of coffee per day. But even more than 5.0 cups of coffee per day were of advantage compared with non-coffee drinkers with a hazard ratio of 0.88 (0.78–0.99), confirming that even higher consumption of total coffee, caffeinated coffee, and decaffeinated coffee was of no harm and associated with lower risk of total mortality [30].

2.4.1.2 Tea

Tea has traditionally a better image concerning the development of cardiovascular disease. The relationship between tea consumption and mortality after acute myocardial infarction was examined in a prospective study. The self-reported tea consumption in the year before myocardial infarction was associated with a lower mortality after myocardial infarction [112].

Short-term and long-term black tea consumption has a potential to reverse endothelial dysfunction in patients with coronary artery disease, which may partly explain the association between tea consumption and decreased cardiovascular disease events in primary and secondary prevention [35]. The addition of milk however counteracted the favorable health effects of tea on flow-mediated dilatation [92].

Similarly, green tea consumption is associated with reduced mortality due to all causes and due to cardiovascular disease, but primarily because of a decreased risk of stroke. The hazard ratios of cancer mortality were not significantly different from non-tea consumers [84]. In the already mentioned large Japanese population study, four or more cups of green tea per day reduced the hazard ratio for stroke by 20 % compared to persons who seldom drank tea [80], but again there was no effect on coronary events. Drinking a cup of tea is frequently associated with relaxation and recovery from stress. Steptoe and coworkers reported in a double-blind (!) randomized trial that regular drinking of tea is associated with less platelet–leukocyte aggregates, platelet–monocyte aggregates, and platelet–neutrophil aggregates. They also found lower post-stress cortisol levels and a stronger subjective feeling of relaxation under the artificial test conditions. The consumption of black tea may have its potential health effects mediated through better recovery from a stress via psycho endocrine and inflammatory mechanisms [152].

Thus, in summary black tea (without milk) has a favorable effect on the flow-dependent vasodilatation. Tea consumption is associated with decreased mortality after myocardial infarction, and green tea reduces the stroke risk, but probably has no effect on the coronary artery risk.

2.4.2   Alcohol and Cardiovascular Morbidity and Mortality

A large number of epidemiological studies of both community and clinical cohorts have associated moderate alcohol consumption with decreased risk for subsequent cardiovascular morbidity and mortality [75, 77].

2.4.2.1 Alcohol and Cardiovascular Morbidity and Mortality

In the INTERHEART case–control study which encompassed 52 countries, low levels of alcohol use were associated in most participants with a moderate reduction in the risk of myocardial infarction; the strength of this association however was not uniform across different countries. An episode of heavy drinking was associated with an increased risk of acute MI in the subsequent 24 h, particularly in older individuals above age 65 [88].

But there are also some dangers of alcohol consumption: alcohol consumption appears to be associated with a higher risk for ischemic stroke among men who consumed >2 drinks per day [113]. In the Atherosclerosis Risk in Communities study, self-reported light-to-moderate alcohol consumption at midlife was not associated with reduced stroke risk compared with abstention over 20 years of follow-up. Heavier consumption increased the risk for ischemic stroke and intracerebral hemorrhage as did moderate intake for intracerebral hemorrhage [69].

The consumption of wine, particularly of red wine, has been associated in cross-sectional studies with a better prognostic outcome than the consumption of beer. This was partially attributed to the content of polyphenols found in red wine, especially resveratrol, which have favorable effects on endothelial function and decreased platelet aggregation even in dealcoholized wine [121]. Johansen et al. examined in a cross-sectional study the food-buying habits of people who buy wine or beer. People buying wine significantly more often also bought olive oil and low-fat milk products or low-fat meat, whereas people buying beer favored sausages, cold cuts, and pork. Thus there is a significant potential for social selection bias by just evaluating the type of alcohol consumed [68].

In the setting after myocardial infarction, the ONSET [111], the Lyon Diet Heart Study [27], and the Stockholm Heart Epidemiology Program (SHEEP) [67] have prospectively compared mortality across alcohol consumption categories in survivors of a recent acute myocardial infarction. The favorable effects of moderate alcohol consumption are reproduced in most of these studies, and the possibility of a "social selection bias" has largely been excluded by multivariate analysis, although unknown confounders in the absence of randomized studies are still a possibility. In the SHEEP study, there was no difference in the beneficial effects between wine and beer consumption, and the benefit started already at a low dose of less than 5 g of alcohol per day [68]. Also in a meta-analysis of eight studies on a total of 16,351 patients with cardiovascular disease, light-to-moderate alcohol consumption (5–25 g/day) was significantly associated with a lower incidence of cardiovascular and all-cause mortality [21].

Alcoholic beverages in small amounts – and it is probably the ethanol itself – have anti-inflammatory effects and reduce fibrinogen. In interventional studies a significant reduction of CRP concentrations and fibrinogen after 3 weeks of diet-controlled consumption of three glasses of beer/day in women or four glasses of beer/day in men have been demonstrated. Moreover, a 4-week consumption of 30 g/day of alcohol in red wine led to a significant decrease in CRP (21 %) in healthy adult men [37].

Alcohol also increases HDL cholesterol, endothelial function, antioxidative effects, and fibrinolysis and leads to a decrease in plasma viscosity and platelet aggregation. The combination of these effects may explain part of the beneficial effects of alcohol on the incidence of CV events [77].

2.4.2.2 Alcohol and Myocardial Function

Moderate alcohol consumption in primary prevention had a beneficial effect on the incidence of ischemia-related heart failure in the Physicians' Health Study [31], where the authors concluded that modest alcohol consumption may lower the risk of heart failure and that this possible benefit may be mediated through beneficial effects of alcohol on coronary artery disease, but the study also showed that moderate alcohol consumption does not prevent nonischemic cardiomyopathy.

2.4.2.3 Alcohol and Atrial Fibrillation

Atrial fibrillation/atrial flutter, the most common cardiac arrhythmia, is accompanied with a four- to fivefold increased risk for stroke, tripling of the risk for heart failure, doubling of the risk for dementia, and 40–90 % increase in the risk for all-cause mortality [8]. In women who consume more than two drinks per day [19] and in men who consume more than five drinks per day, the risk of atrial fibrillation increases [114].

In a large Swedish observational study and in a meta-analysis of seven prospective studies compared with nondrinkers, the hazard ratios increased from 1.08 (95 %

CI, 1.06–1.10) for one drink/day (i.e., 12 g of alcohol) to 1.26 (95 % CI, 1.19–1.33) for three drinks/day and 1.47 (95 % CI, 1.34–1.61) for five drinks/day, indicating that even moderate alcohol consumption is a risk factor for atrial fibrillation [85]. The authors conclude that for each 1 drink/day increase of alcohol consumption, the overall risk of atrial fibrillation increases by 8 %.

2.4.2.4 Alcohol and Abdominal Aortic Aneurysm

In a large Swedish registry of 44,715 men and 35,569 women with an average follow-up of 12.7 years (about one million person-years), moderate alcohol consumption (120 g of alcohol/week for men and 50 g of alcohol for women) specifically wine and beer (but not liquor) was associated with a reduced hazard ratio of 0.8 for men and 0.57 for abdominal aortic aneurysm compared to one drink per week [149].

Women tolerate less alcohol or have similar benefits at a lower dosage of alcohol, probably because of the lower activity of the gastric alcohol dehydrogenase. In women the beneficial effects of alcohol consumption on the heart are mitigated by an increase of breast cancer risk [28].

Despite the theoretically favorable effects of alcohol, e.g., in Germany, 40,000 persons die each year from alcohol consumption, and 2000 children are born with alcohol-induced malformations [146]. Therefore a recommendation for alcohol consumption appears at present not sensible and possibly hazardous – although a recent observation from the ARIC study showed that people who spontaneously begin consuming alcohol in middle age rarely do so beyond recommended amounts. Those who began drinking moderately experienced a relatively prompt benefit of lower rates of cardiovascular disease morbidity with no change in mortality rates after 4 years [75].

In nine nationally representative samples of US adults, light and moderate alcohol consumption were inversely associated with CVD mortality, even when compared with lifetime abstainers, but consumption above recommended limits was not [115].

The findings also support the relative safety of continued light alcohol consumption for ischemic cardiovascular events among adults who have been able to appropriately regulate the quantity, type, and timing of their alcohol use, but there is an increased risk of atrial fibrillation beginning at one alcoholic drink (12 g of alcohol) per day: thus the decision for alcohol consumption has to be individualized.

2.4.3 Soft Drinks and the Risk of Obesity and Cardiovascular Events

Soft drinks are an American development and represent an important nutritional problem worldwide but particularly in the United States. The problem has been analyzed in several studies. Sugar-sweetened soft drinks contribute 7.1 % of total energy intake and represent the largest single food source of calories in the US diet. In children and adolescents, beverages now even account for 10–15 % of the calories consumed. For each extra can or glass of sugared beverage consumed per day, the likelihood of a child's becoming obese increases by 60 % [10].

The regular consumption of soft drinks has been associated with overweight, the metabolic syndrome, and diabetes.

The rise of obesity and type 2 diabetes in the United States paralleled the increase in sugar-sweetened soft drink consumption [96]. In an examination of the Framingham's Third Generation cohort, sugar-sweetened soft drink intake was associated with greater change in visceral adipose tissue volume which increased by 852 cm^3 from nonconsumers to daily consumers (P trend <0.001 after adjustment for multiple confounders). In contrast, diet soda consumption was not associated with change in abdominal adipose tissue [93].

In the longitudinal observation of the Nurses' Health Study, women consuming one or more sugar-sweetened soft drinks or fruit punch per day had an almost two-fold risk to develop a type 2 diabetes compared with those who consumed less than one of these beverages per month.

Similarly regular consumption of sugar-sweetened beverages, i.e., 1 serving per month vs. 2 servings per day during 24 years of follow-up, was associated with a 35 % higher risk of CHD in women, even after other unhealthy lifestyle or dietary factors were accounted for, whereas artificially sweetened beverages were not associated with CHD [48].

2.5   Concluding Remarks

Thus there is strong evidence supporting a protective cardiovascular effect for intake of vegetables, nuts, mono- and polyunsaturated fatty acids and Mediterranean diet as well as a high-quality or a "prudent" dietary pattern. There is good evidence supporting a protective effect for intake of fish (omega-3 fatty acids in primary prevention only), whole grains, fruits, and fibers.

There is indirect evidence for the beneficial effect of a low ratio of saturated/mono- and polyunsaturated fatty acids mostly through the evidence from the Mediterranean diet. Alcohol consumption at low levels appears to be safe with respect to ischemic cardiovascular events, but there is an increased risk for atrial fibrillation beginning even at low daily consumption of alcoholic beverages.

There is good evidence that the so-called Western dietary pattern, the southern US dietary pattern, processed meats, industrially produced trans-fatty acids, and sugar-sweetened beverages increase the risk of cardiovascular disease.

References

1. Aatola H, Koivistoinen T, Hutri-Kähönen N, Juonala M, Mikkilä V, Lehtimäki T, Viikari JSA, Raitakari OT, Kähönen M. Lifetime fruit and vegetable consumption and arterial pulse wave velocity in adulthood the Cardiovascular Risk in Young Finns Study. Circulation. 2010;122:2521–8.
2. Åkesson A, Larsson SC, Discacciati A, Wolk A. Low-risk diet and lifestyle habits in the primary prevention of myocardial infarction in men a population-based prospective cohort study. J Am Coll Cardiol. 2014;64:1299–306.

3. Akin I, Schneider H, Nienaber CA, Jung W, Lübke M, Rillig A, Ansari U, Wunderlich N, Birkemeyer R. Lack of "obesity paradox" in patients presenting with ST-segment elevation myocardial infarction including cardiogenic shock: a multicenter German network registry analysis. BMC Cardiovasc Disord. 2015;15:67–75.

4. Albert CM, Gaziano JM, Willett WC, Manson JAE. Nut consumption and decreased risk of sudden cardiac death in the physicians' health study. Arch Intern Med. 2002;162:1382–7.

5. Bak AA, Grobbee DE. The effect on serum cholesterol levels of coffee brewed by filtering or boiling. N Engl J Med. 1989;321:1432–7.

6. Bao Y, Han J, Hu FB, Giovannucci EL, Stampfer MJ, Willett WC, Fuchs CS. Association of nut consumption with total and cause-specific mortality. N Engl J Med. 2013;369:2001–11.

7. Bastien M, Poirier P, Lemieux I, Després JP. Overview of epidemiology and contribution of obesity to cardiovascular disease. Prog Cardiovasc Dis. 2014;56:369–81.

8. Benjamin EJ, Chen PS, Bild DE, et al. Prevention of atrial fibrillation: report from a national heart, lung, and blood institute workshop. Circulation. 2009;119:606–18.

9. Bouvard V, Loomis D, Guyton KZ, Grosse Y, Ghissassi FE, Benbrahim-Tallaa L, Guha N, Mattock H, Straif K, on behalf of the International Agency for Research on Cancer Monograph Working Group. Carcinogenicity of consumption of red and processed meat. Lancet Oncol. 2015;16:1599–600.

10. Brownell KD, Frieden TR. Ounces of prevention — the public policy case for taxes on sugared beverages. New Engl J Med. 2009;360:1805–8.

11. Bureau of labor statistics; American Time use survey-Time spent in primary activities and percent of the civilian population engaging in each activity, averages per day by sex, 2014 annual averages. http://www.bls.gov/news.release/atus.t01.htm. Accessed 9 Feb 2016.

12. Büttner HJ, Mueller C, Gick M, Ferenc M, Allgeier J, Comberg T, Werner KD, Schindler C, Neumann F-J. The impact of obesity on mortality in UA/non-ST-segment elevation myocardial infarction. Eur Heart J. 2007;28(14):1694–701.

13. Calle EE, Thun MJ, Petrelli J, Rodriguez C, Heath CW. Body-mass index and mortality in a prospective cohort of U.S. adults. N Engl J Med. 1999;341:1097–105.

14. Calle EE, Rodriguez C, Walker-Thurmond K, Thun MJ. Overweight, obesity, and mortality from cancer in a prospectively studied cohort of U.S. adults. N Engl J Med. 2003;348:1625–38.

15. Cholesterol Treatment Trialists' (CTT) Collaboration, Baigent C, Blackwell L, Emberson J, et al. Efficacy and safety of more intensive lowering of LDL cholesterol: a meta-analysis of data from 170,000 participants in 26 randomised trials. Lancet. 2010;376:1670–81.

16. Chow CK, Jolly S, Rao-Melacini P, Fox KAA, Anand SS, Yusuf S. Association of diet exercise, and smoking modification with risk of early cardiovascular events after acute coronary syndromes. Circulation. 2010;121:750–8.

17. Christakis NA, Fowler JH. The spread of obesity in a large social network over 32 years. N Engl J Med. 2007;357:370–9.

18. Clarke R, Frost C, Collins R, Appleby P, Peto R. Dietary lipids and blood cholesterol: quantitative meta-analysis of metabolic ward studies. BMJ. 1997;314:112–7.

19. Conen D, Tedrow UB, Cook NR, Moorthy MV, Buring JE, Albert CM. Alcohol consumption and risk of incident atrial fibrillation in women. JAMA. 2008;300:2489–96.

20. Corti R, Flammer AJ, Hollenberg NK, Lüscher TF. Cocoa and cardiovascular health. Circulation. 2009;119:1433–41.

21. Costanzo S, Di Castelnuovo A, Donati MB, Iacoviello L, de Gaetano G. Alcohol consumption and mortality in patients with cardiovascular disease a meta-analysis. J Am Coll Cardiol. 2010;55:1339–47.

22. Covas M-I, Nyyssönen K, Poulsen HE, Kaikkonen J, Zunft HJF, Holger Kiesewetter, Gaddi A, et al, for the EUROLIVE Study Group (2006) The effect of polyphenols in olive oil on heart disease risk factors. A randomized trial. Ann Intern Med 145:333–41.

23. Crowe FL, Roddam AW, Key TJ, Appleby PN, Overvad K, Jakobsen MU, et al. Fruit and vegetable intake and mortality from ischaemic heart disease: results from the European Prospective Investigation into Cancer and Nutrition (EPIC)-Heart study. Eur Heart J. 2011;32:1235–43.

24. Curb JD, Wergowske G, Dobbs JC, Abbott RD, Huang B. Serum lipid effects of a high–mono-unsaturated fat diet based on macadamia nuts. Arch Intern Med. 2000;160:1154–8.

25. Dai J, Miller AH, Bremner JD, Goldberg J, Jones L, Shallenberger L, Buckham R, Murrah NV, Veledar E, Wilson PW, Vaccarino V. Adherence to the Mediterranean diet is inversely associated with circulating interleukin-6 among middle-aged men. A twin study. Circulation. 2008;117:169–75.

26. de Lorgeril M, Salen P, Martin J-L, Monjaud I, Delaye J, Mamelle N. Mediterranean diet, traditional risk factors, and the rate of cardiovascular complications after myocardial infarction final report of the lyon diet heart study. Circulation. 1999;99:779–85.

27. de Lorgeril M, Sale P. Wine ethanol, platelets, and Mediterranean diet. Lancet. 1999;353:1067. Research letter

28. Di Castelnuovo A, Costanzo S, Bagnardi V, Donati MB, Iacoviello L, de Gaetano G. Alcohol dosing and total mortality in men and women. Arch Intern Med. 2006;166:2437–45.

29. Digenio AG, Mancuso JP, Gerber RA, Dvorak RV. Comparison of methods for delivering a lifestyle modification program for obese patients- a randomized trial. Ann Intern Med. 2009;150:255–62.

30. Ding M, Satija A, Bhupathiraju SN, Hu Y, Sun Q, Han J, Lopez-Garcia E, Willett Wvan Dam RM, Hu FB. Association of coffee consumption with total and cause-specific mortality in three large prospective cohorts. Circulation. 2015;132:2305–15.

31. Djoussé L, Gaziano JM. Alcohol consumption and risk of heart failure in the physicians' health study I. Circulation. 2007;115:34–9.

32. Djoussé L, Gaziano JM. Breakfast cereals and risk of heart failure in the physicians' health study. Arch Intern Med. 2007;167:2080–5.

33. Djousse L, Gaziano JM. Egg consumption and risk of heart failure in the physicians' health study. Circulation. 2008;117:512–6.

34. Djoussé L, Khawaja OA, Gaziano JM. Egg consumption and risk of type 2 diabetes: a meta-analysis of prospective studies. Am J Clin Nutr. 2016;103:474–80.

35. Duffy SJ, Keaney Jr JF, Holbrook M, Gokce N, Swerdloff PL, Frei B, Vita JA. Short- and long-term black tea consumption reverses endothelial dysfunction in patients with coronary artery disease. Circulation. 2001;104:151–6.

36. Eckel RH, Jakicic JM, Ard JD, de Jesus JM, Houston-Miller N, Hubbard VS, Lee IM, Lichtenstein AH, Loria CM, Millen BE, Nonas CA, Sacks FM, Smith SC, Svetkey LP, Wadden TA, Yanovski SZ. 2013 AHA/ACC guideline on lifestyle management to reduce cardiovascular risk: a report of the American College of Cardiology/American Heart Association Task Force on practice guidelines. Circulation. 2014;129:S76–99.

37. Estruch R, Martinez-Gonzalez MA, Corella D, Salas-Salvado J, Ruiz-Gutierrez V, Covas MI, Fiol M, Gomez-Gracia E, Lopez-Sabater MC, Vinyoles E, Aros F, Conde M, Lahoz C, Lapetra J, Saez G, Ros E, for the PREDIMED Study Investigators. Effects of a Mediterranean-style diet on cardiovascular risk factors – a randomized trial. Ann Intern Med. 2006;145:1–11.

38. Estruch R, Ros E, Salas-Salvadó J, Covas MI, Corella D, Arós F, Gómez-Gracia E, Ruiz-Gutiérrez V, Fiol M, Lapetra J, et al, for the PREDIMED Study Investigators (2013) Primary prevention of cardiovascular disease with a Mediterranean diet. N Engl J Med 368:1279–90.

39. Ezzati M, Vander Hoorn S, Rodgers A, Lopez AD, Mathers CD, Murray CJL, the Comparative Risk Assessment Collaborating Group. Estimates of global and regional potential health gains from reducing multiple major risk factors. Lancet. 2003;362:271–80.

40. Farvid MS, Ding M, Pan A, Sun Q, Chiuve SE, Steffen LM, Willett WC, Hu FB. Dietary linoleic acid and risk of coronary heart disease: a systematic review and meta-analysis of prospective cohort studies. Circulation. 2014;130:1568–78.

41. Farzaneh-Far R, Lin J, Epel ES, Harris WS, Blackburn EH, Whooley MA. Association of marine omega-3 fatty acid levels with telomeric aging in patients with coronary heart disease. JAMA. 2010;303(3):250–7.

42. Finucane MM, Stevens GA, Cowan MJ, et al, The Global Burden of Metabolic Risk Factors of Chronic Diseases Collaborating Group (Body Mass Index) (2011) National, regional, and global trends in body-mass index since 1980: systematic analysis of health examination

surveys and epidemiological studies with 960 country-years and 9.1 million participants Lancet 377: 557–67.

43. Fitó M, Guxens M, Corella D, Sáez G, Estruch R, de la Torre R, Francés F, Cabezas C, del Carmen M, López-Sabater MJ, García-Arellano A, Arós F, Ruiz-Gutierrez V, Ros E, Salas-Salvadó J, Fiol M, Solá R, Covas MI, for the PREDIMED Study Investigators. Effect of a traditional Mediterranean diet on lipoprotein oxidation: a randomized controlled trial. Arch Intern Med. 2007;167:1195–203.

44. Fontaine KR, Redden DT, Wang C, Westfall AO, Allison DB. Years of life lost due to obesity. JAMA. 2003;289:187–93.

45. Flammer AJ, Hermann F, Sudano I, Spieker L, Hermann M, Cooper KA, Serafini M, Lüscher TF, Ruschitzka F, Noll G, Corti R. Dark chocolate improves coronary vasomotion and reduces platelet reactivity. Circulation. 2007;116:2376–82.

46. Fraser GE, Sabate J, Beeson WL, TM S. A possible protective effect of nut consumption on risk of CHD the adventist health study. Archives Intern Med. 1992;152:1416–24.

47. Fung TT, McCullough ML, Newby PK, Manson JE, Meigs JB, Rifai N, Willett WC, Hu FB. Diet-quality scores and plasma concentrations of markers of inflammation and endothelial dysfunction. Am J Clin Nutr. 2005;82:163–73.

48. Fung TT, Malik V, Rexrode KM, Manson JAE, Willett WC, Hu FB. Sweetened beverage consumption and risk of coronary heart disease in women. Am J Clin Nutr. 2009;89:1–6.

49. Fung TT, Rexrode KM, Mantzoros CS, et al. Mediterranean diet and incidence of and mortality from coronary heart disease and stroke in women. Circulation. 2009;119:1093–100.

50. Grundy SM, Becker D, Clark LT, Cooper RS , Denke MA, Howard WJ et al (2002) Third report of the National Cholesterol Education Program (NCEP) expert panel on detection, evaluation, and treatment of high blood cholesterol in adults (Adult Treatment Panel III) National Cholesterol Education Program National Heart, Lung, and Blood Institute National Institutes of Health NIH publication no. 02–5215

51. Gruppo Italiano per lo Studio della Sopravivenza nell'Infarto miocardico. Dietary supplementation with n-3 polyunsaturated PUFAs and vitamin E after myocardial infarction: results of the GISSI-Prevenzione trial. Lancet. 1999;354:447–55.

52. Guasch-Ferré M, Bulló M, Martínez-González MA, Ros E, Corella D, Estruch R, et al, PREDIMED Study Group (2013) Frequency of nut consumption and mortality risk in the PREDIMED nutrition intervention trial. BMC Med. 11:164.

53. Hajer GR, van Haeften TW, Visseren FLJ. Adipose tissue dysfunction in obesity, diabetes, and vascular diseases. Eur Heart J. 2008;29:2959–71.

54. Hammer S, Snel M, Lamb HJ, Jazet IM, van der Meer RW, Pijl H, Meinders EA, Romijn JA, de Roos A, Smit JWA. Prolonged caloric restriction in obese patients with type 2 diabetes mellitus decreases myocardial triglyceride content and improves myocardial function. JACC. 2008;52:1006–12.

55. Harcombe Z, Baker JS, Cooper SM, Davies B, Sculthorpe N, DiNicolantonio JD, Grace F. Evidence from randomised controlled trials did not support the introduction of dietary fat guidelines in 1977 and 1983: a systematic review and meta-analysis. Open Heart. 2015;2:e000196. doi:10.1136/openhrt-2014-000196.

56. Harris WS, PhD MD, Rimm E, Kris-Etherton P, Rudel LL, Appel LJ, Engler MM, Engler MB, Sacks F. Omega-6 fatty acids and risk for cardiovascular disease. A science advisory from the American Heart Association Nutrition Subcommittee of the Council on Nutrition, Physical Activity, and Metabolism; Council on Cardiovascular Nursing; and Council on Epidemiology and Prevention. Circulation. 2009;119:902–7.

57. He M, van Dam RM, Rimm E, Hu FB, Qi L. Whole-grain, cereal fiber, bran, and germ intake and the risks of all-cause and cardiovascular disease–specific mortality among women with type 2 diabetes mellitus. Circulation. 2010;121:2162–8.

58. Heiss C, CL K, Kelm M. Flavanols and cardiovascular disease prevention. Eur Heart J. 2010;31:2583–92.

59. Hollenberg NK, Fisher NDL. Is it the dark in dark chocolate? Circulation. 2007;116:2360–2.

60. Howell WH, McNamara DJ, Tosca MA, Smith BT, Gaines JA. Plasma lipid and lipoprotein responses to dietary fat and cholesterol: a meta analysis. Am J Clin Nutr. 1997;65:1747–64.
61. Schweizer Schokoladenindustrie http://www.chocosuisse.ch/chocosuisse/de/documentation/facts_figures.html. Accessed 02-07-2016
62. Hu FB, Stampfer MJ, Rimm EB, Manson JE, Ascherio A, Colditz GA, Rosner BA, Spiegelman D, Speizer FE, Sacks FM, Hennekens CH, Willett WC. A prospective study of egg consumption and risk of cardiovascular disease in men and women. JAMA. 1999;281:1387–94.
63. Huxley R, Barzi F, Woodward M. Excess risk of fatal coronary heart disease associated with diabetes in men and women: meta-analysis of 37 prospective cohort studies. BMJ. 2006;332:73–8.
64. Iqbal R, Anand S, Ounpuu S, Islam S, Zhang X, Rangarajan S, Chifamba J, Al-Hinai A, Keltai M, Yusuf S, on behalf of the INTERHEART Study Investigators. Dietary patterns and the risk of acute myocardial infarction in 52 countries: results of the INTERHEART study. Circulation. 2008;118:1929–37.
65. Jakes RW, Day NE, Khaw KT, et al. Television viewing and low participation in vigorous recreation are independently associated with obesity and markers of cardiovascular disease risk: EPIC-Norfolk population-based study. Eur J Clin Nutr. 2003;57:1089–96.
66. Jakulj F, Zernicke K, Bacon SL, van Wielingen LE, Key BL, West SG, TS C. A high-fat meal increases cardiovascular reactivity to psychological stress in healthy young adults. J Nutr. 2007;137:935–9.
67. Janszky RL, Ahnve S, Hallqvist J, Bennet AM, Mukamal KJ. Alcohol and long-term prognosis after a first acute myocardial infarction: the SHEEP study. Eur Heart J. 2008;29: 45–53.
68. Johansen D, Friis K, Skovenborg E, Ml G. Food buying habits of people who buy wine or beer: cross sectional study. Br Med J. 2006;332:519–24.
69. Jones SB, Loehr L, Avery CL, Gottesman RF, Wruck L, Shahar E, WD R. Midlife alcohol consumption and the risk of stroke in the atherosclerosis risk in communities study. Stroke. 2015;46:3124–30.
70. Joshipura KJ, Ascherio A, Manson JE, Stampfer MJ, Rimm EB, Speizer FE, et al. Fruit and vegetable intake in relation to risk of ischemic stroke. JAMA. 1999;282:1233–9.
71. Joshipura KJ, Hu FB, Manson JE, Stampfer MJ, Rimm EB, Speizer FE, Colditz GA, Ascherio A, Rosner B, Spiegelman D, Willett WC. The effect of fruit and vegetable intake on risk for coronary heart disease. Ann Intern Med. 2001;134:1106–14.
72. Katan MB. Weight loss diets for prevention and treatment of obesity. N Engl J Med. 2009;360:923–5.
73. Keys A. Seven countries: a multivariate analysis of death and coronary heart disease. Cambridge: Harvard University Press; 1980.
74. Keys A, Menotti A, Karvonen MJ, Aravanis C, Blackburn H, Buzina R, Djordjevic BS, Dontas AS, Fidanza F, Keys MH, Kromhout D, Nedeljkovic S, Punsar S, Seccareccia F, Toshima H. The diet and 15 year death rate in the Seven Countries Study. Am J Epidemiol. 1986;124:903–15.
75. King DE, Mainous AG, Geesey ME. Adopting moderate alcohol consumption in middle age: subsequent cardiovascular events. Am J Med. 2008;121:201–6.
76. Kleber ME, Delgado GE, Lorkowski S, März W, von Schacky C. Trans fatty acids and mortality in patients referred for coronary angiography: the Ludwigshafen Risk and Cardiovascular Health Study. Eur Heart J. 2016;37:1072–8.
77. Kloner RA, Rezkalla SH. To drink or not to drink? That is the question. Circulation. 2007;116:1306–17.
78. Knoops KT, de Groot LC, Kromhout D, et al. Mediterranean diet, lifestyle factors, and 10-year mortality in elderly European men and women: the HALE project. JAMA. 2004;292:1433–9.
79. Köhler A, Bittner D, Löw A, von Schacky C. Effects of a convenience drink fortified with n-3 fatty acids on the n-3 index. Br J Nutr. 2010;104:729–36.
80. Kokubo Y, Iso H, Saito I, Yamagishi K, Yatsuya H, Ishihara J, Inoue M, Tsugane S. The impact of green tea and coffee consumption on the reduced risk of stroke incidence in Japanese population the Japan public health center-based study cohort. Stroke. 2013;44:1369–74.

81. Kris-Etherton PM, Harris WS, Appel LJ, for the Nutrition Committee. Fish consumption, fish oil, omega-3 fatty acids, and cardiovascular disease. Circulation. 2002;106:2747–57.
82. Kris-Etherton PM, Hu FB, Ros E, Sabaté J. The role of tree nuts and peanuts in the prevention of coronary heart disease: multiple potential mechanisms. J Nutr. 2008;138:1746S–51S. Supplement: 2007 Nuts and Health Symposium
83. Kumanyika SK, Obarzanek E, Stettler N, Bell R, Field AE, Fortmann SP, Franklin BA, Gillman MW, Lewis CE, Poston WC, Stevens J, Hong Y. Population-based prevention of obesity: the need for comprehensive promotion of healthful eating, physical activity, and energy balance: a scientific statement from American Heart Association Council on Epidemiology and Prevention, Interdisciplinary Committee for Prevention (formerly the expert panel on population and prevention science). Circulation. 2008;118:428–64.
84. Kuriyama S, Shimazu T, Ohmori K, Kikuchi N, Nakaya N, Nishino Y, Tsubono Y, Tsuji I. Green tea consumption and mortality due to cardiovascular disease, cancer, and all causes in Japan: the Ohsaki study. JAMA. 2006;296:1255–65.
85. Larsson SC, Drca N, Wolk A. Alcohol consumption and risk of atrial fibrillation a prospective study and dose-response meta-analysis. J Am Coll Cardiol. 2014;64:281–9.
86. Lavie CJ, Milani RV, Mehra MR, Ventura HO. Omega-3 polyunsaturated fatty acids and cardiovascular diseases. J Am Coll Cardiol. 2009;54:585–94.
87. Lavie CJ, McAuley PA, Church TS, Milani RV, Blair SN. Obesity and cardiovascular diseases implications regarding fitness, fatness, and severity in the obesity paradox. J Am Coll Cardiol. 2014;63:1345–54.
88. Leong DP, Smyth A, Teo KK, McKee M, Rangarajan S, Pais P, Liu L, Anand SS, Yusuf S, on behalf of the INTERHEART Investigators. Patterns of alcohol consumption and myocardial infarction risk observations from 52 countries in the INTERHEART case–control study. Circulation. 2014;130:390–8.
89. Li Y, Hruby A, Bernstein AM, Ley SH, Wang DD, Chiuve SE, Sampson L, Rexrode KM, Rimm EB, Willett WC, Hu FB. Saturated fats compared with unsaturated fats and sources of carbohydrates in relation to risk of coronary heart disease: a prospective cohort study. J Am Coll Cardiol. 2015;66:1538–48.
90. Lim SS, Vos T, Flaxman AD, Danaei G, Shibuya K, Adair-Rohani H, Al Mazroa MA, Amann M, et al (2012) A comparative risk assessment of burden of disease and injury attributable to 67 risk factors and risk factor clusters in 21 regions, 1990-2010: a systematic analysis for the Global Burden of Disease Study 2010. Lancet. 380:2224–60.
91. Lopez-Garcia E, Rodriguez-Artalejo F, Rexrode KM, Logroscino G, Hu FB, van Dam RM. Coffee consumption and risk of stroke in women. Circulation. 2009;119:1116–23.
92. Lorenz M, Jochmann N, von Krosigk A, Martus P, Baumann G, Stangl K, Stangl V. Addition of milk prevents vascular protective effects of tea. Eur Heart J. 2007;28:219–23.
93. Ma J, McKeown NM, Hwang S-J, Hoffmann U, Jacques PF, Fox CS. Sugar-sweetened beverage consumption is associated with change of visceral adipose tissue over 6 years of follow-up. Circulation. 2016;133:370–7.
94. Madala MC, Franklin BA, Chen AY, Berman AD, Roe MT, Peterson ED, Ohman EM, Smith SC, Gibler WB, McCullough PA, for the CRUSADE Investigators. Obesity and age of first non–ST-segment elevation myocardial infarction. J Am Coll Cardiol. 2008;52:979–85.
95. Mahajan R, Lau DH, Brooks AG, Shipp NJ, Manavis J, Wood JPM, Finnie JW, Samuel CS, Royce SG, Twomey DJ, Thanigaimani S, Kalman JM, Sanders P. Electrophysiological, electroanatomical, and structural remodeling of the atria as consequences of sustained obesity. J Am Coll Cardiol. 2015;66:1–11.
96. Malik VS, Popkin BM, Bray GA, Despres J-P, Hu FB. Sugar-sweetened beverages, obesity, type 2 diabetes mellitus, and cardiovascular disease risk. Circulation. 2010;121:1356–64.
97. Martınez-Gonzalez de la Fuente-Arrillaga C, Nunez-Cordoba JM, Basterra-Gortari FM, Beunza JJ, Vazquez Z, Benito S, Tortosa A, Bes-Rastrollo M. Adherence to Mediterranean diet and risk of developing diabetes: prospective cohort study. Br Med J. 2008;336:1348–51.
98. McGillicuddy FC, de la Llera MM, Hinkle CC, Joshi MR, Chiquoine EH, Billheimer JT, Rothblat GH, Reilly MP. Inflammation impairs reverse cholesterol transport in vivo. Circulation. 2009;119:1135–45.

99. Mente A, de Koning L, Shannon HS, Anand SS. A systematic review of the evidence supporting a causal link between dietary factors and coronary heart disease. Arch Intern Med. 2009;169:659–69.

100. Micha R, Wallace S, Mozaffarian D. Red and processed meat consumption and risk of incident coronary heart disease, stroke, and diabetes: a systematic review and meta-analysis. Circulation. 2010;121:2271–83.

101. Miedema MD, Petrone A, Shikany JM, Greenland P, Lewis CE, Pletcher MJ, Gaziano JM, Djousse L. Association of fruit and vegetable consumption during early adulthood with the prevalence of coronary artery calcium after 20 years of follow-up the coronary artery risk development in young adults (CARDIA) study. Circulation. 2015;132:1990–8.

102. Mitrou PN, Kipnis V, Thiébaut ACM, Reedy J, Subar AF, Wirfält E, Flood A, Mouw T, Hollenbeck AR, Leitzmann MF, Schatzkin A. Mediterranean dietary pattern and prediction of all-cause mortality in a US population. Results from the NIH-AARP diet and health study. Arch Int Med. 2007;167:2461–8.

103. Mokdad AH, Marks JS, Stroup DF, Gerberding JL. Actual causes of death in the United States, 2000. JAMA. 2004;291:1238–45.

104. Mozaffarian D, Ascherio A, Hu FB, Stampfer MJ, Willett WC, Siscovick DS, Rimm EB. Interplay between different polyunsaturated fatty acids and risk of coronary heart disease in men. Circulation. 2005;111:157–64.

105. Mozaffarian D, Katan MB, Ascherio A, Stampfer MJ, Willett WC. Trans-fatty acids and cardiovascular disease. N Engl J Med. 2006;354:1601–13.

106. Mozaffarian D, Marfisi R, Levantesi G, Silletta MG, Tavazzi L, Tognoni G, et al. Incidence of new-onset diabetes and impaired fasting glucose in patients with recent myocardial infarction and the effect of clinical and lifestyle risk factors. Lancet. 2007;370:667–75.

107. Mozaffarian D, Appel LJ, Van Horn L. Components of a cardioprotective diet -new insights. Circulation. 2011;123:2870–91.

108. Mozaffarian D, Hao T, Rimm EB, Willett WC, Hu FB. Changes in diet and lifestyle and long term weight gain in women and men. N Engl J Med. 2011;364:2392–404.

109. Mozaffarian D, Afshin A, Benowitz NL, Bittner V, Daniels SR, Franch HA, et al, American Heart Association Council on Epidemiology and Prevention, Council on Nutrition, Physical Activity and Metabolism, Council on Clinical Cardiology, Council on Cardiovascular Disease in the Young, Council on the Kidney in Cardiovasc (2012) Population approaches to improve diet, physical activity, and smoking habits: a scientific statement from the American Heart Association. Circulation.126:1514–63.

110. Mozaffarian D. Dietary and policy priorities for cardiovascular disease, diabetes, and obesity a comprehensive review. Circulation. 2016;133:187–225.

111. Mukamal KJ, Maclure M, Muller JE, Sherwood JB, Mittleman MA. Prior alcohol consumption and mortality following acute myocardial infarction. JAMA. 2001;285:1965–70.

112. Mukamal KJ, Maclure M, Muller JE, Sherwood JB, Mittleman MA. Tea consumption and mortality after acute myocardial infarction. Circulation. 2002;105:2476–81.

113. Mukamal KJ, Ascherio A, Mittleman MA, Conigrave KM, Camargo Jr CA, Kawachi I, Stampfer MJ, Willett WC, Rimm EB. Alcohol and risk for ischemic stroke in men: the role of drinking patterns and usual beverage. Ann Intern Med. 2005;142:11–9.

114. Mukamal KJ, Psaty BM, Rautaharju PM, et al. Alcohol consumption and risk and prognosis of atrial fibrillation among older adults: the Cardiovascular Health Study. Am Heart J. 2007;153:260–6.

115. Mukamal KJ, Chen CM, Rao SR, Breslow RA. Alcohol consumption and cardiovascular mortality among U.S. adults, 1987 to 2002. JACC. 2010;55:1328–35.

116. Nicholls SJ, Lundman P, Harmer JA, Cutri B, Griffiths KA, Rye K-A, Barter PJ, Celermajer DS. Consumption of saturated fat impairs the anti-inflammatory properties of high-density lipoproteins and endothelial function. JACC. 2006;48:715–20.

117. Nöthlings U, Schulze MB, Weikert C, Boeing H, van der Schouw YT, Bamia C, Benetou V, Lagiou P, Krogh V, Beulens JWJ, Peeters PHM, Halkjær J, Tjønneland A, Tumino R, Panico S, Masala G, Clavel-Chapelon F, de Lauzon B, Boutron-Ruault M-C, Vercambre M-N, Kaaks

R, Linseisen J, Overvad K, Arriola L, Ardanaz GCA, Tormo M-J, Bingham S, Khaw K-T, Key TJA, Vineis P, Riboli E, Ferrari P, Boffetta P, Bueno-de-Mesquita HB, der A DL v, Berglund G, Wirfält E, Hallmans G, Johansson I, Lund E, Trichopoulo A. Intake of vegetables, legumes, and fruit, and risk for all-cause, cardiovascular, and cancer mortality in a European diabetic population. J Nutr. 2008;138:775–81.

118. O'Keefe JH, Gheewala NM, O'Keefe JO. Dietary strategies for improving post-prandial glucose, lipids, inflammation, and cardiovascular health. JACC. 2008;51:249–55.

119. Oh K, Hu FB, Manson JE, Stampfer MJ, Willett WC. Dietary fat intake and risk of coronary heart disease in women: 20 years of follow-up of the Nurses' Health Study. Am J Epidemiol. 2005;161:672–9.

120. Okie S. New York to trans fats: you're out! N Engl J Med. 2007;356:2017–21.

121. Opie LH, Lecour S. The red wine hypothesis: from concepts to protective signalling molecules. Eur Heart J. 2007;28:1683–93.

122. Pai JK, Cahill LE, Hu FB, Rexrode KM, Manson JE, Rimm EB. Hemoglobin A1c is associated with increased risk of incident coronary heart disease among apparently healthy, nondiabetic men and women. J Am Heart Assoc. 2013;2:e000077. doi:10.1161/ AHA.112.000077.

123. Pathak RK, Middeldorp ME, Meredith M, Mehta AB, Mahajan R, Wong CX, Twomey D, Elliott AD, Kalman JM, Abhayaratna WP, Lau DH, Sanders P. Long-term effect of goal-directed weight management in an atrial fibrillation cohort a long-term follow-up study (LEGACY). J Am Coll Cardiol. 2015;65:2159–69.

124. Peeters A, Barendregt JJ, Willekens F, Mackenbach JP, Mamun AA, Bonneux L, for NEDCOM, the Netherlands Epidemiology and Demography Compression of Morbidity Research Group. Obesity in adulthood and its consequences for life expectancy: a life-table analysis. Ann Intern Med. 2003;138:24–32.

125. Pereira MA, O'Reilly E, Augustsson K, Fraser GE, Goldbourt U, Heitmann BL, Hallmans G, Knekt P, Liu S, Pietinen P, Spiegelman D, Stevens J, Virtamo J, Willett WC, Ascherio A. Dietary fiber and risk of coronary heart disease: a pooled analysis of cohort studies. Arch Intern Med. 2004;164:370–6.

126. Pereira MA, Parker ED, Folsom AR. Coffee consumption and risk of type 2 diabetes mellitus: an 11-year prospective study of 28 812 postmenopausal women. Arch Intern Med. 2006;166:1311–6.

127. Perk J, De Backer G, Gohlke H, Graham I, Reiner Z, Verschuren WM, et al. European guidelines on cardiovascular disease prevention in clinical practice (version 2012): the fifth joint task force of the European society of cardiology and other societies on cardiovascular disease prevention in clinical practice (constituted by representatives of nine societies and by invited experts). Eur Heart J. 2012;33(13):1635–701.

128. Pouliopoulos J, Chik WW, Kanthan A, et al. Intramyocardial adiposity after myocardial infarction: new implications of a substrate for ventricular tachycardia. Circulation. 2013;128:2296–308.

129. Pischon T, Boeing H, Hoffmann K, et al. General and abdominal adiposity and risk of death in Europe. N Engl J Med. 2008;359:2105–20.

130. Rauch B, Schiele R, Schneider S, Diller F, Victor N, Gohlke H, Gottwik M, Steinbeck G, Del Castillo U, Sack R, Worth H, Katus H, Spitzer W, Sabin G, Senges J, OMEGA Study Group. OMEGA, a randomized, placebo-controlled trial to test the effect of highly purified omega-3 fatty acids on top of modern guideline-adjusted therapy after myocardial infarction. Circulation. 2010;122:2152–9.

131. The Risk and Prevention Study Collaborative Group. n–3 fatty acids in patients with multiple cardiovascular risk factors. N Engl J Med. 2013;368:1800–8.

132. Roberto CA, Swinburn B, Hawkes C, Huang TT-K, Costa SA, Ashe M, Zwicker L, Cawley JH, Brownell KD. Patchy progress on obesity prevention: emerging examples, entrenched barriers, and new thinking. Lancet. 2015;385:2400–9.

133. Romon M, Lommez A, Tafflet M, et al. Downward trends in the prevalence of childhood overweight in the setting of 12-year school- and community-based programmes. Public Health Nutr. 2009;12:1305–6.

134. Ros E, Núñez I, Pérez-Heras A, Serra M, Gilabert R, Casals E, Deulofeu R. A walnut diet improves endothelial function in hypercholesterolemic subjects a randomized crossover trial. Circulation. 2004;109:1609–14.
135. Sabate J, Fraser GE, Burke K, Knutsen SF, Bennett H, KD L. Effects of walnuts on serum lipid levels and BP in normal Men. N Engl J Med. 1993;328:603–7.
136. Sacks FM, Bray GA, Carey VJ, Smith SR, Ryan DH, Anton SD, McManus K, Champagne CM, Bishop LM, Laranjo N, Leboff MS, Rood JC, de Jonge L, Greenway FL, Loria CM, Obarzanek E, Williamson DA. Comparison of weight loss diets with different compositions of fat, protein, and carbohydrates. N Engl J Med. 2009;360:859–73.
137. Sacks FM, Carey VJ, Anderson CAM, Miller III ER, Copeland T, Charleston J, Harshfield BJ, Laranjo N, McCarron P, Swain J, White K, Yee K, Appel LJ. Effects of high vs low glycemic index of dietary carbohydrate on cardiovascular disease risk factors and insulin sensitivity. The OmniCarb randomized clinical trial. JAMA. 2014;312(23):2531–41.
138. Sala-Vila A, Guasch-Ferre M, Hu FB, Sanchez-Tainta A, Bullo M, Serra-Mir M, Lopez-Sabater C, Sorli JV, Aros F, Fiol M, Munoz MA, Serra-Majem L, Martınez JA, Corella D, Fito M, Salas-Salvado J, Martınez-Gonzalez M, Estruch R, Ros E, for the PREDIMED Investigators. Dietary a-linolenic acid, marine x-3 fatty acids, and mortality in a population with high fish consumption: findings from the PREvencion con DIeta MEDiterranea (PREDIMED) Study. J Am Heart Assoc. 2016;5:e002543. doi:10.1161/JAHA.115.002543.
139. Salas-Salvado J, Fernandez-Ballart J, Ros E, Martınez-Gonzalez M-A, Fito M, Estruch R, Corella D, Fiol M, Gomez-Gracia E, Aros F, Flores G, Lapetra J, Lamuela-Raventos R. Effect of a Mediterranean diet supplemented with nuts on metabolic syndrome status-one-year results of the PREDIMED randomized trial. Arch Intern Med. 2008;168:2449–58.
140. Sarwar N, Gao P, Seshasai SR, Gobin R, Kaptoge S, Di Angelantonio E, Ingelsson E, Lawlor DA, Selvin E, Stampfer M, Stehouwer CD, Lewington S, Pennells L, Thompson A, Sattar N, White IR, Ray KK, Danesh J. Diabetes mellitus, fasting blood glucose concentration, and risk of vascular disease: a collaborative Metaanalysis of 102 prospective studies. Lancet. 2010;375:2215–22.
141. Shai I, Schwarzfuchs D, Henkin Y, Shahar DR, Witkow S, Greenberg I, Golan R, Fraser D, Bolotin A, Vardi H, et al for the Dietary Intervention Randomized Controlled Trial (DIRECT) Group (2008) Weight loss with a low-carbohydrate, Mediterranean, or low-fat diet. N Engl J Med 359:229–41
142. Shai I, Spence JD, Schwarzfuchs D, Henkin Y, Parraga G, Rudich A, Fenster A, Mallett C, Liel-Cohen N, Tirosh A, Bolotin A, Thiery J, Fiedler GM, Buher M, Stumvoll M, Stampfer MJ, for the DIRECT Group (2010) Dietary intervention to reverse carotid atherosclerosis. Circulation 121:1200–8
143. Shikany JM, Safford MM, Newby PK, Durant RW, Brown TM, Judd SE. Southern dietary pattern is associated with hazard of acute coronary heart disease in the reasons for geographic and racial differences in stroke (REGARDS) study. Circulation. 2015;132:804–14.
144. Shin JY, Xun P, Nakamura Y, He K. Egg consumption in relation to risk of cardiovascular disease and diabetes: a systematic review and meta-analysis. Am J Clin Nutr. 2013;98(1):146–59.
145. Shinmura K, Tamaki K, Saito K, Nakano Y, Tobe T, Bolli R. Cardioprotective effects of short-term caloric restriction are mediated by adiponectin via activation of AMP-activated protein kinase. Circulation. 2007;116:2809–17.
146. Singer MV, Teyssen S. Alcohol associated somatic hazards. Dtsch Ärztebl. 2001;98:A2109–20.
147. Sofi F, Cesaro F, Abbate R, Gensini GF, Casini A. Adherence to Mediterranean diet and health status: meta-analysis. Br Med J. 2008;337:a1344.
148. Spence JD, Jenkins DJ, Davignon J. Egg yolk consumption and carotid plaque. Atherosclerosis. 2012;224:469–73.
149. Stackelberg O, Björck M, Larsson SC, Orsini N, Wolk A. Alcohol consumption, specific alcoholic beverages, and abdominal aortic aneurysm. Circulation. 2014;130:646–52.

150. Stamatakis E, Hirani V, Rennie K. Moderate-to-vigorous physical activity and sedentary behaviours in relation to body mass index defined and waist circumference-defined obesity. Br J Nutr. 2009;101:765–73.
151. Steffen LM, Folsom AR, Cushman M, et al. Greater fish, fruit, and vegetable intakes are related to lower incidence of venous thromboembolism. The longitudinal investigation of thromboembolism etiology. Circulation. 2007;115:188–95.
152. Steptoe A, Gibson EL, Vounonvirta R, Williams ED, Hamer M, Rycroft JA, Erusalimsky JD, Wardle J. The effects of tea on psychophysiological stress responsivity and post-stress recovery: a randomized double-blind trial. Psychopharmacology. 2007;190:81–90.
153. Stewart RAH, Wallentin L, Benatar J, Danchin N, Hagström E, Held C, Husted S, Lonn E, Stebbins A, Chiswell K, Vedin O, Watson D, White HD, on Behalf of the STABILITY Investigators. Dietary patterns and the risk of major adverse cardiovascular events in a global study of high-risk patients with stable coronary heart disease. Eur Heart J. 2016; doi:10.1093/eurheartj/ehw125.
154. Streppel MT, Ocke MC, Boshuizen HC, Kok FJ, Kromhout D. Long-term fish consumption and n-3 fatty acid intake in relation to (sudden) coronary heart disease death: the Zutphen study. Eur Heart J. 2008;29:2024–30.
155. Sun Q, Ma J, Campos H, Hankinson SE, Manson JE, Stampfer MJ, Rexrode KM, Willett WC, Hu FB. A prospective study of trans fatty acids in erythrocytes and risk of coronary heart disease. Circulation. 2007;115:1858–65.
156. Tang G, Wang D, Long J, Yang F, Si L. Meta-analysis of the association between whole grain intake and coronary heart disease risk. Am J Cardiol. 2015;115:625–9.
157. Tognon G, Lissner L, Sæbye D, Walker KZ, Heitmann BL. The Mediterranean diet in relation to mortality and CVD: a Danish cohort study. Br J Nutr. 2014;111:151–9.
158. Toledo E, Salas-Salvadó J, Donat-Vargas C, Buil-Cosiales P, Estruch R, Ros E, Corella D, Fitó M, Hu FB, Arós F, Gómez-Gracia E, Romaguera D, Ortega-Calvo M, Serra-Majem L, Pintó X, Schröder H, Basora J, Sorlí JV, Bulló M, Serra-Mir M, Martínez-González MA. Mediterranean diet and invasive breast cancer risk among women at high cardiovascular risk in the PREDIMED trial -a randomized clinical trial. JAMA Intern Med. 2015;175(11): 1752–60.
159. Trichopoulou A, Costacou T, Bamia C, Trichopoulos D. Adherence to a Mediterranean diet and survival in a Greek population. N Engl J Med. 2003;348:2599–608.
160. Trichopoulou A, Orfanos P, Norat T, et al. Modified Mediterranean diet and survival: EPIC-elderly prospective cohort study. Br Med J. 2005;330:991–7.
161. US Department of Health and Human Services. Scientific report of the 2015 dietary guidelines advisory committee dietary guidelines for Americans. Washington, DC; 2015.
162. Valls-Pedret C, Sala-Vila A, Serra-Mir M, Corella D, de la Torre R, Martinez-Gonzalez MA, Martinez-Lapiscina E-H, Fito M, Perez-Heras A, Salas-Salvado J, Estruch R, Ros E. Mediterranean diet and age-related cognitive decline a randomized clinical trial. JAMA Intern Med. 2015;175:1094–103.
163. Van Dam RM, Willett WC, Manson JE, Hu FB. Coffee, caffeine, and risk of type 2 diabetes. A prospective cohort study in younger and middle-aged U.S. women. Diabetes Care. 2006;29:398–403.
164. Virtanen JK, Mursu J, Tuomainen T-P, Virtanen HEK, Voutilainen S. Egg consumption and risk of incident type 2 diabetes in men: the Kuopio Ischaemic Heart Disease Risk Factor Study. Am J Clin Nutr. 2015; doi:10.3945/ajcn.114.104109.
165. von Schacky C, Harris WS. Cardiovascular benefits of omega-3 fatty acids. Cardiovasc Res. 2007;73:310–5.
166. Wang DD, Li Y, Chiuve SE, Stampfer MJ, Manson JE, Rimm EB, Willett WC,Hu FB Association of specific dietary fats with total and cause-specific mortality. JAMA Intern Med. Published online 2016. doi:10.1001/jamainternmed.2016.2417
167. Whitlock G, Lewington S, Sherliker P, Clarke R, Emberson J, Halsey QN, Collins R, Peto R. Body-mass index and cause-specific mortality in 900 000 adults: collaborative analyses of 57 prospective studies Prospective Studies Collaboration. Lancet. 2009;373:1083–96.

168. Yusuf S, Hawken S, Ounpuu S, Dans T, Avezum A, Lanas F, McQueen M, Budaj A, Pais P, Varigos J, Lisheng L, INTERHEART Study Investigators. Effect of potentially modifiable risk factors associated with myocardial infarction in 52 countries (the INTERHEART study): case-control study. Lancet. 2004;364:937–52.
169. Zong G, Gao A, Hu FB, Sun Q. Whole grain intake and mortality from all causes, cardiovascular disease, and cancer – a meta-analysis of prospective cohort studies. Circulation. 2016;133:2370–80.

Psychological Care of Cardiac Patients

3

Paul Bennett

3.1 Introduction

This chapter addresses the impact and rehabilitation needs of patients following diagnosis with acute coronary syndrome (ACS) and how psychologically based interventions may benefit such patients. It considers a range of approaches that can be used with individuals or in group contexts, all of which are targeted at two key goals:

- Changing risk behaviours, such as smoking and low levels of exercise
- Helping people adjust emotionally to their illness

These goals may be achieved through a variety of means: participation in an exercise programme, for example, may both improve cardiovascular fitness and reduce emotional distress as the individual feels they are gaining control over their illness and life. Likewise, changes in depression or anxiety may improve adherence to medication or exercise regimens. Nevertheless, any interventions can be divided roughly into those that address behavioural change and those that address emotional issues. Accordingly, this chapter will introduce a number of intervention approaches targeted at each outcome. The interventions discussed are not specialist interventions to be used only with a minority of patients. Rather, they, or the principles on which they are based, can usefully be incorporated into any rehabilitation programme. Before addressing these issues, however, the chapter briefly examines the psychological impact an acute coronary event can have on the individual.

P. Bennett, PhD
Department of Psychology, University of Swansea, Singleton Park,
Swansea SA2 8PP, UK
e-mail: p.d.bennett@swansea.ac.uk

© Springer International Publishing AG 2017
J. Niebauer (ed.), *Cardiac Rehabilitation Manual*,
DOI 10.1007/978-3-319-47738-1_3

3.2   The Impact of Acute Coronary Events

Cardiac events can trigger significant emotional reactions, but surprisingly modest behavioural change, at least in the long term. Hajek et al. [14], for example, found that 6 weeks following a myocardial infarction (MI), 60 % of those who smoked before their MI no longer did so. One year after MI, the percentage of those remaining a non-smoker fell to 37 %. Diet may also change in the short term although, again, old habits may creep back over time. Leslie et al. [23], for example, found that 65 % of participants in their nutritional educational programme were eating five portions of fruit or vegetables a day at its end: a figure that fell to 31 % over the following year. Levels in fitness may change markedly following participation in specific exercise programmes (e.g. [15]). However, the duration of any changes in the absence of continued follow-up is not clear. Lear et al. [22], for example, reported minimal changes from the baseline on measures of leisure time exercise and treadmill performance 1 year following MI despite participants taking part in a general rehabilitation programme.

Of concern also is that even modest behavioural change may be confined to a subgroup of patients. Bennett et al. [3] found that in the 6 months following acute coronary syndrome (ACS), levels of exercise rose only among patients already engaging in meaningful levels of exercise and did not change in those engaging in low levels of exercise. More encouragingly, people with relatively poor diets before the event did show more improvement than those with good diets, although they still did not reach the dietary scores achieved by the latter group at any time. Those with good dietary habits showed no improvement at all.

The psychological consequences of MI may be profound and persistent. Osler et al. [28] reported that 20 % of patients became depressed in the 2 years following the event. Lane et al. [21] found a 31 % prevalence rate of elevated depression scores during hospitalisation. The 4- and 12-month prevalence rates were 38 and 37 %. The same group reported the prevalence of elevated state anxiety to be 26 % in hospital, 42 % at 4-month follow-up and 40 % at the end of 1 year. They also reported high levels of comorbidity between anxiety and depression. Interest in the rates of post-traumatic stress disorder as a consequence of MI has recently increased, with prevalence rates typically being around 8–10 % up to 1 year following infarction (e.g. [5]). Poor emotional outcomes may be predicted by a range of psychosocial factors, including age (younger is worse), gender (female is worse), previous psychiatric history, lacking the availability of a confidant, the experience of ongoing life problems and personality factors including type D personality (e.g. [35, 18]).

Each of these emotional reactions can also influence important outcomes. Depression, and to a lesser extent anxiety, independently predicts re-infarction (e.g. [37]) as well as having a number of emotional and behavioural implications. Depressed and anxious individuals are least likely to attend cardiac rehabilitation classes [20]. Paradoxically, they are more likely to contact doctors and have more readmissions in the year following infarction [35]. Many of these appointments will be due to worry and health concerns rather than cardiac problems. The impact of mood on health behaviour change is modest. Huijbrechts et al. [16] reported that depressed and anxious patients were less likely to have stopped smoking 5 months after their MI than their less distressed counterparts. Bennett et al. [4] reported a modest association between low levels of exercise and depression, but no differences between depressed and nondepressed individuals on measures of smoking, alcohol consumption or diet. Finally, Shemesh et al. [31] found that high levels of PTSD symptoms, but not depression, were significant predictors of non-adherence to aspirin.

More importantly, perhaps, depression has consistently been associated with delayed or failure to return to work, reduced work hours and low ratings of work or social satisfaction (e.g. [32]). Delay in returning to work has been predicted by greater concerns about health and low social support. Resuming work at a lower activity level than before infarction is associated with older age, higher health concerns and patients' expectations of lower working capacity (independently of actual capacity). Indeed, patient's beliefs about their condition, which will be influenced by mood, appear critical in determining their behavioural response to it. Petrie et al. [30], for example, found that attendance at cardiac rehabilitation was significantly related to a stronger belief during admission that the illness could be cured or controlled. Return to work within 6 weeks was significantly predicted by the perception that the illness would last a short time and have less negative consequences. Patients' belief that their heart disease would have serious consequences was significantly related to later disability in work around the house, recreational activities and social interaction.

Finally, the partners of patients also experience high levels of distress, often greater than that reported by the patient [26]. Such anxieties may be increased by fears for the patient's health linked to a poor prognosis and non-compliance with treatment or behaviour change programmes [6]. Many wives also appear to inhibit angry or sexual feelings and become overprotective of their husbands [33].

3.3   Changing Risk Behaviour

A key component of any cardiac rehabilitation programme should address behaviour change designed to reduce risk for further disease progression and enhance quality of life. Achieving this goal can best be considered to involve two sets of processes:

- Increasing motivation to change
- Developing strategies of change

As the evidence reviewed above suggests, not everyone is motivated to change risk behaviours, even after acute events such as an MI. This group of individuals can be particularly challenging to health professionals as they are unlikely to respond to exhortations to change their behaviour, nor are they likely to benefit from interventions designed to show them how to change their behaviour. The best approach to use with such individuals is one that increases their *intrinsic* motivation to change.

3.3.1 Information Provision

One apparently simple approach to increasing motivation to change involves the provision of information. If individuals are unaware of the advantages of change, they are unlikely to be motivated to attempt to make change. The logic is clear. Unfortunately, while clear information may be of benefit when it is completely novel, does not contradict previous understandings of issues, is highly relevant to the individual and is relatively easy to act on, health-related information rarely meets all these criteria. And even when it does, it may well not impact on behaviour.

Reasons for these failures are complex and involve social, psychological and situational factors. Even relatively simple behavioural changes, such as improvements to diet, may involve quite complex barriers to change including negotiations within families, potential expense and lack of cooking skills. For this reason, a number of specific strategies have been used in attempts to influence motivation to change. One guide to relevant strategies is provided by the UK National Institute for Health and Care Excellence Guidelines on Behavioural Change (NICE 2014). These identify, for example, several ways of framing information through conversation or leaflets and similar outputs in order to increase the motivation of smokers to quit. Key messages should target psychological factors known to influence behaviour and include:

- *Outcome expectancies*: Smoking causes people to die on average 8 years earlier than the average.
- *Personal relevance*: If you were to stop smoking, you could add 6 years to your life and be fitter over that time.
- *Positive attitude*: Life is good and worth living. Better to be fit as you get older than unable to engage in things you would like to do.
- *Self-efficacy (confidence)*: You have managed to quit before. With some support there is no reason why you cannot sustain change now.
- *Descriptive norms*: Around 30 % of people of your age have successfully given up smoking.
- *Subjective norms*: Your wife and children will appreciate it if you were to give up smoking.
- *Personal and moral norms*: Smoking is anti-social and you do not want your kids to start smoking.

3.3.2 Motivational Interview

A more formal, technique-based approach to increasing motivation is afforded by the so-called motivational interview [25]. As its name suggests, its goal is to increase an individual's motivation to consider change – not to show them how to change. If the interview succeeds in motivating change, only then can any intervention proceed to considering ways of achieving that change. The approach is designed to help people to explore and resolve any ambivalence they may have about changing their behaviour. It assumes that when an individual is facing the need to change, they may have beliefs and attitudes that both support and counterchange. Prior to the interview, thoughts that counterchange probably predominate, or else the person would be actively making change. Nevertheless, the goal of the interview is to elicit both sets of beliefs and attitudes and to bring them into sharp focus, perhaps for the first time: 'I know smoking does damage my health', 'I enjoy smoking', and so on. This is thought to bring the individual to a decision point which is resolved by rejecting one set of beliefs in favour of the other. These may (or may not) favour behavioural change. If an individual decides to change their behaviour, the intervention will then focus on consideration of how to achieve change. If the individual still rejects the possibility of change, they would typically not continue in any programme of behavioural change, although the possibility of future motivational change should not completely preclude such continuation.

The motivational interview is deliberately non-confrontational. Miller and Rollnick consider the process to be a philosophy of supporting individual change and not attempting to persuade an individual to go against their own wishes. When the intervention was first developed, it was based on exploration of two key issues:

- 'What are the good things about your present behaviour?'
- 'What are the not so good things about your present behaviour?'

The first question is important as it acknowledges the individual is gaining something from their present behaviour and is intended to reduce the potential for resistance and argument. This process of exploration is not simply a one-question approach. Both the questions above are leads into a wider detailed exploration of these issues. However, once the individual has considered each issue (both for and against change), they are summarised by the health professional in a way that highlights the contradiction between the two sets of issues: 'So, smoking helps you cope with stress, but it causes trouble at home because your wife doesn't want you to smoke'. Once this has been fed back to the individual, they are invited to consider how this information makes them feel. Only if they express some interest in change should the interview then go on to consider how to change. More recently, Miller and Rollnick have suggested that patients may be encouraged to consider more actively the benefits of change and how things may be different were change achieved. Other key strategies include:

- *Expressing empathy through the use of reflective listening*: this involves engaging with the individual and trying to see things from their perspective rather than that of a health professional trying to encourage change. This helps develop an alliance between patient and health professional rather than a potentially adversarial relationship.
- *Avoiding arguments by assuming the individual is responsible for the decision to change*: this removes the onus of the health professional to actively persuade. In the end, it is up to the individual whether they change their behaviour, not the health professional.

- *'Rolling with resistance' rather than confronting or opposing it*: again, this means avoiding arguments and attempts at direct persuasion.
- *Supporting beliefs in the ability to change an optimism for change*: if the individual is unwilling to contemplate change because they are not sure they can achieve it, then part of the conversation could usefully look for evidence of the person's ability to change and feed this back to them, to increase their confidence in achieving change.

The motivational approach can be extremely powerful, even where people show high levels of resistance. Take the (true) example of Mr Jones, who had continued smoking despite having had two infarctions and being told that he may require two below-the-knee amputations due to ischaemia in his lower legs if he continued smoking:

Mr Jones: I know you want me to give up smoking. The doctors have told me that I have to give up, but I'm not going to. I know it's your job, but you can't persuade me! It's the one pleasure that I have, and I'm not giving it up.

Nurse: OK. OK. I'm not going to try and persuade you to stop smoking. In the end it is your choice. However, I am interested in why you smoke and why you are so firmly against changing despite all the hassle you have had from the doctors. So, what do you get out of smoking?

Mr Jones: Oh! (looks surprised and relieved and starts talking in a much more non-confrontational manner). Well, I've smoked all my life, ever since I was a kid really. It's difficult to give up something you've done for so long. It's part of my life. In a way, that's the main thing really – it's just part of my life. I can't see life without smoking. It helps me keep calm, and most of my mates are smokers – so it's part of my social life.

Nurse: So, it's difficult to see how to give up and how life would be without smoking....

Mr Jones: That's about it, really. I've tried to give up in the past and it's been really difficult. I've been back to smoking pretty quickly, so it's difficult to see myself giving up, even if I wanted to....

Nurse: Oh, so you've tried in the past to quit. What led you to that?

Mr Jones: Well, I know it really does make my heart bad, and I get out of breath when I smoke. So, it really makes it obvious the harm I'm doing to myself. But it's one thing to say you want to quit and another to actually do it. And I know I can't quit, so what's the point of even trying?

Note at this point that by not challenging or actively trying to persuade Mr Jones, the conversation has shifted from his not *wanting* to give up to not *feeling able* to give up – although because of the confrontational way this had been discussed previously, this had not been clear. So, the nurse moves from highlighting the pros and cons of behavioural change and takes this as a cue to look at how and why things have gone wrong before, in the hope that this may lead to consideration of behavioural change:

Nurse:	You say you have tried to stop smoking in the past. How did you set about this?
Mr Jones:	Well, I just tried to do it…. What do you call it? Will power?
Nurse:	How well did that work? Not too good from what you say….
Mr Jones:	No, not very well. I started to feel awful, sweaty, shaky, and I had to have a cigarette. And once you give in, then it's back to smoking, isn't it.
Nurse:	It sounds like you were having withdrawal symptoms from the nicotine. Did you take any nicotine replacements like Nicorette or something like that?
Mr Jones:	No, just tried on my own.
Nurse:	That may be why you had problems. It's possible that if you used something to help the withdrawal, it may have been easier to quit.
Mr Jones:	Oh right, what does that involve then?

Note here that the nurse did not try to persuade Mr Jones that he could stop smoking, but rather began to search for evidence of why things went wrong in the past. False reassurance with no basis in fact will not encourage change. Here, however, there were some clues as to why things went wrong previously and how they could be changed to increase Mr Jones's chances of successfully quitting. This was subtly fed back to him, and he is now beginning to think about stopping smoking, despite the nurse making no attempt at active persuasion through the conversation. In fact, Mr Jones did go on to state he wanted to quit smoking and was successful in stopping smoking using nicotine replacement therapy.

3.3.3 Changing Behaviour

Changing behaviours such as smoking, exercise or food choices can be difficult within the context of our complex lives. We frequently know what we should be doing, but still fail to put these intentions into action. So frequent is this failure, it has been bestowed a name: the intention-behaviour gap. One way to increase the chances of intentions actually leading to actions involves planning and thinking through how any desired changes can be made. One of the earlier approaches to this process was developed by Egan [11]. His model of problem-focused counselling involves three phases, through which the identification and change of any factors that are inhibiting behavioural change can be achieved:

- Problem exploration and clarification
- Goal setting
- Facilitating action

3.3.4   Problem Exploration and Clarification

The goal of the first stage is to help an individual identify the problems he or she is facing that may be contributing to their problems or interfering with attempts at behavioural change. The goal of this stage is to clarify *exactly* what difficulties the individual is facing, and in some detail, only then can appropriate problem-solving strategies be applied. The most obvious way of eliciting this type of information is to ask direct questions. Egan also suggests the use of prompts ('Tell me about…') and probes ('How did that cause problems…?') requesting information. A further, and important, method of encouraging problem exploration is through the use of what Egan termed empathic feedback: 'So, you felt very frustrated when your partner refused to talk about…'.

3.3.5   Goal Setting

Once particular problems have been identified, some people may feel they are able to deal with them and need no further help in making appropriate changes. Others, however, may need further support in determining what they want to change and how to change it. The first stage in this process is to help the individual to decide the goals he or she wishes to achieve and to frame his or her goals in specific rather than general terms (e.g. 'I will try to relax more' versus 'I will take 20 minutes out each day to practise some yoga'). If the final goal seems too difficult to achieve in one step, the identification of sub-goals working towards the final goal should be encouraged.

Some goals may be apparent following the problem exploration phase. However, should this not be the case, Egan identified a series of strategies designed to help the patient identify and set goals. One of the most important is to encourage the individual to explore new perspectives – to think about new ways of doing things. At this stage, direct challenges or advice giving ('Well, why don't you take some time out each day to relax?') is likely to result in resistance or feelings of defeat. The individual should be encouraged to explore their own solutions rather than them being provided by the health professional.

3.3.6   Facilitating Action

Once goals have been established in the second phase, some individuals may feel they need no further support in achieving them. However, some people may not be able to plan how they could achieve any goals they wish to achieve. Accordingly, the final stage is to plan ways of achieving the identified goals. It can be helpful to work towards relatively easy goals at the beginning of any attempt at change, before working towards more difficult to change goals as the individual gains skills or confidence in their ability to change.

The following case study provides an example of problem-focused counselling and how the appropriate assessment of a problem can ensure that any attempts at change are successful.

Following an infarction at a relatively early age, Mrs T was found to be obese and to have a raised serum cholesterol level. After seeing a dietician, she agreed to lose a kilogramme a week over the following months. She was given a leaflet providing information about the fat and calorific content of a variety of foods and a leaflet describing a number of 'healthy' recipes.

On her follow-up visits, her cholesterol level and weight remained unchanged. So, the dietician changed her tactics and began to explore why Mrs T had not made use of the advice she had been given. Mrs T explained that she already knew which were 'healthy' and 'unhealthy' foods. Indeed, she had been on many diets before – with little success. They then began to explore why this was the case. At this point, the key problem became apparent.

Mrs T's husband supported her attempts to lose weight and was prepared to change his diet to help her. However, her sons often demanded meals late at night when they got back from the 'pub' (bar), often relatively drunk. As a consequence, Mrs T often started to cook late at night at the end of what may have been a successful day of dieting. She then nibbled high-calorie food while cooking. This had two outcomes. Firstly, she increased her calorie input. Secondly, she frequently 'catastrophised' ('I've eaten so much; I may as well abandon my diet for today') and ate a full meal at this time. It also reduced her motivation to follow her diet the following day.

Once this specific problem had been identified, Mrs T set a goal of not cooking late-night fry-ups for her sons. She decided that if her sons wanted a fry-up, they could cook it themselves. Once the goal was established, Mrs T felt a little concerned about how her sons would react to her no longer cooking for them. So, she and the dietician explored ways in which she could set about telling them – and sticking to her resolution. She finally decided she would tell them in the coming week, explaining why she felt she could no longer cook for them at that time of night. She even rehearsed how she would say it. This she did, with good effect, as she stopped cooking for them and did start to lose weight.

If nothing else, this vignette shows the danger of making implicit assumptions about what is preventing change (in this case, the dietician initially assumed it was lack of knowledge about healthy foodstuffs). Time spent assessing the precise cause of any problems an individual is experiencing is time well spent and ensures that the rest of any intervention is focusing on appropriate issues.

3.3.7   Implementing Plans and Intentions

A simpler approach to that of Egan, but compressed into a period of minutes rather than hours, involves simply planning change. According to Gollwitzer [13], we frequently fail to translate our intentions into behaviours for a number of reasons, including:

- *Failing to start*: the individual does not remember to start, they do not seize the opportunity to act, or they have second thoughts at the critical moment.
- *Becoming 'derailed' from goal striving*: the individual is derailed by enticing stimuli, they find it difficult to suppress habitual behavioural responses, or many are adversely affected by negative mood states or expectations of negative mood if they implement change.

To overcome these obstacles, a relatively simple procedure may be utilised. This approach involves specifying a relatively simple goal ('I will eat less fatty food') and how this will be achieved ('I will buy healthy food options at the supermarket'). This link between goal and behaviour may take 5 min of planning; it is not complex. The approach can take a number of slightly more complex forms, one of which is known as the 'if-then' approach: '*If* I find myself bored and hungry, *then* I will try to find something active to do/eat a health snack'. Ideally, the behaviour is specified in terms of when, where and how. Although simple, the premise of this approach is that this process will result in a mental association between representations of specified cues (feeling bored) and means of attaining goals (engaging in non-boring activities, not eating), which will become activated when the cue is encountered. Developing appropriate implementations is simple in practice, particularly for one-off simple behaviours: 'If I have an urge to smoke in the house, I will play a game on the Xbox to take my mind of it', 'If I am offered a cigarette by a friend...', and so on. Establishing these if-then associations may promote the initiation of goal-relevant behaviours, stabilise them over time and shield the individual from alternatives and obstacles. By considering times or situations of particular salience to the individual, they have a preformed plan of what to do when in this situation. Through planning, the individual should not find themselves in a challenging or difficult situation without a plan to engage in, a context which makes the likelihood of resort to previous behaviours associated with that situation highly likely.

3.4   Emotional Adjustment

While any negative emotional outcome following the onset of disease is worthy of treatment in itself, the adverse impact that emotional distress can have on rehabilitation or even the prognosis of the disease should make the treatment of such problems key to any rehabilitation programme (e.g. [8]). The chapter introduces one well-known approach to reducing emotional distress and one that is perhaps less well known:

- Cognitive-behavioural interventions
- Written emotional expression

3.4.1   Cognitive-Behavioural Interventions

Cognitive-behavioural interventions assume that emotional distress results not just from the things that happen to us, but how we interpret them. They consider distress often to involve misinterpretations of events or exaggerations of the negative elements within them and a loss of focus on any positive aspects of the situation. The most basic cognitive intervention is to identify such distorted thinking and to help the individual look at the situation from a different perspective. See, for example, in the dialogue below, how Tom exaggerates the negative consequences of his MI and how the nurse encourages him to consider other ways of looking at the situation:

Tom: Well, that's it. I've had a heart attack. And I know I'll lose my job now... and what's going to happen about money. I can see we're going to have to sell the house or at least the cars....

Nurse: That's a lot of things to be worrying about.... Tell me, why do you think you'll lose your job?

Tom: Well, heart attacks are bad news, aren't they? Most people have to stop work when they have one, don't they?

Nurse: Some people do – but most people can go back to work. Having a heart attack doesn't have to disable you and stop you working.... Most people get back to the same or a similar lifestyle to the one they had before their heart attack.... What sort of job do you have?

Tom: I'm a manager in a large marketing company.

Nurse: So, your job is not very physically demanding.... It doesn't put a lot of strain on the heart. So, going back to work isn't going to be difficult from a physical point of view.

Tom: No, I guess not....

Nurse: I wonder.... You must have known a number of people who have had a serious illness in your line of work. How does the company treat them? Do they have to leave?

Tom: In some ways that would be crazy, if they are a good worker and can still work, the company would keep them on.

Nurse: So as far as you know, the company tries to keep people on even if they
           are ill.
Tom: So there's no real need for the company to have a problem with me?
Nurse: Perhaps not....
Tom: So, things might not be that bad after all. Wow, I feel better after thinking
           that through....

Here, Tom is encouraged to rethink some of the assumptions he has made about
the company's response to his illness and not simply to accept them as true. Note
that the nurse did not try to reassure him directly, but gave him some relevant information and then encouraged him to look for evidence to challenge his own errone-
ous assumptions – a much more powerful procedure. In a more formal
cognitive-behavioural programme, the health professional may talk through any
inappropriate assumptions that the individual may make and teach them to challenge them as they occur in real life. The educational approach of Petrie and colleagues described above also adopts this type of approach in a formal and systematic
manner, identifying the types of beliefs that are likely to affect how engaged an
individual is in any rehabilitation programme and providing evidence to challenge
them [29].

3.4.2   Relaxation Training

A second cognitive-behavioural approach – usually used in stress management programmes – involves teaching relaxation skills. The goal of teaching relaxation skills
is to enable the individual to relax as much as possible and appropriate both throughout the day and at times of particular stress. This contrasts with procedures such as
meditation, which provide a period of deep relaxation and 'time out', as sufficient
in themselves. Relaxation skills are best learned through three phases:

- Learning basic relaxation skills
- Monitoring tension in daily life
- Using relaxation at times of stress

The first stage of learning relaxation skills is to practise them under optimal conditions such as a quiet room in a comfortable chair – where there are no distractions
and it is relatively easy to relax. Initially, the patient should be led through the relaxation process by an experienced practitioner. This can then be added to by continued
practice at home, typically using taped instructions. The relaxation process most
commonly taught is based on Jacobson's deep muscle relaxation technique. This
involves alternately tensing and relaxing muscle groups throughout the body in an
ordered sequence. Over time, the emphasis of practice shifts towards relaxation
without prior tension, or relaxing specific muscle groups while using others, to
mimic the use of relaxation in the 'real world'.

At the same time as practising relaxation skills, individuals can begin to monitor
their levels of physical tension throughout the day. Initially, this serves as a learning

process, helping them to identify how tense they are at particular times of the day and what triggers any excessive tension. Such monitoring may also help identify future triggers to stress and provide clues as to when the use of relaxation procedures may be particularly useful. After a period of learning relaxation techniques and monitoring tension, individuals can begin to integrate relaxation into their daily lives. At this stage, relaxation involves reducing tension to appropriate levels while engaging in everyday activities. Initially, this may involve trying to keep as relaxed as possible and appropriate at times of relatively low stress and then, as the individual becomes more skilled, using relaxation at times of increasing stress. The goal of relaxation at these times is not to escape from the cause of stress, but to remain as relaxed as possible while dealing with the particular stressor. An alternative strategy involves relaxing at regular intervals (such as coffee breaks) throughout the day.

3.4.3   Mindfulness

A relatively new, but increasingly popular, approach to helping people cope with stress involves the use of a technique known as mindfulness. This involves the individual learning to recognise the presence of stressful thoughts while remaining emotionally disengaged from them. Mindfulness has a long history and is central to Buddhist philosophy. It can be achieved through meditation, but can also be evoked, with practice, while engaged in day-to-day activities. Mindfulness may be considered to have two elements:

- *Self-regulation of attention*: Mindfulness involves being fully aware of our current experience – observing and attending to our changing thoughts, feelings and sensations as they occur. This allows us to be aware of these phenomena, but not to elaborate on them. Rather than getting caught up in ruminative thoughts, mindfulness involves a direct non-judgmental experience of events in the mind and body.
- *An orientation towards experiences in the present moment characterised by curiosity, openness and acceptance*: The lack of cognitive effort given to the engagement and elaboration of our experiences allows us to focus on our present experience. Rather than observing experience through the filter of our beliefs and assumptions, mindfulness involves a direct, unfiltered awareness of our experiences.

In essence, mindfulness involves a focus on our whole experience at any one time, not just focusing on panicky, anxious or depressed thoughts. These become just part of our experience, and we can learn to observe them rather than allow them to dominate our consciousness. Achieving this level of simultaneous awareness and disengagement is not easy, and most programmes that teach mindfulness do so over sessions spread over many weeks or months.

One of the most widely recognised training programmes is the mindfulness-based stress reduction programme of Kabat-Zinn (e.g. [17]). This involves an

8–10-week course for groups of participants who meet weekly for practice in mindfulness meditation skills, together with discussion of stress, coping and homework assignments. An all-day mindfulness training session is also included. Several mindfulness meditation skills are taught. These include the 'body scan', involving a 45-min exercise in which attention is directed sequentially to numerous areas of the body while lying down with eyes closed. Sensations in each area are carefully observed. In sitting meditation, participants are instructed to sit in a relaxed and wakeful posture with eyes closed and to direct attention to the sensations of breathing. Hatha yoga postures are used to teach mindfulness of bodily sensations during gentle movements and stretching. Participants also practise mindfulness during ordinary activities like walking, standing and eating. For all mindfulness exercises, participants are instructed to focus attention on the target of observation and to be aware of it in each moment. When emotions, sensations or cognitions arise, they are observed non-judgmentally. If participants notice their mind has wandered into thoughts, memories or fantasies, their nature or content is briefly noted, and then attention is returned to the present moment. An important consequence of mindfulness practice is the realisation that most sensations, thoughts and emotions fluctuate, or are transient, passing by 'like waves in the sea'.

Mindfulness can act as a 'stand-alone' intervention. It can also be integrated into other therapies and used to help people cope with challenging behavioural experiments or distressing thoughts as part of the treatment of mood and anxiety disorders. While mindfulness training may be beyond the remit of most rehabilitation programmes, patients may usefully be signposted to the many self-help interventions available on the Internet and books, such as Stahl and Goldstein [34] and Alinda [1].

3.5 Concluding Remarks

Cardiac rehabilitation works. We know that appropriate interventions can effectively change behaviour and emotional consequences of the experience of an acute cardiac event. We also know that more complex interventions work better than simpler approaches. Those, for example, that involve the development of personal strategies of change are more effective than less complex educational programmes [2], although the latter can be highly effective if conducted in appropriate manner. These relatively complex interventions need not necessarily be provided in complex ways, however. The 'self-help' intervention developed by Lewin and colleagues [24] provides a graduated programme of behavioural change and emotional regulation over a period of six weekly instalments and has proven as effective as the same programme provided 'live' in cardiac rehabilitation centres [10]. Intriguingly, we have still to find out what type of intervention works best for which patients. Nevertheless, there is consistent evidence that either live interventions or the Internet- or other media-based interventions are most effective if they apply the principles considered in this chapter [7, 9, 12, 19, 27, 36]. Ultimately, a triaged system in which patients are enrolled in programmes of varying complexity and cost may ultimately provide the most effective and cost-effective approach, with simple educational provision being the basic intervention and more complex interventions being initiated as appropriate.

References

1. Alinda S. The mindful way through stress: the proven 8-week path to health, happiness, and well-being. New York: Guildford Press; 2015.
2. Bennett P. Psychological interventions in secondary care. In: Kaptein A, Weinman J, editors. Introduction to health psychology. London: BPS Blackwell; 2006.
3. Bennett P, Gruszczynska E, Marke V. Dietary and exercise change following acute cardiac syndrome: a latent class growth modelling analysis. J Health Psychol. 2015; doi:10.1177/1359105315576351.
4. Bennett P, Mayfield T, Norman P, Lowe R, Morgan M. Affective and social cognitive predictors of behavioural change following myocardial infarction. Br J Health Psychol. 1999;4:247–56.
5. Bennett P, Owen R, Koutsakis S, Bisson J. Personality, social context, and cognitive predictors of post-traumatic stress disorder in myocardial infarction patients. Psychol Health. 2002;17:489–500.
6. Bennett P, Connell H. Dyadic responses to myocardial infarction. Psychol Health Med. 1999;4:45–55.
7. Black JL, Allison TG, Williams DE, Rummans TA, Gau GT. Effect of intervention for psychological distress on rehospitalization rates in cardiac rehabilitation patients. Psychosomatics. 1998;39:134 43.
8. British Association of Cardiovascular Prevention and Rehabilitation. BAPCR standards and core components for cardiovascular disease prevention and rehabilitation 2012. London: BACPR; 2012.
9. Burke BL, Arkowitz H, Menchola M. The efficacy of motivational interviewing: a meta-analysis of controlled clinical trials. J Consult Clin Psychol. 2003;71:843–61.
10. Clark M, Kelly T, Deighan C. A systematic review of the Heart Manual literature. Eur J Cardiovasc Nurs. 2011;10:3–13.
11. Egan G. The skilled helper: models, skills, and methods for effective helping. Brooks Cole: Monterey; 1998.
12. Esterling BA, L'Abate L, Murray EJ, Pennebaker J. Empirical foundations for writing in prevention and psychotherapy: mental and physical health outcomes. Clin Psychol Rev. 1999;19:79–96.
13. Gollwitzer PM. Implementation intentions: strong effects of simple plans. Am Psychol. 1999;54:493–503.
14. Hajek P, Taylor TZ, Mills P. Brief intervention during hospital admission to help patients to give up smoking after myocardial infarction and bypass surgery: randomised controlled trial. Br Med J. 2002;324:87–9.
15. Hevey D, Brown AS, Cahill A, Newton H, Kierns M, Horgan JH. 4-week cardiac rehabilitation produces similar improvements in exercise capacity and quality of life to a 10-week programme. J Cardpulm Rehabil. 2003;23:17–21.
16. Huijbrechts IP, Duivenvoorden HJ, Deckers JW. Modification of smoking habits five months after myocardial infarction: relationship with personality characteristics. J Psychosom Res. 1999;40:369–78.
17. Kabat-Zinn J. Full catastrophe living, revised edition: how to cope with stress, pain and illness using mindfulness meditation. London: Piatkus; 2013.

18. Keegan C, Conroy R, Doyle F. Longitudinal modelling of theory-based depressive vulnerabilities, depression trajectories and poor outcomes post-ACS. J Affect Disord. 2016;191:41–8.
19. Lacey EA, Musgrave RJ, Freeman JV, Tod AM, Scott P. Psychological morbidity after myocardial infarction in an area of deprivation in the UK: evaluation of a self-help package. Eur J Cardiovasc Nurs. 2004;3:219–24.
20. Lane D, Carroll D, Ring C, Beevers DG, Lip GY. Predictors of attendance at cardiac rehabilitation after myocardial infarction. J Psychosom Res. 2001;51:497–501.
21. Lane D, Carroll D, Ring C, Beevers DG, Lip GY. The prevalence and persistence of depression and anxiety following myocardial infarction. Br J Health Psychol. 2002;7:11–21.
22. Lear SA, Ignaszewski A, Linden W, Brozic A, Kiess M, Spinelli JJ, et al. The Extensive Lifestyle Management Intervention (ELMI) following cardiac rehabilitation trial. Eur Heart J. 2003;24:1920–7.
23. Leslie WS, Hankey CR, Matthews D, Currall JE, Lean ME. A transferable programme of nutritional counselling for rehabilitation following myocardial infarction: a randomised controlled study. Eur J Clin Nutr. 2004;58:778–86.
24. Lewin B, Robertson IH, Irving JB, Campbell M. Effects of self-help post-myocardial-infarction rehabilitation on psychological adjustment and use of health services. Lancet. 1992;339: 1036–40.
25. Miller W, Rollnick S. Motivational interviewing: preparing people to change addictive behaviour. 3rd ed. New York: Guilford Press; 2012.
26. Moser DK, Dracup K. Role of spousal anxiety and depression in patients' psychosocial recovery after a cardiac event. Psychosom Med. 2004;66:527–32.
27. Oldenburg B, Allam R, Fastier G. The role of behavioral and educational interventions in the secondary prevention of heart disease. Clin Abnorm Psychol. 1989;27:429–38.
28. Osler M, Mårtensson S, Wium-Andersen IK, Prescott E, Andersen PK, Jørgensen TS, et al. Depression after first hospital admission for acute coronary syndrome: a study of time of onset and impact on survival. Am J Epidemiol. 2016;183:218–26.
29. Petrie KJ, Cameron LD, Ellis CJ, Buick D, Weinman J. Changing illness perceptions after myocardial infarction: an early intervention randomized controlled trial. Psychosom Med. 2002;64:580–6.
30. Petrie KJ, Weinman J, Sharpe N, Buckley J. Role of patients' view of their illness in predicting return to work and functioning after myocardial infarction: longitudinal study. Br Med J. 1996;312:1191–4.
31. Shemesh E, Yehuda R, Milo O, Dinur I, Rudnick A, Vered Z, et al. Posttraumatic stress, nonadherence, and adverse outcome in survivors of a myocardial infarction. Psychosom Med. 2004;66:521–6.
32. Soderman E, Lisspers J, Sundin O. Depression as a predictor of return to work in patients with coronary artery disease. Soc Sci Med. 2003;56:193–202.
33. Stewart M, Davidson K, Meade D, Hirth A, Makrides L. Myocardial infarction: survivors' and spouses' stress, coping, and support. J Adv Nurs. 2000;31:1351–60.
34. Stahl B, Golsdtein E. A mindfulness-based reduction workbook. Oakland: New Harbinger Publications; 2010.
35. Strik JJ, Lousberg R, Cheriex EC, Honig A. One year cumulative incidence of depression following myocardial infarction and impact on cardiac outcome. J Psychosom Res. 2004;56: 59–66.
36. Whalley B, Rees K, Davies P, Bennett P, Ebrahim S, Liu Z, et al. Psychological interventions for coronary heart disease. Cochrane Database Syst Rev. 2011;(8):CD002902.
37. Whooley MA, Wong JM. Depression and cardiovascular disorders. Ann Rev Clin Psychol. 2013;9:327–54.

Part II

Cardiac Rehabilitation in Specific Cases

Exercise Training in Cardiac Rehabilitation

4

Birna Bjarnason-Wehrens and Martin Halle

Physical activity counseling and individually prescribed and supervised exercise training are core components of a comprehensive cardiac rehabilitation (CR) program, compromising 30–50 % (up to >70 %) of all cardiac rehabilitation activities. This applies to phase II as well as to phase III cardiac rehabilitation for patients post-acute coronary syndrome and post-primary coronary angioplasty (PCI), post-cardiac surgery (coronary artery bypass, valve heart surgery, cardiac transplantation), as well as in chronic heart failure patients.

Within a large meta-analysis of Cochrane database, exercise-based cardiac rehabilitation has been shown to reduce overall mortality rate by 13 %, cardiovascular mortality rate by 26 %, and hospital admission rate by 18–31 % in patients with coronary heart disease (CHD) [1–3]. Moreover meta-analysis has revealed CR programs with exercise training interventions as only content to be even more effective, demonstrating exercise only to reduce overall mortality rate by 27–28 %, mortality rate due to cardiovascular disease by 31 % (Fig. 4.1), and the re-infract rate by 43 % [3–5]. These results emphasize the impact of exercise interventions as a core component of CR program. However, so far epidemiological studies have not been able to provide sufficient statistically significant evidence linking the incidence of nonfatal heart attacks and sudden cardiac death to exercise training-based rehabilitation measures [1–5].

B. Bjarnason-Wehrens (✉)
Institute for Cardiology and Sports Medcine, German Sportuniversity Cologne, Am Sportpark Müngersdorf 6, Cologne 50933, Austria
e-mail: bjarnason@dshs-koeln.de

M. Halle
Department for Prevention, Rehabilitation and Sports Medicine, Georg-Brauchle-Ring 56 (Campus C), D-80992 Munich, Germany

© Springer International Publishing AG 2017
J. Niebauer (ed.), *Cardiac Rehabilitation Manual*,
DOI 10.1007/978-3-319-47738-1_4

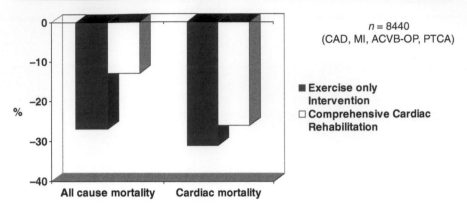

Fig. 4.1 Effectiveness of exercise only or exercise as part of a comprehensive cardiac rehabilitation program on all-cause mortality and cardiac mortality (According to Jolliffe et al. [3])

4.1 Definition of Terms

Any muscle contraction resulting in an energy metabolism above basal metabolic rate is characterized as *physical activity* [6]. *Exercise or exercise training* is any physical activity that is planned, structured, performed repeatedly, and specifically aimed at improving the physical fitness level [6]. *Physical fitness* comprises the ability of performance including cardiopulmonary endurance, muscle strength, flexibility, and coordination [6, 7]. *Cardiorespiratory fitness* is determined by the maximal cardiovascular exercise capacity and is dependent on oxygen transport via lung diffusion, cardiocirculation to the muscle fiber, where it is used in the mitochondria for energy production (ATP synthase). Assessment of maximal oxygen uptake ($VO_{2peak/max}$) is the gold standard for evaluating cardiorespiratory fitness, typically assessed during a maximal exercise tolerance test performed on a bicycle or treadmill ergometer [8]. *Maximal exercise capacity* is the highest power output a person can sustain during an exercise tolerance [8]. *Exercise tolerance* is defined as the highest power output possible before any pathological symptoms and/or medical indications occur [9]. In a healthy person both terms can be used interchangeably, but in a patient the range can differ substantially [8]. For the definition of the amount of physical activity or exercise, the interrelation between the *total dose* of activity and the *intensity* at which the activity is performed have to be considered (volume of exercise = duration × intensity). While the dose refers to the total energy expended, intensity reflects to the rate of energy expenditure during the physical activity. *Absolute intensity* reflects the rate of energy expenditure during exercise, usually expressed in metabolic equivalent tasks (MET). One MET is the energy expenditure or oxygen consumption (VO_2) measured during sitting, which equals 3.5 mL O_2 kg^{-1} min^{-1}. MET-hours are the product of exercise intensity and exercise time [6]. *Relative intensity* refers to the percent of aerobic power utilized during exercise. It is expressed as percent of maximal heart rate or percent of VO_{2peak}. In this context, activities performed at a relative intensity of <40 % VO_{2peak} are considered to be of light intensity, those performed at 40–60 % VO_{2peak} to be of moderate intensity, and those performed at relative intensity of >60 % VO_{2peak} to be of vigorous intensity [6]. For the estimation of intensity, the person's individual premises have to be taken into account. For example, brisk walking at 4.8 km h^{-1} has an absolute intensity of ~4 MET. For a young and healthy person, this intensity is low in relative terms, but represents a vigorous intensity for an 80-year-old person.

Exercise therapy "is medically indicated and prescribed exercise, planned and dosed by therapists, controlled together with the physician and carried out with the patient either alone or in a group" [10]. *Sport and exercise therapy* "is an exercise based therapeutic measure which compensates for destroyed physical, mental and social functions with suitable sports remedies, regenerates, guards against secondary damage and supports health oriented behaviour. Sport therapy is based on biological principles; especially includes physiological, medical, pedagogic-psychological as well as social therapeutic elements and attempts to create enduring health competence" [10].

4.2   Objective of Exercise-Based Training Intervention

The primary objective of an exercise-based training intervention in cardiac rehabilitation is to positively influence disease progression and prognosis. This is most successfully achieved in coronary heart disease (CHD) and its pathological consequences (acute coronary syndrome, sudden death, ischemic heart failure) and in nonischemic chronic heart failure [1, 2, 6, 11–17]. The main secondary objectives are an improvement in the symptom-free exercise tolerance and overall quality of life [6, 12–14]. Further secondary objectives are overcoming cardiovascular and musculoskeletal limitations caused by inactivity (in particular in chronic heart failure and after open-heart surgery), as well as to improve mobility, independence, psychological well-being, social and occupational reintegration, and cardiovascular risk factors and thereby reduce the need for future home care, enhance participation, and enable the patient to take up his further life. In order to achieve these objectives, an extensive physical activity counseling including individual instructions is of crucial importance, in addition to the supervised exercise training [6, 11, 12, 14, 16–19].

Individual objectives should be based on the patient's cardiac diagnosis, exercise capacity, possible exercise-limiting comorbidities, age, gender, exercise experience, as well as the patient's motivation, personal exercise goals, and preferences. Respecting somatic, psychosocial, and educative objectives, they should aim to support the patient's health-oriented behavior, to create his/her persistent health competence, and to improve his/her self-efficacy (Table 4.1 and Fig. 4.2).

Table 4.1 Somatic, psychosocial, and educative objectives of individually prescribed and supervised exercise training in cardiac rehabilitation

Somatic objectives:
To positively influence disease progression and prognosis
To overcome cardiovascular and musculoskeletal limitations caused by inactivity
To improve symptom-free exercise tolerance
    To improve cardiopulmonary exercise tolerance
    To improve coordination, flexibility, agility, and muscular strength
To positively influence cardiovascular risk factors
Psychosocial objectives:
To improve body awareness and perception, especially the patient's perception of stress during exercise training
To reduce the patient's anxiety for overload during exercise training
To improve the patient's realistic judgment of his/her individual exercise tolerance
To improve overall well-being
To improve psychosocial well-being and coping with the disease
To improve overall social integration
To increase level of independency
To improve quality of life
Educative objectives:
To improve knowledge in the impact and health benefits of regular physical activity and exercise training
To improve practical skills of self-control and adequate handling during physical activity and/or exercise training to the patient
To improve long-term compliance to lifestyle changes
To implement a physically active lifestyle

Modified after Bjarnason-Wehrens et al. [20]

4.3 How to Set Up an Exercise Training Program in Cardiac Rehabilitation

Exercise training in cardiac rehabilitation should be medically supervised and led by an experienced exercise therapist (or physiotherapist). During the initial phase after an acute event, the exercise program should be started under careful medical supervision. The supervision should include physical examination, monitoring of heart rate, blood pressure, and rhythm before, during, and after the exercise training [12, 14, 17]. A careful supervision allows to verify individual responses and tolerability, clinical stability, and promptly identifying signs and symptoms indicating necessary modification or termination of the program. The supervision should be prolonged in patients with high risk of cardiovascular events (severe coronary heart disease, heart failure NYHA III, ventricular arrhythmias, implantable cardioverter defibrillator (ICD), heart transplantation). In these patients an inpatient cardiac rehabilitation setting is recommended [12].

Exercise training in cardiac rehabilitation should be prescribed on an individualized approach after a careful clinical evaluation including: risk stratification, symptom-limited exercise testing (either on bicycle or on treadmill),

Fig. 4.2 Objectives of exercise-based training intervention

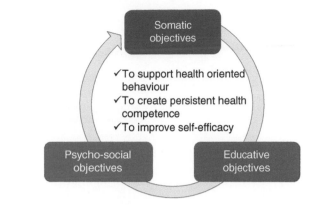

Fig. 4.3 Contents of comprehensive exercise based training intervention in cardiac rehabilitation

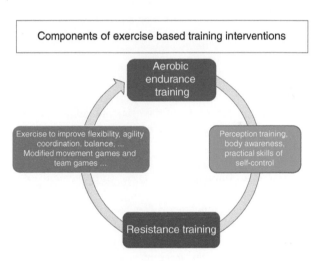

assessment of possible exercise-limiting comorbidities, assessment of functional capacity (especially in groups at risk to have reduced functional capacity, e.g., older patients, females, and/or heart failure patients), assessment of behavioral characteristics (movement and exercise experiences, physical activity level, readiness to change behavior, self-confidence, barriers to increase physical activity, as well as social support in making positive changes), and patient's personal goals and exercise preferences. The type and severity of the disease also have to receive similar attention such as personal characteristics like age and gender [12, 14, 17] (Fig. 4.3).

Exercise training in cardiac rehabilitation should be based on aerobic endurance training. On its basis, further components such as resistance exercise and gymnastics including exercises for coordination (inclusive balance and sensorimotoric), flexibility, agility, and strength as well as perceptional training, are to be added. In frail and older patients, special exercise elements for preventing falls should be a part of the exercise program (Fig. 4.4).

Fig. 4.4 Components
that have to be considered
by planning and
implementation of an
individually dosed,
adapted and controlled
exercise program in
cardiac rehabilitation

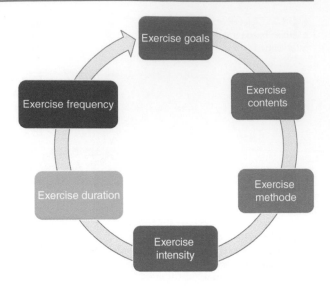

Based on the results of the clinical evaluation, every person should receive *individualized exercise training recommendations* containing the following information [14] (Fig. 4.5):

- Exercise training goals (i.e., improvement of exercise capacity, muscular strength)
- Exercise training mode (i.e., aerobic endurance training, moderate resistance training)
- Exercise training content, with reference to the preferred type of exercise (i.e., bicycle ergometer, treadmill, walking, Nordic walking, etc.; resistance training using weight machines, elastic bands, etc.)
- Exercise training method (steady-state training, interval training, etc.)
- Exercise training intensity (i.e., % HR_{peak}, % VO_{2peak}, % of one repetition maximum)
- Exercise training duration (duration of the individual training unit [i.e., 30–60 min] and the supervised training program [i.e., 3–6 months])
- Exercise training frequency (i.e., 3–7 exercise units per week) [12]

Exercise training duration, intensity, and frequency should start at a low level and be increased incrementally. Especially in patients taking up an exercise training after a long period of inactivity, it is important to pay close attention to the variation in time each organ system needs in order to adapt to the training process. While the cardiovascular and muscular systems show a fast adaptation, bones, tendons, ligaments, and joints adapt very slowly. The primary goal should be to increase training duration and frequency [12]. If these are well tolerated, then the intensity can also be increased.

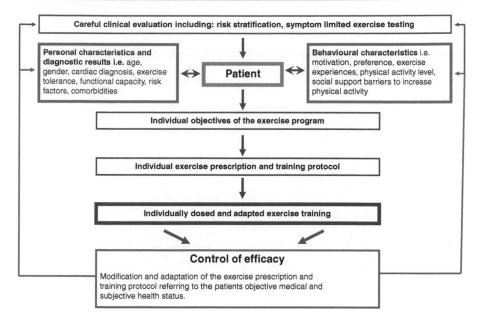

Fig. 4.5 How to set up an individually dosed and adapted, and controlled exercise training program in cardiac rehabilitation

Exercise training should be planned in three stages: initial stage, improvement stage, and maintaining stage (Fig. 4.6) [12, 14, 17].

The objectives of the *initial stage* are to prepare the patient for the exercise training and to verify the individual response and tolerability to a low-intensity exercise program. This phase also includes improvement of coordination and flexibility as well as developing the patient's perception for exercise intensity. Previously physically inactive people and older patients have to receive special attention. In the initial stage the intensity of exercise should be kept at a low level. According to perceived symptoms and clinical status, the duration of the exercise unit can be prolonged (i.e., from 15 to 30 min). The duration of the initial stage depends on the patient's clinical status and exercise tolerance, but should not exceed 4–6 exercise units during 1–2 weeks, respectively.

The objectives of the *improvement stage* are to gradually increase exercise capacity and other components of physical fitness such as coordination, flexibility, muscular strength, and endurance capacity. During this stage, the exercise intensity should be gradually increased according to the patient's exercise prescription and exercise goals. Likewise, each exercise session can be prolonged up to 30–60 min and even beyond as well as exercise frequency can be increased up to daily sessions. However, this has to be adapted to the patient's objective medical status and subjective health status.

The objectives of the *maintenance stage* are to stabilize and preserve the improvements achieved as well as extend them over a long period of time. Exercise intensity, exercise duration, and exercise frequency can be gradually increased if tolerated. In this stage, special attention has to be paid to the patient's motivation as

Stages of exercise training

| **The initial stage**
 4–6 exercise units during 1–2 weeks

 Exercise duration: short (i.e. 15–30 min)

 Exercise intensity: low | - Preparation,
 - Adaptation,
 - Verifying the individual response and
  tolerability |

↓

| **The improvement stage**

 Exercise duration: gradually prolonged up <br> to ≥ 30–60 min

 Exercise intensity: gradually increase <br> exercise capacity up to target values | - Increase exercise capacity and
  physical fitness
 - Improve muscular strength and
  endurance
 - Improve flexibility and coordination |

↓

| **The maintenance stage**

 Gradually increase exercise intensity and <br> or exercise time if tolerated | - Long term stabilisation of improvements
  achieved
 - Stabilize adherence to regular physical
  activity and exercise training |

Fig. 4.6 Stages of exercise training in cardiac rehabilitation

well as education to increase and or stabilize adherence to regular physical activity and exercise training. It is mandatory to provide the patient with the necessary practical skills of self-control and adequate handling during physical activity and/or exercise training. Careful instruction about the impact and health benefits of regular physical activity and exercise training might be helpful to improve his/her adherence to a physically active lifestyle.

Overall, during cardiac rehabilitation the individual exercise training recommendations have to be adapted individually and reevaluated after change of medical status, change of medication, hospitalization, or other illnesses.

4.4 Physical Activity Counseling: Motivation to a Physically Active Lifestyle

Provided they are performed on a regular and a long-term basis, physical activity and exercise training are valuable sources of multiple health benefits. The patient's motivation to take up an active lifestyle and start regular exercise training on a sustained basis is therefore an important goal of the cardiac rehabilitation program. Investigations have shown that the patient's thorough information and motivation provided by the attending physician is the most effective instrument to achieve such behavioral changes [21]. Based on this initial encouragement by the physician, the motivation achieved has to be stabilized and augmented through individual as well as group counseling during the rehabilitation process.

The primary preventive role of regular physical activity is well established by large epidemiological studies. Results of meta-analyses demonstrate regular physical activity compared with sedentary behavior to be associated with reduction of overall mortality rate by 22–36 % and reduction of cardiovascular mortality rate by 25–35 % [22–25]. The impact of regular physical activity in the secondary prevention of CHD is less well established. The results of smaller prospective studies demonstrate the prognostic importance of regular physical activities after diagnosis of the CHD, showing regular physical activity to be associated with a relative risk reduction of overall mortality by 19–58 % and cardiovascular mortality and/or morbidity by 20–62 % [26–35]. These prospective cohort studies [27, 32] also showed that it is never too late to take up an active lifestyle. They found reduced overall mortality rate by 29–50 % in former inactive CHD patients that increased their activity levels after the diagnosis of the disease [27, 32]. A relative reduction for overall mortality by 34–79 % was found in anciently physically active patients that maintained active, compared to those who were sedentary before and after the diagnosis of the disease [27, 32]. These results have to be established by studies with greater cohorts. Thereby in cardiac rehabilitation, it is important to emphasize sedentary lifestyle as an independent risk factor and explain the health benefits achieved by any increase in physical activity to the patients. However, the exercise therapist should keep in mind that it is not sufficient to inform the patient about the achievable health benefits. During the rehabilitation process, the patient's perceptions, attitude, and health esteem regarding physical activity and exercise training have to be influenced positively. It is important that he/she experiences the exercise training provided during cardiac rehabilitation as a convenient task that he/she can cope with as well as an activity that is associated with well-being, fun, and social contacts. On a long-term basis, the patient will only integrate physical activity and exercise training into his/her daily life, if medical benefits are associated with personal values. The motivation to be physically active for health benefits usually only lasts for few months [36]. It is essential to change the patient's secondary motivation (exercise training for health) into a primary motivation (e.g., I like exercise training, it is associated with fun, well-being, and/or meeting friends); otherwise he/she will return to his/her inactive lifestyle within a short period of time.

During the cardiac rehabilitation program, the patient should receive individual advices and exercise prescription for his/her physical activity and exercise training after the termination of the program and get the opportunity to put those into practice under supervision. These individual advises should take into consideration the patient's age, gender, past habits, comorbidities, preferences, and goals. The patient's readiness to change behavior, his/her self-confidence, and/or social support in making positive changes as well as possible barriers to increase and take up independent exercise training should be addressed. The participation in long-term maintenance programs like heart groups should be recommended if available.

4.5   Perception Training, Body Awareness, and Practical Skills of Self-Control

After an acute cardiac event (acute coronary syndrome, PCI, or cardiac surgery), most of the patients are uncertain regarding physical activity overall and, particularly, how much physical stress they are able to tolerate and what kind of physical activity they are allowed to perform. This uncertainty in combination with the experience of the vulnerability of the heart results in the avoidance of any physical strain and foster physical inactivity. Other patients rather tend to mentally suppress the cardiac event that might assimilate a danger of overload. During the exercise training, the patient has to learn the limit of his/her exercise tolerance and his/her exercise limits. The goal is to achieve the patient's realistic judgment as well as his/her acceptance of the often considerable reduced exercise tolerance. The exercise training is an optimal instrument to improve the patient's body awareness and perception. The experience of subjective and objective symptoms that occur during exercise training should be used to help the patient to recognize such symptoms as well as estimate their relevance for the load achieved. Improving body awareness and perception should therefore be an integral component of each exercise training, explaining the exercise procedure and its beneficial as well as possible adverse effects on the body to the patient. Through the exercise training, the patient should learn to perceive and observe his/her local and systemic reactions (i.e., increased heart rate, respiration, level of exertion of the muscle, subjective well-being, etc.) and to interconnect them to the objective exertion performed. By gradually increased exercise intensity, the patient should perceive the limit of his/her exercise tolerance in order to be able to recognize it. The exercise therapist should communicate with the patient asking him/her to prescribe his/her perceptions of objective and subjective symptoms during exercise. These practical skills of self-control are the fundamental instruments for the patient's safe and effective approach to physical activity and training. This will reduce anxiety and improve a certainty regarding physical exertion during occupation, recreation, or daily life (Fig. 4.7).

4.6   Aerobic Endurance Training

Oxygen consumption (VO_{2peak}) assessed by means of cardiopulmonary exercise testing is one of the strongest predictors of disease prognosis in patients with coronary artery disease and chronic heart failure [36–42] (Fig. 4.8). In CHD patients every 1.0 ml/kg^1 min^1 increase in VO_{2peak} is associated with 15 % decrease in risk of death, 14 % (in women) and 17 % (in men) decrease in risk of overall mortality, and 10–14 % (in women) and 9–16 % (in men) decrease in risk of cardiovascular mortality [42]. Martin et al. [43] demonstrated in a retrospective analysis of a cohort of 5641 CHD patients that improvements in VO_{2peak} achieved during cardiac rehabilitation have prognostic value. They found every increase in exercise capacity in one MET achieved during 12-week CR to be associated with 13 % reduction of overall mortality. In patients who started the CR program in the lowest fitness group, the

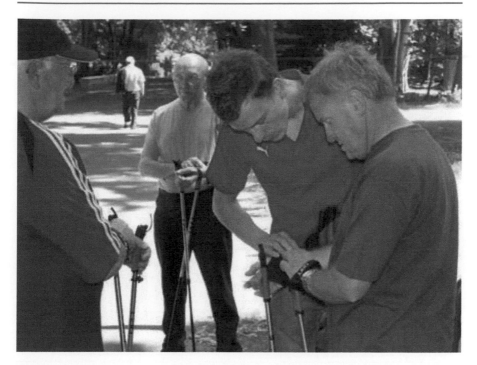

Fig. 4.7 Patient should learn to perceive and observe his/her local and systemic reactions, i.e. increased heart rate

benefit on exercise capacity was even of greater value. In this group an increase in one MET was associated with 30 % reduction of overall mortality.

A systematically carried out aerobic endurance exercise program leads to an increase in exercise capacity and symptom-free exercise tolerance [13, 42–46]. In patients with cardiovascular disease, the increase in exercise capacity gained has been reported to range between 11 and 36 % [13, 45, 46] depending on the patient's exercise tolerance, clinical status, as well as intensity and dose of the exercise training [13, 47–49]. Sedentary untrained and deconditioned patients have been shown to achieve the greatest benefits [13, 47–49]. In addition, long-term regular aerobic endurance training positively influences well-known cardiovascular risk factors such as hypertension, type 2 diabetes mellitus, dyslipidemia, and abdominal obesity [50–59] (Fig. 4.9).

4.6.1 Exercise Prescription and Definition of Individual Exercise Intensity

Based on careful clinical evaluation and risk stratification, including symptom-limited exercise testing, aerobic endurance training can be performed in a safe and an effective manner [3, 4, 46].

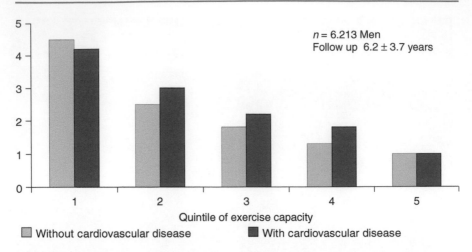

Fig. 4.8 The relative risk of death from any cause according to quintile of exercise capacity among subjects with and without cardiovascular disease (According to Myers et al. [41])

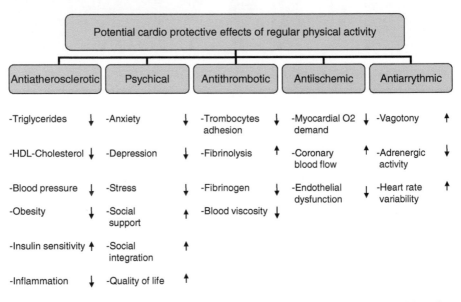

Fig. 4.9 Potential cardioprotective effects of regular physical activity, especially aerobic endurance training

In addition to the maximal achieved exercise capacity, the intensity that the patient is able to tolerate without any pathology (exercise tolerance) is to be well defined and taken into account when exercise prescription is given.

Absolute contraindications to aerobic endurance training are summarized in Table 4.2 [14].

Table 4.2 Contraindications for aerobic endurance training [14]

Acute coronary syndrome (ACS)
Malignant hypertension with systolic blood pressure >190 mmHg during exercise training despite exhaustive antihypertensive medication therapy
Drop in systolic blood pressure by ≥20 mmHg during exercise, in particular in patients with CHD
Severe secondary mitral valve insufficiency or more specifically moderate mitral valve insufficiency with evidence of increased regurgitation during exercise
Heart failure NYHA IV
Supraventricular and ventricular arrhythmias causing symptoms or hemodynamic compromise, continual ventricular tachycardia
Frequent ventricular extrasystoles, noncontinual ventricular tachycardia in advanced left ventricular dysfunction or more specifically after myocardial infarct as well as in response to exercise or during the postexercise regeneration phase
Cardiovascular diseases that have not been risk evaluated and that have not been treated according to guideline requirements in terms of best possible prognosis outcome (i.e., beta-blocker in patients with CHD, angiotensin-converting enzyme inhibitor in patients with heart failure) or, more specifically, hemodynamic control (i.e., maximal medication therapy for blood pressure regulation in severe arterial hypertension). Patients with contraindications to exercise training due to malignant arrhythmias, on the other hand, can be introduced to a training program after antiarrhythmic measures have been taken (i.e., implantable cardioverter defibrillator (ICD), proven efficacy of medication therapy)

4.6.1.1 How to Define Exercise Intensity

Training intensity should be established and controlled based on the results of a maximal exercise stress test done on a bicycle/treadmill ergometer including ECG and blood pressure monitoring. This should yield maximal heart rate, maximal exercise load in watts, possible ischemic threshold, and blood pressure response to exercise. These data will form the basis for determining the individual training load and training heart rate. Additional cardiovascular examinations or improvement of therapy has to be included, if cardiac complaints and/or symptoms arise during the exercise stress test. If complaints or symptom limitations persist, despite maximal therapeutic efforts, it is advised to keep the exercise load at a level free of symptoms and ischemia. It is generally recommended that the training intensity should be clearly below the ischemic threshold [11–13, 17].

The *heart rate* is an objective, easily determined parameter used to regulate and control exercise load in cardiac rehabilitation. The *maximal heart rate (HRpeak)* is the highest heart rate achieved prior to termination of an incremental exercise tolerance test due to subjective exhaustion or objective indications [8]. The training heart rate can be determined as percent of maximal heart rate (HR_{peak}). In cardiac rehabilitation a training heart rate of 65–75 % (if tolerated 80–85 %) HR_{peak} is recommended [17]. It is important to keep in mind that only the heart rate response to an exercise stress test performed under the patients actual medication can be used for exercise prescription. This applies especially to the use of ß-receptor blockers (Fig. 4.10).

The training heart rate can also be determined mathematically by using the Karvonen formula, in which the heart rate reserve (HRR) is calculated. The heart

Patient: 52 years old man post acute coronary syndrome and PCI

Medication: ß-receptor-blocker, statins and ASS

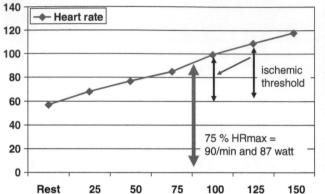

Maximal heart rate
118 beats/min

Heart rate at threshold
109 beats /min

Exercise heart rate
ischemic clearly below
the ischemic threshold
(at least 10 beats/min)
maximal at 99
beats/min

Target heart rate 75 %
of maximal heart rate at
90 beats/min

Fig. 4.10 How to determine a target heart rate and exercise load (watt) for exercise training in cardiac rehabilitation

rate reserve is the difference between maximal heart rate and resting heart rate, as determined in maximal exercise stress test (Fig. 4.11).

In cardiac patients training heart rate of 40–60 % (if tolerated 65–70 %) of heart rate reserve is recommended [17]. The heart rate reserve method should especially be used in patients with chronotropic incompetence. The training heart rate should always be determined clearly below the ischemic threshold (i.e., 10 beats/min).

Maximal exercise capacity measured in watt is a reliable and reproducible parameter in order to regulate exercise training performed on a bicycle ergometer [11]. In cardiac rehabilitation exercise intensity at 40–60 % (if tolerated up to 70–80 %) of maximal load (watt) achieved in a symptom limited exercise test is recommended [17]. In patients with very low exercise tolerance, very low heart rate reserve, as well as with the inability of the sinus node to react adequately to exercise stress by increasing heart rate (i.e., patients with chronotropic incompetence, atrial fibrillation, pacemakers, and post-heart transplant), training intensity should be controlled according to exercise load in watts and by using the Borg scale.

The *Borg scale* (rate of perceived exertion (RPE)) is used to subjectively assess how the individual perceives the intensity of the performed exercise on a scale from 6 to 20 points [60] (Fig. 4.12). It is not advisable, however, to solely rely on the Borg scale to advise on training load as it contains too many influencing factors from the patient's perspective (i.e., unfamiliar method, poor body awareness, over motivation, and peer pressure) [61]. The Borg scale can be used as a supplement to other training regulation options, as well as to facilitate developing body awareness to the exercise load. Target values are RPE 11–14, comparable to light to moderate exercise intensity [17].

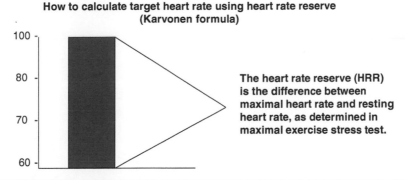

Fig. 4.11 How to determine the target heart rate for exercise training in cardiac rehabilitation using the Karvonen formula

Fig. 4.12 The Borg scale – rate of perceived exertion (RPE)

20	
19	**Extremely hard**
18	
17	**Very hard**
16	
15	Hard / heavy
14	
13	Somewhat hard
12	
11	**Light**
10	
9	**Very light**
8	
7	**Extremely light**
6	

The Borg-scale
(Rate of perceived exertion, RPE)

RPE < 12   < 40 % VO2peak

RPE 12–13 40-60 % VO2peak

RPE 14–16 60-85 % VO2peak

The *maximal oxygen consumption (VO₂peak)* reached during an exercise stress test and the oxygen consumption at the anaerobic threshold (VO_2-AT) are meaningful parameters in regulating exercise load during training [62]. The latter can also be determined during submaximal exercise testing, independent of the individual's motivation level [63]. If a cardiopulmonary exercise test is used to determine aerobic training intensity then 40–70 % of VO_{2peak} (up to 80 % if tolerated) should be targeted, close to the individual's anaerobic threshold (1st VAT) [17, 64] (Fig. 4.13).

4.6.1.2 Aerobic Endurance Training Duration and Frequency

Health benefits can only be reached and maintained with long-term aerobic endurance training done on a regular basis. Aerobic endurance training should be performed for ≥30 min 3–5 times per week, preferably everyday, resulting in a total exercise time of ≥150 min per week (or 21/2 h/week). Ideally, exercise time should

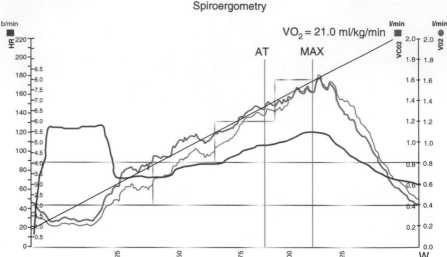

Fig. 4.13 An exemplary result from a cardiopulmonary exercise testing in a 62-year-old man with coronary artery disease and type 2 diabetes

be around 3–4 h/week. The initial aerobic endurance exercise phase should last around 5–10 min in untrained individuals and gradually increase to ≥30 min per training session during the course of the training program. Low-intensity physical activities, such as walking in plane, can and should be done on a daily basis (preferably more than once a day) [12, 14, 17].

4.6.1.3 How to Perform Aerobic Exercise Training

The most common training forms used in cardiac rehabilitation to improve aerobic endurance are ergometer training on a cycle or treadmill. Additional common aerobic exercise modes include walking, Nordic walking, and biking. Jogging may be performed in those with good exercise capacity. This holds also true for swimming, as only those with stable cardiac condition without ischemia or potential for life-threatening should perform swimming. The decisive factors in choosing an appropriate training form in cardiac rehabilitation should be the ability to exactly dose, control, and gradually increase the appropriate exercise intensity, and the availability to monitor vital parameters (i.e., ECG, heart rate, blood pressure) is necessary.

When choosing a training form, an individual's baseline characteristics (such as age, gender, exercise experience, exercise tolerance, and concomitant diseases) as well as preference and motivation must be considered. For overweight and obese individuals, non-weight-bearing exercise modes should be chosen (i.e., biking, bicycle ergometer training, and swimming). Walking and Nordic walking can be considered, if there are no pre-existing joint problems.

Aerobic Endurance Training on a Cycle Ergometer

In phase II of cardiac rehabilitation, aerobic endurance training on a cycle ergometer is recommended as standard procedure. The advantages of this training form are that it is non-weight bearing and enables the exercise load to be precisely dosed, independent of the patient's body weight. Moreover, the minimal upper body motion enables blood pressure and ECG to be monitored at a high-quality standard during exercise. This type of exercise can be performed in an upright or supine position, and special safety equipment is available to facilitate patients with special needs, for example, extremely obese subjects, elderly insecure patients, or patients with history of stroke (Fig. 4.14). Computer-controlled cycle ergometer training and monitoring systems, specially designed for the use in cardiac rehabilitation, are available. Cycle ergometry can be performed as group training or at an individual basis. Training should be performed on an electrically braked cycle ergometer 3–5 times per week. If possible, it should be taken advantage of everyday the cardiac rehabilitation program is offered.

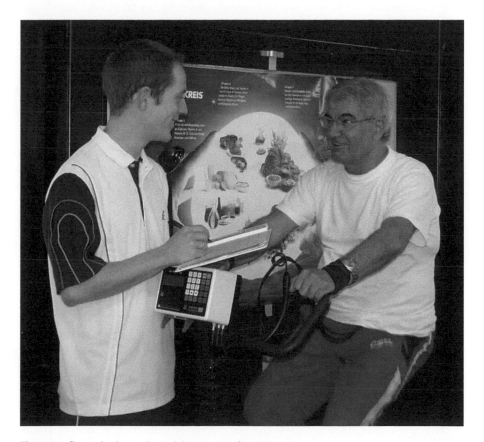

Fig. 4.14 Supervised exercise training on a cycle ergometer

Endurance training (i.e., 10–30 min) is the most effective method to improve aerobic endurance capacity. Every exercise unit on the cycle ergometer should be constructed in four phases (Table 4.3 and Fig. 4.15).

Table 4.4 shows the recommendation for the implementation of moderate-intensity-continuous-endurance training in cardiac rehabilitation [17].

The safety and efficiency of moderate-intensity-continuous-aerobic training in patients with cardiac diseases is well established and therefore recommended as a standard training modality in cardiac rehabilitation in international guidelines and position papers. In primary prevention it is well known that higher exercise volume aerobic exercise training is more effective to improve exercise capacity and to reduce overall mortality. On the other hand by increasing the intensity similar effects can be achieved by shorter exercise boots [66]. Results of a meta-analyses [22] demonstrate an inverse relationship between exercise intensity and overall mortality, which was independent of age and gender. The question is if vigorous aerobic exercise training is also safe, effective, and well tolerated in cardiac patients. An interval-training mode would allow to exercise with at least short high-intensity bouts alternating to bouts of low or moderate intensity. In fact in the last decade, some studies with high-intensity interval training (HIIT) in cardiac patients have been carried out. The results prove HIIT to be beneficial [67, 68] and safe [69] in CHD patients [67–75] as well as in patients with markedly reduced exercise capacity (i.e., severe chronic heart failure) [76–80]; however long-term effects are still equivocal. In cardiac rehabilitation mainly two types of interval trainings protocols have been in focus of science and implementation: *sprint or short-term interval training* and *high-intensity interval training (HIIT)*.

The type of *sprint or short (term) interval training* mostly used in cardiac rehabilitation is characterized by alternating short bouts of high-intensity exercise (20–30s) followed by a long recovery phase at minimal load typically twice the

Table 4.3 Recommendations for moderate-intensity-continuous-endurance training on a cycle ergometer

Phase I (warm-up phase I)	
Exercise intensity:	<50 % of target exercise intensity
Exercise duration:	>2 min
Phase II (warm-up phase II)	
Exercise intensity:	Gradually increase in exercise load by 1–10 watt/min (depending on patient's exercise tolerance) until target exercise intensity has been reached
Exercise duration:	5–10 min
Phase III (exercise phase)	
Exercise intensity:	100 % of the target exercise intensity in watt and/or of the target training heart rate
Exercise duration:	>5 min and gradually prolong the exercise duration up to 20–30 min (up to 45–60 min)
Phase IV (cool down phase)	Gradually reduce the exercise load to 0 watt within the time of 3 min.

Modified after Bjarnason-Wehrens et al. [14])
The composition of one exercise session

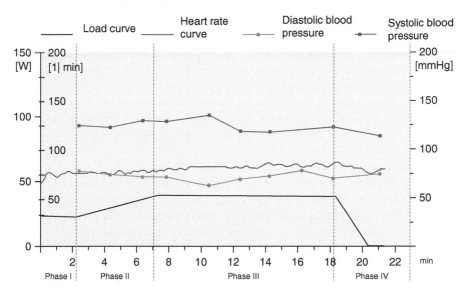

Fig. 4.15 Aerobic endurance training on a cycle ergometer. The graphic shows the composition of an exemplary exercise session

Table 4.4 Recommendations for moderate-intensity-continuous-endurance training on a cycle ergometer

Aerobic endurance training on a cycle ergometer training with monitoring			
Stages	Exercise intensity	Exercise duration	Exercise frequency
Initial stage	Low intensity, that is, 40–50 % VO_{2peak}, 60 % HR_{peak} 40 % HRR Below 1st VAT RPE < 11	Starting with ca. 5 min (in the exercise phase) and gradually increase to 10 min	3–5 days/week Target: daily
Improvement stage	Gradually increase the exercise intensity from low to moderate up to target values, depending on the patient's exercise tolerance and clinical status, that is, 50, 60, 70, (80 %) VO_{2peak} 65, 70, 75 (80–85 %) HR_{peak} 45, 50, 55, 60 % (65–70 %) HRR RPE 12–14	Gradually prolong the exercise training from 10 to 20 (up to 30–45) min	3–5 days/week Target: ≥5 days/week
Maintenance stage	Long-term stabilization of the exercise intensity and exercise duration achieved during the improvement stage; gradually increase exercise intensity and especially exercise duration and frequency if intended and well tolerated	Gradually prolong the exercise training from 20–45 (up to >60) min if tolerated	3–5 days/week Target: most days/week

Modified after [17, 18, 49, 65]
A long-term exercise training program should be composed of three stages: initial stage, improvement stage, and maintenance stage
HR heart rate, *HRR* heart rate reserve, *RPE* rate of perceived exertion, *VAT* ventilator (an)aerobic threshold

length of the exercise bout (ratio of exercise time: recovery time = 1:2) (Fig. 4.16 and Table 4.5). The advantage of this type of training is that the short bout of high-intensity exercise stimulates peripheral adaptations in the leg muscles to take place without compromising an overload in central mediation. The exercise intensity can be determined as a percentage of maximum load (watt$_{peak}$) achieved during a symptom-limited exercise stress test. An intensity as high as 85–90 % of watt$_{peak}$ is usually recommended. Conclusive evidence base concerning the safety and effi-ciency of this type of training is only preliminary and must be confirmed by ran-domized controlled studies [14, 17].

Within the last few years, the safety and the efficacy of the 4 × 4 min *high-intensity interval training protocol (HIIT)* (Table 4.5 and Fig. 4.17) has been in the scientific focus for its use in cardiac rehabilitation. Meta-analysis including the results of few small, randomized controlled studies comparing the efficacy of HIIT to *moderate-intensity-continuous-endurance training* has revealed HIIT to be more effective in improving exercise capacity measured as a VO$_{2peak}$. A meta-analysis of nine studies (206 CHD patients) [67] revealed HIIT to increase VO$_{2peak}$ a 1.60 mL/kg^{-1}/min^{-1} more than moderate continuous training. High-intensity interval training resulted in a significant larger benefit in VO$_{2peak}$ compared to moderate continuous training (MCT) in patients with CHD (HIIT 20.5 % vs. MCT 12.8 %; $p < 0.001$). A second meta-analysis of six studies (229 CHD patients; EF < 40; 99 were random-ized to HIIT) confirms these results [68]. Patients in the HIIT group improved their VO$_{2peak}$ by 1.53 mL/kg^{-1}/min^{-1} more than those in the MCT group. The authors point out that small sample sizes and the large inconsistency and heterogeneity

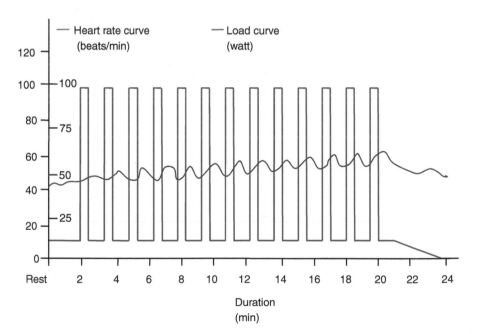

Fig. 4.16 Interval training on a cycle ergometer. The graph shows the composition of an exem-plary exercise session

Table 4.5 Exercise protocol commonly used for interval training in cardiac rehabilitation: *sprint or short (term) interval training* and *high-intensity interval training* to be performed on a cycle or treadmill ergometer

Sprint or short (term) interval training[a]	High-intensity interval training (HIIT)
Phase I (warm-up phase)	*Phase I (warm-up phase)*
> 2 min without or with very low load	10 min with 60 % of the heart rate$_{peak}$
Phase II (exercise phase)	*Phase II (exercise phase)*
Alternating short (20–30 s) exercise bouts with 100 % of the target exercise intensity and twice as long (40–60 s) recovery bouts without or with very low load ≥10 repetitions of the intervals – to be prolonged up to ≥20 repetitions.	Alternating 4 × 4 min exercise bouts with 85–95 of HR$_{peak}$ and 3 × 3 min recovery bouts with 60–70 % of HR$_{peak}$
Phase III (recovery phase)	*Phase III (recovery phase)*
< 3 min without or with very low load	3–5 min with 60–70 % of HR$_{peak}$

The construction of an exercise unit
[a]Modified after Refs. [64, 76, 82]

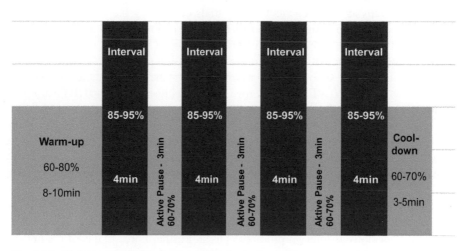

Fig. 4.17 High-intensity interval training. The 4 × 4 min aerobic interval-training model. Intensity is given in peak heart rate (HR$_{peak}$) (Modified after Refs. [64, 77])

between the study results in the included studies limit the informational value of this meta-analysis. On the other hand, a recently published larger randomized controlled study (200 CHD patients; EF > 40 %) comparing HITT versus MCT does not confirm these results [74]. The results show no advantage for one of the exercise modalities (HIIT: 23.5 ± 5.7 vs. 28.6 ± 6.9 mL/kg^{-1}/min^{-1}; +22.7 %; MCT: 22.4 ± 5.6 vs.

26.8 ± 6.7 mL/kg^{-1}/min^{-1}; +20.3 %; p (time) =0.001; p (interaction) = ns) [74]. Both 12-week interventions equally improved VO$_{2peak}$, peripheral endothelial function, as well as quality of life in CHD patients. Both programs seem to be safe for CHD patients, and no adverse events were reported during the exercise sessions. The authors' experience was that the implementation of the 4×4 HIIT protocol with the target intensity of 90–95 % of HR$_{peak}$ is hardly feasible in CHD patients. The mean intensity achieved in the HIIT group was 88 % of HR$_{peak}$ compared to mean intensity of 80 % HR$_{peak}$ in MCT group. These results demonstrate the impact of sufficient training intensity in continuous exercise training, which may, if tolerated, be more than the generally recommended 65–75 % of the HR$_{peak}$. Rogmore et al. [69] evaluated the risk of cardiovascular events during organized high-intensity interval exercise training (HIIT 85–95 % HR$_{peak}$) and moderate-intensity training (MCT 60–70 % HR$_{peak}$) among 4846 patients, primary with coronary heart disease. The results indicate that the risk of a cardiovascular event is overall low during both high-intensity exercise and moderate-intensity exercise in a cardiovascular rehabilitation setting (MCT, one fatal cardiac arrest (1 per 129,456 exercise hours); HIIT, two nonfatal cardiac arrests (1 per 23,182 exercise hours)). In a recently published study, a significant correlation between the changes in physical fitness during the intervention and the physical activity levels after the 1-year follow-up was found, indicating that patients who improved their physical fitness more had a higher motivation to adopt a physically active lifestyle following cardiac rehabilitation [80, 81].

A meta-analysis of seven randomized trials comparing the results of HIIT vs. MCT in heart failure patients (mean LVEF 32 %) showed high-intensity interval training (HIIT) to be more effective for improving VO$_{2peak}$ than traditionally prescribed moderate-intensity continuous aerobic training (MCT) (WMD 2.14 mL VO$_2$/kg/min, 95 % CI 0.66–3.63). The comparison of the effects on the left ventricular ejection fraction (LVEF) at rest revealed inconclusive results (HIIT vs. MCT: WMD 3.3 %, 95 % CI −0.7–7.3 %) [79]. An interesting meta-analysis stratified aerobic exercise studies in heart failure patients by activity intensity [80]. The results revealed the magnitude of improvements in cardiorespiratory fitness to be greater with increasing intensity, unrelated to baseline fitness levels or exercise volume. The largest improvement in VO$_{2peak}$ was observed with high-intensity training (23 %) showing a linear decrease in effect size with decreasing exercise intensity (vigorous intensity 16 %, moderate intensity 13 %, low intensity 7 %, respectively). Exercising with high or vigorous intensity seems to be well tolerated in heart failure patients, especially if interval protocol is used. Furthermore studies of continuous exercise training used a greater volume (duration) of exercises and some of them multiple daily sessions. In high-intensity exercise programs, the volume of work is completed in shorter time and may therefore require shorter session duration and lower exercise frequency that might influence the patient's adherence to the exercise program [80]. Moreover this analysis also demonstrated exercising with higher intensity in heart failure patients to be safe, showing no increased risk of death, adverse events, or hospitalization in the high- and vigorous-intensity exercise groups [80]. These interesting results must be confirmed by more prospective randomized controlled studies, with greater cohorts and longer follow-up period, though, before definite recommendations can be given [14, 17]. Furthermore until now the prognostic value of high-intensity interval training have not yet been evaluated neither in CHD nor in heart failure patients.

For the implementation in cardiac rehabilitation, the more scientific discussion of intensity and exercise mode allows to derive the knowledge that aerobic exercise of any intensity of continuous or interval mode seems to be effective to improve exercise capacity in cardiac patients. Exercising with high or vigorous intensity leads to greater improvements than exercising with moderate or low intensity. Higher intensity seems to be better tolerated, if the exercise training is carried out with an interval mode, which allows resting periods between the high or vigorous exercise bouts. In the general praxis of cardiac rehabilitation, it is in the responsibility of the exercise therapist in agreement with the CR physician to decide, which exercise intensity and exercise mode fits best for the individual patient. Rigid interval protocols might not be optimal for every patient. The exercise specialist should consider modification in order to adapt the program to the individual capability of the patient.

Thus high-intensity interval training is not an alternative for continuous aerobic exercise training but could be an effective and well-tolerated supplementary approach for aerobic endurance training in cardiac rehabilitation.

Other Forms of Aerobic Endurance Training in Cardiac Rehabilitation

To further improve aerobic endurance, other forms of exercise such as walking, Nordic walking, slow jogging, and cycling can be added to the individual's training program depending on the patient's preference and exercise tolerance. This also applies to phase II of cardiac rehabilitation.

Endurance training in form of walking improves the physical fitness and has a positive influence on numerous cardiovascular risk factors [83–85]. Going for a walk or walking in general (brisk walking with deliberate arm movement) are ideal types of aerobic endurance exercise for getting started for unfit individuals, the elderly, and/or postmenopausal women, without risking an overload of the cardiopulmonary system.

Organized rehabilitation programs should provide the opportunity for all patients to take part in supervised walks and walking programs provided that patients meet necessary exercise tolerance criteria and are without adverse comorbidities. The walking terrain, walking pace, and duration should be tailored to the needs of the participating patients. The benefit of walking programs is their applicability in everyday life, which makes them ideal to motivate patients to increase their daily physical activity. They also offer an excellent opportunity to improve the patient's body perception and self-awareness. By becoming familiar with exercise parameters like heart rate, breathing frequency, well-being, and level of exhaustion, the individual can translate this experience into his/her every day activities. Exercise intensity can be controlled by the target heart rate for aerobic endurance training. This approach is applicable to most types of endurance exercise.

The use of walking poles ("Nordic walking") can somehow increase exercise intensity by increasing muscle recruitment. This translates into higher oxygen uptake (up to + 4.4 ml.kg^{-1}.min^{-1}) and overall energy expenditure (up to +1.5 kcal. min^{-1}) [86]. Further advantages of Nordic walking include a reduction in weight bearing on the joints and an increase in body stabilization due to the walking poles (especially during downhill walking) [87, 88]. During recent years Nordic walking has become extremely popular and is well tolerated especially by elderly and female patients. To utilize the advantages of this exercise form, correct technique should be emphasized. Exercise intensity can be controlled by means of target heart rate for aerobic endurance training [88] (Fig. 4.18).

Biking is an ideal endurance and recreational sport for persons of all age groups. Organized rehabilitation programs typically provide biking tours and can be applied in cardiac rehabilitation as well. Special attention should be paid to the suitability of the bike (i.e., touring bike with many gears, e-bike, good transmission, suspension, and a comfortable saddle), the terrain (solid leveled surface), as well as the safety (helmet). The experience gained from supervised biking tours during the rehabilitation program can be motivating to the patient in order to implement this activity into his/her everyday life. Biking on a solid leveled surface is a non-weight-bearing activity and is well suited for patients with low exercise tolerance. Alternatively, a motor-assisted pedal cycle can be used; however lower exercise intensity has to be taken into account. Exercise intensity can be controlled by the target heart rate for aerobic endurance training.

In patients with very good exercise tolerance, endurance running (*jogging*) is one option to improve aerobic endurance capacity and to positively influence cardiovascular risk factors. Even this mode of exercise can be modified regarding intensity from slow to rather fast jogging, the former also termed "wogging." Maximal adaptations can be achieved with minimal efforts during this type of exercise [8]. Exercise intensity can be controlled by the target heart rate for aerobic endurance training.

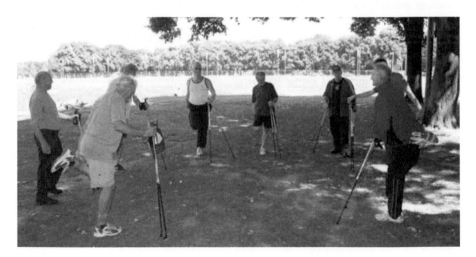

Fig. 4.18 Nordic walking has become popular and is well tolerated especially by elderly and female patients

4.7   Resistance Exercise Training

The objective of resistance exercise training is to increases muscular strength by performing *static* or *dynamic* muscle contractions. While *dynamic* (isotonic) exercise is performed by movement of the joint, *static* (isometric) exercise does not result in movement of the joint. Most physical activities comprise both dynamic and static contractions and are therefore classified based on their dominant characteristics.

In cardiac rehabilitation resistance training programs include primarily dynamic repetitions with both *concentric* (muscle shortening) and *eccentric* (muscle lengthening) muscle actions. Isometric muscle actions play a secondary role [89].

Muscular hypertrophy is defined as the increase in total muscle mass. Hypertrophy training is intensity dependent and dominated by isometric contractions (muscle contraction without changes in muscle length), which is not in focus in cardiac rehabilitation. *Muscular endurance* is the ability to sustain muscular strength over an extended period of time with minimal decrease in power output and is composed of dynamic contractions [8].

The exercise intensity of dynamic resistance training is determined using the *one-repetition maximum (1-RM)* method [90], often not assessing 100 % but rather submaximal values in cardiac patients (Sect. 4.7.5).

4.7.1   The Impact of Resistance Exercise in Cardiac Rehabilitation

Resistance exercise can lead to an increase in muscular strength and muscular endurance by increasing muscle mass and/or improving coordination and muscle metabolism [91–93]. It is known to have diversified health benefits, i.e., reduced loss in muscle mass and strength associated with heart disease or old age, as well as increased exercise and functional capacity, to positively influence several cardiovascular risk factors, to improve mobility, participation, and quality of life [17] (Table 4.6).

In many cases (especially in elderly patients) the loss in muscle mass and strength is associated with heart disease or old age, the essential reason for reduced everyday activity levels, mobility, and participation. Thus in these patients the improved ability to develop muscular strength can influence the quality of life decisively. Adequate individualized resistance training positively influences the ability to carry out everyday activity; improve the patient's self-confidence, independency, and psychosocial well-being; as well as avert or reduce the need of nursing care. Improved proprioception mediated by adequate resistance training positively influence coordination and balance. Combined resistance and balance training improve stability and gait ability, enhance security of movement, and thus play a major role in preventing falls [92, 98].

Individualized and adequately dosed dynamic resistance training has been demonstrated to be safe and effective in cardiac patients and is encouraged by the current recommendations on exercise training in cardiac rehabilitation [1–13, 17, 49] (Fig. 4.19). This particularly applies to patients with coronary artery disease who

Table 4.6 Objectives and possible effects of a resistance exercise as a part of a cardiac rehabilitation program [17]

The impact of resistance exercise as a part of a cardiac rehabilitation program
Objectives:
To improve muscular strength and muscular endurance by increasing muscle mass and/or improving coordination and metabolism (including improved insulin resistance and peripheral lipolysis)
To work against loss in skeletal muscle mass and strength caused by
old age [91–93]
Long-term bed confinement or inactivity due to illness
Skeletal muscle atrophy (e.g., in heat failure patients) [94, 95]
Long-lasting immunosuppressive therapy (heart transplant recipients) [96]
To reduce and/or prevent decrease in bone mass (age related, postmenopausal, or due to long-lasting immunosuppressive therapy (heart transplant recipients)) [97]
To improve proprioception (positively impact coordination and balance; preventing falls) [92, 98]
To improve mobility, participation, and quality of life [17]
An increase in muscular strength and muscular endurance mediated by adequately dosed resistance training can:
Increase exercise capacity [90, 99]
Increase functional capacity [100]
Reduce functional impairment
Improve everyday activity levels [101, 102]
Positively influence self-confidence and psychosocial well-being, social readaptation, and reintegration
Improve quality of life
Positively influence cardiovascular risk factors
Enhance weight reduction and stabilization [59, 103]
Improve insulin sensitivity (independent from changes in body weight and endurance capacity) [104–107]
Reduce of blood pressure [50]

possess good exercise tolerance and preserved left ventricular function. The results of a meta-analysis evaluating the efficacy of aerobic endurance training compared to combined programs of aerobic and resistance training in CHD patients revealed combined programs to be more effective in improving lower and upper body strength, body composition (decreased percent body fat and trunk fat and increased fat-free mass), and peak working capacity [99].

Resistance training has also been shown to be well tolerated and effective in the elderly and/or female patients [108–112].

The efficacy and safety of resistance exercise in high-risk patients, that is, patients with chronic heart failure, has remained an ongoing discussion over the last decade. Numerous studies have been conducted exploring this topic, most of them including only a small cohort differing markedly in their research approach and research question. However, none of these previous studies has shown any increased cardiac risk associated with resistance training, which has proven overall effective. According to new scientific evidence, supervised individualized dynamic resistance

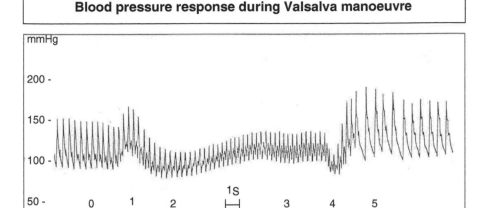

Fig. 4.19 Blood pressure response during Valsalva maneuver (modified according to Graf [125])

exercise training at low-to-moderate intensity is a safe and effective training mode and should be prescribed in addition to aerobic exercise training. This helps to counteract muscle atrophy and peripheral changes typically seen in heart failure patients [17, 113–117].

It has to be noted though that only aerobic endurance training has shown to improve clinical prognosis. Comparable prospective studies focusing on surrogate endpoints do not exist for resistance exercise [17, 118]. In cardiac rehabilitation the implementation of adequately dosed resistance training is recommended to compliment aerobic endurance exercise training [17, 49] (Fig. 4.20). Absolute contraindications to resistance training are the same as absolute contraindications for aerobic endurance training (Table 4.2).

4.7.2 Blood Pressure Response During Resistance Exercise

It is well known that resistance exercise can result in an extreme increase in blood pressure, but it is also recognized that this does not necessarily have to be the case, if an appropriate training volume (weight, number of repetitions, sets) is chosen. It should be taken into account, when prescribing exercise, that the actual blood pressure response to resistance exercise is dependent on the amount of static (isometric) muscle contraction, the actual load (% of individual's 1-RM) [119, 120], and the amount of muscle mass involved [121]. Blood pressure response is also dependent on the number of repetitions and total duration of muscular contraction [122] as well as repetition speed and rest periods [122]. The highest blood pressure response is reached, when multiple repetitions are performed at 70–95 % of 1-RM to exhaustion, since it is equally affected by both intensity and duration. Exercise load below 70 % of 1RM as well as duration of muscular contraction above 95 % of 1-RM are insufficient to elicit a significant rise in blood pressure response [124].

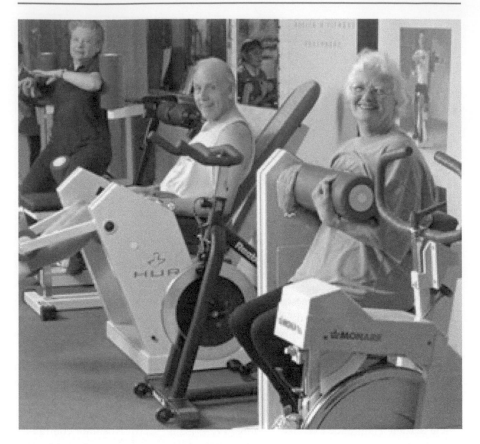

Fig. 4.20 Resistance training

A dynamic resistance training with low-to-moderate intensity allows a high number of repetitions (muscular endurance training (15–30 reps), moderate hypertrophy training (10–15 reps)) without evoking any major rise in blood pressure. The blood pressure response during this type of training is lower compared to the increase in blood pressure seen during moderate endurance training.

If the *Valsalva maneuver* (a forced expiration is invoked against the closed glottis) is carried out during resistance exercise, the rise in blood pressure is more pronounced. The Valsalva maneuver leads to an increase in intrathoracic pressure, which, in turn, leads to a decrease in venous return and potentially reduction in cardiac output [124]. The physiological response includes an increase in heart rate to maintain cardiac output and peripheral vasoconstriction to maintain blood pressure, which otherwise may decrease with decreasing cardiac output. Once the imposed strain is released, there is a dramatic increase in venous return and subsequently an increase in cardiac output being forced through a constricted arterial vascular system. The dramatic rise and drop in blood pressure can limit myocardial oxygen delivery resulting in potentially dangerous arrhythmias and/or reduced

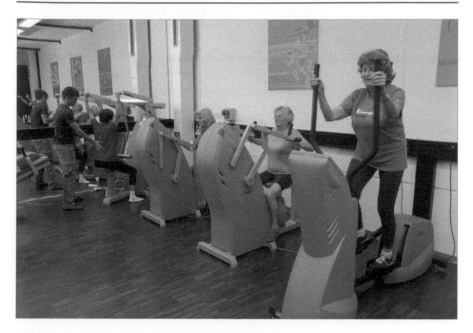

Fig. 4.21 Combined aerobic and resistance training

perfusion of the coronary arteries leading to ischemia [124]. A rapid fall in blood pressure after straining at maximal workload sometimes results in syncope even in healthy persons [125] (Fig. 4.21).

Special attention should be paid to the Valsalva maneuver during resistance exercise training. Before starting the resistance exercise program, the patient should be educated about the complications potentially associated with the Valsalva maneuver. He/she should learn to pay attention to his/her breathing while exercising and learn to combine exercise and breathing in a way that enables him/her to avoid Valsalva maneuver. This should be a part of the preparation in the initial exercise stage.

4.7.3 Implementation of Resistance Training in Cardiac Rehabilitation

Exercise training in cardiac rehabilitation should be started by means of aerobic endurance training. Resistance training may be considered in phase II and phase III cardiac rehabilitation, but is contraindicated in phase I (hospital phase). Resistance training should be implemented as an alternative training mode, supplementary to aerobic exercise, and can be integrated into the training program after one or two sessions of continuous endurance trainings at the earliest.

In the absence of any adverse comorbidity, moderate-intensity dynamic resistance training is recommended for all low-risk patients with stable cardiovascular disease and good exercise tolerance (including myocardial infarction and/or interventional revascularization), moderate to good left ventricular function, no clinical signs of heart failure, and without symptoms of angina pectoris or ischemic ST segment depression during exercise stress test. Low-intensity resistance exercise training should not be started earlier than 2 weeks post-myocardial infarction and/or 7 days post-interventional revascularization. Combined endurance and resistance training (up to 60 % of 1-RM), delivered early after myocardial infarction, does not induce negative left ventricular remodeling and is associated with an increase in VO_{2peak} and muscle strength [126].

In women with CHD, both aerobic endurance training and resistance training delivered within a cardiac rehabilitation program improve physical quality of life and VO_{2peak}. However, within 1 year of follow-up, physical quality of life is significantly higher in women who participated in a combined training regime [127].

In patients recovering from coronary artery bypass surgery (CABG) and other open-heart surgery, exercise capacity can be extremely limited. After a thoracotomy and/or saphenectomy, the wound healing takes approximately 4–6 weeks. Physical exercise inducing tangential vector forces in or around the sternum (pressure or sheer stress) should be avoided for at least 3 months postoperatively. Before resistance training is started, the treating physician must confirm that the sternum is stable. If there are no complications during the postoperative course and the patient has a good exercise tolerance, a low-intensity resistance exercise training for the lower limbs can be carried out earlier, provided a stable trunk positioning is ensured. This may also be true for selected exercises of the upper body.

In *heart transplant recipients*, the continuous immunosuppressive therapy including cortisone often leads to muscle atrophy and decrease in bone mass. In addition, these patients usually have a poor musculoskeletal structure due to the long history of preceding severe cardiac disease and subsequent inactivity. Resistance exercise training has been demonstrated to show good effects in these patients [97, 98]. In clinically stable patients, individualized moderate dynamic resistance training should be started as soon as possible in the postoperative phase and should be continued on a long-term basis, to counteract the negative side effects associated with immunosuppressive therapy.

In patients with stable chronic heart failure, left ventricular function remains stable during moderate-intensity resistance training [128]. In these patients, the amount of exercise intolerance does not correlate with the degree of left ventricular dysfunction. It is well recognized that the reduction in exercise tolerance is also related to morphological, metabolic, and functional changes in the patient's peripheral musculature. Several studies have demonstrated that adequate dynamic resistance training with low-to-moderate intensity may help to counteract the muscle atrophy typically associated with chronic heart failure. In stable patients with chronic heart failure (NYHA I-III), adequate resistance training is recommended in addition to aerobic endurance training [17, 113–117].

4.7.4   How to Perform Resistance Exercise Training

In cardiac rehabilitation resistance training should be medically supervised and led by an experienced exercise therapist/physiotherapist. Objective training goals should be modulated for each patient individually. The use of elastic exercise bands and/or small weights for resistance training is very suitable. This equipment is easy to use and allows individually tailored resistance training as well as group training. Further advantages are the easy storage and their low costs. However, particularly the use of elastic exercise bands must be carefully instructed to each patient to ensure that they are used in a safe manner.

More precise training with less risk of overloading can be achieved through the use of weight machines. They allow for higher precision in implementing individualized training programs and safe movement execution. For this type of training individual supervision is mandatory.

Resistance training is prescribed according to dosage parameters such as intensity (resistance), number of repetition, volume, frequency, and duration as well as rate of progression [89]. A lower repetition range with a heavier weight/resistance may better optimize strength and power, while a higher repetition range with a lighter weight/resistance may better enhance muscular endurance. Weight loads that permit 8–15 repetitions will generally facilitate improvements in muscular strength and endurance [124].

Table 4.7 shows recommendations for the implementation of resistance training in cardiac rehabilitation.

In the initial stage all patients should start training at very low intensity (< 30 % 1-RM) to learn and practice correct movement execution (familiarization). In the improvement stage I, the load should be increased gradually from 30 to 50 %. While elderly patients and/or patients with low exercise tolerance (i.e., heart failure patients) should start training at very low intensity (< 30 % 1-RM), trained patients with good exercise tolerance can start training at moderate intensity (50 % 1-RM), increasing first the number of repetitions and series and thereafter the intensity. In the improvement stage II, the load should be gradually increased (30–50 %1-RM and further up to 60 % 1-RM) based on the patient's exercise tolerance and response to the resistance training. Higher training intensities (stage III) may be considered in well-trained patients with good exercise tolerance and low cardiac risk, who have already completed a 4–6 week resistance exercise training program [17, 124, 130].

After each set of exercises, a resting time of at least 1 min should be implemented [122]. In novice a frequency of three sessions per week is considered most effective. Once trained, and in order to maintain the desired level of strength, frequency can be reduced to two sessions per week [130, 131]. Between each session, there should be 1 day of abstinence from resistance training.

4.7.5 How to Determine the Appropriate Load of Resistance Training

The evaluation of muscle strength is indicated to prescribe individualized safe and effective resistance training intensities, to track the progress of an individual, as well as to evaluate the efficacy of resistance training regime. A number of methods for determining the intensity for resistance training exist. Laboratory-based methods include the use of isometric dynamometers and isokinetic dynamometers. In chronic heart failure patients, the use of isokinetic versus one-repetition maximum

Table 4.7 Recommendation for the implementation of a resistance training in cardiac rehabilitation

Training stage	Training objective	Training method	Training intensity	Repetitions per muscle group	Training volume
Initial stage (pre-training; familiarization)	Implementation of exercise; improvement of self-perception and coordination; learning to correctly perform exercise	Dynamic	<30 % 1-RM RPE ≤11	5–10	2–3 training units per week, 1–3 sets each unit 1–2 min rest between sets
Improvement stage I	Improvement of aerobic endurance and coordination	Dynamic	30–50 % 1-RM RPE 12–13	12–25	2–3 training units per week, 1–3 sets each unit 1–2 min rest between sets
Improvement stage II	Increase in muscle cross-sectional area (hypertrophy), improve intermuscular coordination	Dynamic	40–60 % 1-RM (> 60 % in selected patients)RPE ≤15	8–15	2–3 training units per week, 1–3 sets each unit 1–2 min rest between sets
Improvement stage III	Increase in muscle cross-sectional area (hypertrophy), improve intermuscular coordination	Dynamic	60–80 % 1-RM (in selected patients in good clinical condition and with heavy physical employment or those returning to sport) RPE <15	8–15	2–3 training units per week, 1–3 sets each unit 1–2 min rest between sets

Special directions for training:

Standardized exercises for mobilization and stretching for warming up, preparation, and cooling down

Emphasize familiarization with the learning of how the movement is executed correctly

One to three sets of 6–10 exercises should be performed

Perform varied training covering the major muscle groups: chest, shoulders, arms, back, abdomen, thigh, lower legs (some of the exercises may be performed unilateral)

Involve the major muscle groups of the upper and lower extremities

Avoid a continuous, tensed-up grip

Perform the resistance training in a rhythmical manner at a moderate to slow controlled speed through a full range of motion

Avoid breath holding and straining (Valsalva maneuver) by exhaling during the contraction or exertion phase of the lift and inhaling during the relaxation phase

If symptoms occur, discontinue the training immediately (vertigo, arrhythmias, dyspnea, angina pectoris)

Modified after Refs. [17, 124–129]

strength assessment has been demonstrated to be more accurate to assess changes in muscular strength with exercise training [132]. On the other hand, these methods require sophisticated laboratory equipment and personal trained in their use and in addition are not very specific for the types of movement patterns commonly used in typical cardiac rehabilitation regimes. The one repetition maximum test has been shown to be reliable for various populations, also in untrained middle-aged as well as old individuals [90]. The one repetition maximum is defined as *"the maximum amount of weight/resistance that can be performed for only a single repetition for a given exercise, with a proper lifting technique, without compensatory movements and without breath holding"* [90]. The evaluation of the 1-RM is the gold standard in dynamic resistance exercise testing. This method is comparatively simple and requires relatively inexpensive non-laboratory equipment (Table 4.8). The 1-RM test can be performed using the same patterns as those undertaken by the exercising individuals during their normal training. Numerous studies have reported that the 1-RM method to assess muscle strength is safe for patients with cardiovascular diseases [133, 134].

The maximum strength a person can produce, the maximum weight a person can lift (i.e., the one repetition maximum), is not an absolute value and can be influenced by several factors, i.e., by psychological factors (i.e., motivation and/or external encouragement) and the testing protocol (i.e., with or without familiarization). The

Table 4.8 One repetition maximum test, standard protocol

Perform exercise test optimally at the machine used later on for training; *avoid Valsalva maneuver*
Perform a light warm-up of 5–10 repetitions at 40–60 % of assumed 1RM
Rest period ≥1 min
Perform 3–5 repetitions at 60–80 % of assumed 1RM
Rest period of ≥2–3 min
Gradually increase the weight in small steps
After 3–5 attempts the weight one can lift in a single repetition should be identified
Communication between supervisor and test person is of particular importance
The 1-RM value is reported as the weight of the last successfully completed lift
Special directions for testing
A familiarization process prior to 1-RM strength testing is essential to avoid injury and for ensuring reliable test results and minimize learning effect or systematic bias
Always use standardized protocol for 1-RM testing
Always perform 1-RM testing using the same equipment to be used later on for resistance training
Measured results on the one type of equipment cannot be transferred to training to be performed on another type of equipment
In old and weak patients, the equipment need to have a low starting load and small increments
All lifts should be conducted throughout the full range of motion. If the full range of motion is limited by musculoskeletal problems and/or overweight, the evaluated possible pain-free range of movement prior to testing is mandatory to define an individual successfully performed repetition.

Modified after Kraemer et al. [90]

result may further be influenced by the quality of the test execution (proper lifting technique, range of motion, speed of movement, control for compensatory movements and breath holding, rest periods, and more) as well as the testing possibilities and equipment used [89, 133, 135]. Thus, it has to be kept in mind that the testing of 1-RM may have significant practical problems, making results unreliable. Many cardiac patients are old and weak. Thus the equipment used needs to have a low starting load and options for small increments in order to be able to test this population at all. It must also be considered that different types (manufacturer) of machines/equipment show variable results due to differences in the load transmission. Measured results on the one type of equipment cannot be transferred to training performed on another. Therefore it is strongly recommended always to perform the 1-RM test using the same equipment to be used for resistance training. A familiarization process prior to 1-RM strength testing is essential to avoid injury, for ensuring reliable test results, and minimize learning effect or systematic bias. This includes teaching (and practicing) correct lifting and breathing technique at very low load and/or using submaximal loads. In younger and experienced individuals, one session is sufficient; in older and/or inexperienced patients, multiple sessions are often necessary. Without a familiarization process prior to strength testing, there is a significant increase in the expression of muscle strength between two consecutive strength tests performed a few days apart [133]. Furthermore familiarization may reduce the risk of injury especially in patients, who have no previous lifting experience.

The results of one repetition maximum test can be used to determine the appropriate exercise load for resistance exercise training in cardiac patients. The intensity of training is specified according to a percentage of the one repetition maximum (1-RM).

An alternative, often used in cardiac patients, is the evaluation of a predictive one repetition maximum (testing 10 or fewer repetitions to fatigue) using the Brzycki's equation to determine max load [136]. The use of a prediction equation for older adults appears also to be a valid measure of 1-RM. In older patients, the prediction equation have been shown to underestimate the actual 1-RM, but the error is small [133]. The use of the indirect method to estimate 1-RM is practical and safe and may even produce more accurate result especially in older unexperienced cardiac patients.

To avoid a maximal strength test (1-RM), which might lead to Valsalva maneuver and blood pressure evaluation, the correct intensity can also be found by using a graded exercise testing. Here, the patient begins with very low intensity that does not require much effort, and the resistance load is gradually increased to the point at which the patient can maximally achieve 10–15 repetitions in a correct manner without abdominal strain and symptoms [129]. The Borg scale can be used to assess the patient's perceived exertion in addition to measuring objective physiologic parameters. In patients with moderate risk, perceived exertion (RPE) should be 12–13, not exceeding 15 (Table 4.9; Fig. 4.22).

In summary in exercise-based cardiac rehabilitation, the therapists do not need absolute maximal values of muscular strength, but need reliable values of strength performance to be able to set up an individualized safe and effective resistance exercise program.

Table 4.9 The Borg scale, rate of perceived exertion

20	
19	Extremely hard
18	
17	Very hard
16	
15	Hard/heavy
14	
13	Somewhat hard
12	
11	Light
10	
9	Very light
8	
7	Extremely light
6	

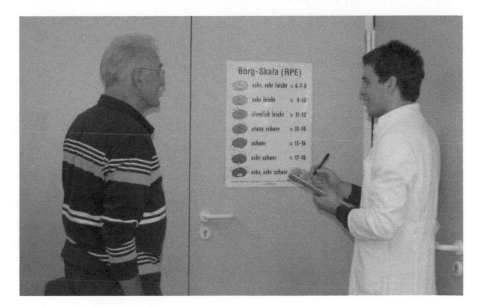

Fig. 4.22 Using the Borg scale for improving patients' body awareness and perception

4.8   Additional Contents of Exercise Training Program in Cardiac Rehabilitation

Physical exercises to improve flexibility, agility, coordination balance, muscular strength, and endurance should be an essential part of all comprehensive exercise training program in cardiac rehabilitation. The main objectives are to provide the premises for effective exercise training and prevent musculoskeletal injuries. Balance is required in many activities of daily living as well as recreational physical activities. Exercises to improve balance, kinesthetic differentiation ability, as well as other coordinative skills are of special importance to prevent falls in the elderly as well as in untrained individuals that are starting exercise after a long period of physical inactivity. Complimentary to resistance training especially balance training for static and dynamic balance is recommended. The balance training should be adapted to the patient's abilities, starting with low levels of difficulty and include various progressions. The different level of difficulty and progression can be achieved by modifying the exercises used, for instance, as follows: decrease/increase the base of support (three separate stances: double leg, single leg, tandem), use different surfaces (ueven and/or uneven surface and medium density balance pad with even and or uneven surfache, etc.), use instable surfaces (use of tilt boards), modify optical control (eyes are open/eyes are closed), prevent the use of arms to help balance (arms crossed), and do supplementary task while balancing (i.e., catching ball).

To prevent overload and the risk of musculoskeletal injury, special attention should be paid to the appropriate exercise choices as well as to correct movement execution. All exercises performed have to be individually dosed and controlled by the exercise therapist. As the determination of the right exercise intensity is far more difficult in these exercises than in aerobic exercise, when the exercise therapist can use heart rate monitoring to control intensity, improving the patient's body perception and awareness is of particular importance. For the supervision a careful control of adequate respiration and observation of symptoms of overload (i.e., exudation, blushing, incorrect execution of the exercise) as well as the use of subjective perceived rate of exertions (Borg scale) in combination with communication between patient and therapist are the instruments of choice. The avoidance of Valsalva maneuver is mandatory to prevent dangerous elevations in blood pressure.

The patient should be integrated into therapy groups according to their exercise tolerance, physical condition, existence of relevant exercise and/or mobility limitations, and/or comorbidities, age, and experience with physical activity and exercise.

According to the exercise tolerance, most rehabilitation centers differentiate at least between so-called chair groups (>0.3–0.5 watt/kg body weight), low-intensity exercise group (>0.5–1.0 watt/kg body weight), and moderate-intensity exercise group (>1.0 watt/kg body weight). In larger centers more distinctive differentiation according to exercise tolerance and rehabilitation indication, age, and gender groups can be followed.

In special indications, i.e., in patients after a thoracotomy and/or saphenectomy, special groups for the treatment of the postoperative consequences are needed. This special program should include breathing exercises and careful mobilization of the thorax to avoid and work against reliving postures and improve breathing quality as well as exercises to improve venous return. Physical exertion which causes tangential vector forces in the sternal area (pressure or sheering stress, i.e., caused by dissymmetric exercises) should be avoided. Due to the limited physical activity early after heart surgery, these exercises are usually performed in seated position.

Exercise intensity can be differentiated by changing individual speed of motion, exercise duration, muscle mass involved, amplitude of the movement, and the flexibility, strength, and coordination demand necessary to perform the exercise in an adequate and correct manner (Table 4.10).

To enhance motivation and interaction within the therapy group, the integration of modified movement games and team games into the exercise program is to be recommended. Small movement games with simple modifiable rules, which can be played in small groups with low organizational demand, are appropriate. If modified team games are to be integrated, games played on separated playing fields are most suitable. Due to the separate radius of activity, the exercise intensity as well as the risk of injury can be reduced. In general the intensity of movement and team games can be modified by changing the rules, reducing/increasing the playground, changing the number of players, reducing/increasing the distances to overcome, reducing/increasing the speed of movement, varying play equipments, etc. This allows adapting the game to the premises of the group and to integrate the playing activities into the exercise program without danger of overload. Because of the inadequate possibility to control the intensity, movement games with higher demand of muscular strength or aerobic endurance are unsuitable (Fig. 4.23).

Table 4.10 Factors influencing exercise intensity while performing exercise to improve flexibility, agility, coordination, and strength

High	Fast	Long	Great	High	High	High	High
Intensity	Speed of motion	Exercise duration	Muscle mass involved	Amplitude of movement	Flexibility demands	Strength demands	Coordination demands
Low	Slow	Short	Small	Low	Low	Low	Low

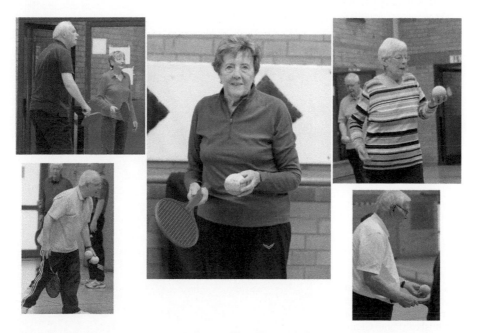

Fig. 4.23 To enhance motivation and interaction within the therapy group, the integration of modified games can be integrated into the exercise program (Photo German Sport University Cologne)

4.9   Patient–Therapist Relationship

Exercise therapy is a core component of the cardiac rehabilitation process that usually is led by a specially educated therapist. He/she works with the patient at every visit to the rehabilitation center, often for several hours every week. Thus, of all therapists he/she learns to know the patient best during the rehabilitation phase. While exercising together a special patient–therapist relationship can be established. This opens the opportunities for informal talks about familiar and/or occupational pleasures and/or problems. The patients do not seldom open themselves to the exercise therapist about his/her problems coping with the disease, his/her insecurity, anxiety, motivation, preferences for lifestyle changes, as well as problems and barriers he/she experiences to fulfill the demands of the CR and lifestyle changes he/she is confronted with during CR program. Furthermore, the supervision of the exercise intervention gives the therapist the best opportunity to observe how the patient reacts. Is the program meeting his/her needs, interests, preferences, and/or motivation? Is he/she enjoying the participation, having fun? Is he/she relaxed, anxious, or depressed? Is the exercise intensity, volume, as well as the contents of the exercise program adequate? Do any symptoms, i.e., arrhythmia, ischemia, musculoskeletal problems, and problems related to comorbidities during exercise occur? Thus the exercise therapist captures a special role within the interdisciplinary cardiac rehabilitation team and can serve as an important connector between the patient and other members of the team, including the CR physician. As a "person of trust," his information and "diagnosis" should be considered invaluable (Fig. 4.24).

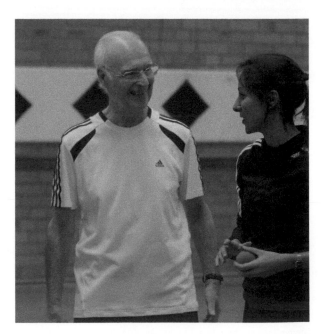

Fig. 4.24 While exercising together, a special patient–therapist relationship can be established (Photo German Sport University Cologne)

In summary the therapist responsible for exercised-based intervention for cardiac rehabilitation has to keep in mind that exercise training is more than a matter of evidence-based medicine, endurance and/or resistance training, intensity, and volume of exercise. On a long-term basis, the benefit strived for will only be achieved if the rehabilitation team manages to motivate the patient to change her/his attitude and take up a regular physical activity and exercise training and optimally to continue this lifelong. In this regard the precondition for a self-controlled exercise training and the basic for the patient's health competence are the improved patient's body awareness and his/her practical skills of self-control. During the rehabilitation process, the patient's perceptions, attitude, and health esteem regarding physical activity and exercise training have to be influenced positively. It is important that he/she experiences the exercise training provided during cardiac rehabilitation as a convenient task that he/she can cope with as well as an activity that is associated with well-being, fun, and social contacts. On a long-term basis, the patient will only integrate physical activity and exercise training into his/her daily life, if medical benefits are associated with personal values.

References

1. Heran BS, Chen JM, Ebrahim S, Moxham T, Oldridge N, Rees K, DR T, RS T. Exercise-based cardiac rehabilitation for coronary heart disease. Cochrane Database Syst Rev. 2011;(8):CD001800.
2. Anderson L, Oldridge N, Thompson DR, Zwisler AD, Rees K, Martin N, Taylor RS. Exercise-based cardiac rehabilitation for coronary heart disease cochrane systematic review and meta-analysis. J Am Coll Cardiol. 2016;67:1–12.
3. Jolliffe JA, Rees K, Taylor RS, Thompson D, Oldridge N, Ebrahim S. Exercise-based rehabilitation for coronary heart disease. Cochrane Database Syst Rev Update. 2001;(1):CD001800. Update Software.
4. Taylor RS, Brown A, Ebrahim S, Jolliffe J, Noorani H, Rees K, Skidmore B, Stone JA, Thompson DR, Oldridge N. Exercise-based rehabilitation for patients with coronary heart disease: systematic review and meta-analysis of randomized controlled trials. Am J Med. 2004;116:682–92.
5. Clark AM, Hartling L, Vandermeer B, McAlister FA. Meta-analysis: secondary prevention programs for patients with coronary artery disease. Ann Intern Med. 2005;143:659–72.
6. Thompson PD, Buchner D, Pina IL, Balady GJ, Williams MA, Marcus BH, Berra K, Blair SN, Costa F, Franklin B, et al. Exercise and physical activity in the prevention and treatment of atherosclerotic cardiovascular disease: a statement from the Council on Clinical Cardiology (Subcommittee on Exercise, Rehabilitation, and Prevention) and the Council on Nutrition, Physical Activity, and Metabolism (Subcommittee on Physical Activity). Circulation. 2003;107:3109–16.
7. U.S. Department of Health and Human Services, Rdt. Physical activity and health: a report of the surgeon general. Atlanta: U.S Department of Health and Human Services. Centers for Disease Control and Prevention National Center for Chronic Disease and Health Promotion; 1996.
8. Hollmann W, Hettinger TH. Sportmedizin. Grundlagen für Arbeit, Training und Präventivmedizin, völlig neu bearbeitete und erweiterte Auflage ed, vol. 4. Stuttgart/New York: Schattauer; 2000.
9. Gielen S, Hambrecht R. Trainingstherapie – Theoretische Grundlagen und Evidenz. In: Rauch B, Middeke M, Bönner G, Karoff M, Held K, editors. Kardiologische rehabilitation. Stuttgart: Thieme; 2007. p. 70–8.

10. Deutcher Verband für Gesundheitssport und Sporttherapie. www.dvgs.de. [Web Page] 2016.
11. Balady GJ, Williams MA, Ades PA, Bittner V, Comoss P, Foody JM, Franklin B, Sanderson B, Southard D. Core components of cardiac rehabilitation/secondary prevention programs: 2007 update: a scientific statement from the American Heart Association Exercise, Cardiac Rehabilitation, and Prevention Committee, the Council on Clinical Cardiology; the Councils on Cardiovascular Nursing, Epidemiology and Prevention, and Nutrition, Physical Activity, and Metabolism; and the American Association of Cardiovascular and Pulmonary Rehabilitation. Circulation. 2007;115:2675–82.
12. Piepoli MF, Corra U, Benzer W, Bjarnason-Wehrens B, Dendale PAC, Gaita D, McGee H, Mendes M, Niebauer J, Olsen-Zwisler AD, Schmid JP. Secondary prevention trough cardiac rehabilitation. 2008. Update. From knowledge to implementation. A position paper from the cardiac rehabilitation section of the European Association of Cardiac Rehabilitation and Prevention. Eur J Cardiovasc Prev Rehabil. 2010;17:1–17.
13. Leon AS, Franklin BA, Costa F, Balady GJ, Berra KA, Stewart KJ, Thompson PD, Williams MA, Lauer MS. Cardiac rehabilitation and secondary prevention of coronary heart disease : an American Heart Association scientific statement from the Council on Clinical Cardiology (Subcommittee on Exercise, Cardiac Rehabilitation, and Prevention) and the Council on Nutrition, Physical Activity, and Metabolism (Subcommittee on Physical Activity), in collaboration with the American association of Cardiovascular and Pulmonary Rehabilitation. Circulation. 2005;111:369–76.
14. Bjarnason-Wehrens B, Schulz O, Gielen S, Halle M, Dürsch M, Hambrecht R, Lowis H, Kindermann W, Schulze R, Rauch B. Leitlinie körperliche Aktivität zur Sekundärprävention und Therapie kardiovaskulärer Erkrankungen. Clin Res Cardiol. 2009;4(Suppl. 3): 1–44.
15. Sagar VA, Davies EJ, Briscoe S, Coats AJS, Dalal HM, Lough F, Rees K, Singh S, Taylor RS. Exercise-based rehabilitation for heart failure: systematic review and meta-analysis. Open Heart. 2015;2:e000163. doi:10.1136/openhrt-2014-000163.
16. Bjarnason-Wehrens B, Held K, Hoberg E, Karoff M, Rauch B. Deutsche Leitlinie zur Rehabilitation von Patienten mit Herz-Kreislauferkrankungen (DLL-KardReha). Clin Res Cardiol. 2007;(Suppl 2):III/1–III/54.
17. Vanhees L, Rauch B, Piepoli M, van Buuren F, Takken T, Börjesson M, Bjarnason-Wehrens B, Doherty P, Dugmore D, Halle M and (on behalf of the writing group of the EACPR). Importance of characteristics and modalities of physical activity and exercise in the management of cardiovascular health in individuals with cardiovascular disease (Part III). Eur J Prev Cardiol 2012;19:1326–1332.
18. Corra U, Giannuzzi P, Adamopoulos S, Bjornstad H, Bjarnason-Weherns B, Cohen-Solal A, Dugmore D, Fioretti P, Gaita D, Hambrecht R, et al. Executive summary of the Position Paper of the Working Group on Cardiac Rehabilitation and Exercise Physiology of the European Society of Cardiology (ESC): core components of cardiac rehabilitation in chronic heart failure. Eur J Cardiovasc Prev Rehabil. 2005;12:321–5.
19. Pina IL, Apstein CS, Balady GJ, Belardinelli R, Chaitman BR, Duscha BD, Fletcher BJ, Fleg JL, Myers JN, Sullivan MJ. Exercise and heart failure: a statement from the American Heart Association Committee on exercise, rehabilitation, and prevention. Circulation. 2003;107: 1210–25.
20. Bjarnason-Wehrens B. Trainingsmaßnahmen. Rauch B, Middeke M, Bönner G, Karoff M, Held K. (Edt.). Kardiologische rehabilitation. Stuttgart: Thieme; 2007. p. 78–89.
21. Eden KB, Orleans CT, Mulrow CD, Pender NJ, Teutsch SM. Does counseling by clinicians improve physical activity? A summary of the evidence for the U.S. Preventive Services Task Force. Ann Intern Med. 2002;137:208–15.
22. Löllgen H, Böckenhoff A, Knapp G. Physical activity and all-cause mortality: An updated meta-analysis with different intensity categories. Int J Sports Med. 2009;30:213–24.
23. Nocon M, Hiemann T, Muller-Riemenschneider F, Thalau F, Roll S, Willich SN. Association of physical activity with all-cause and cardiovascular mortality: a systematic review and meta-analysis. Eur J Cardiovasc Prev Rehabil. 2008;15:239–46.

24. Samitz G, Egger M, Zwahlen M. Domains of physical activity and all-cause mortality: systematic review and dose-response meta-analysis of cohort studies. Int J Epidemiol. 2011;40:1382–400.
25. Löllgen H, Löllgen D. Risikoreduktion kardiovaskulärer Erkrankungen durch körperliche Aktivität. Internist. 2011;53:20–9.
26. Blumenthal JA, Babyak MA, Carney RM, Huber M, Saab PG, Burg MM, et al. Exercise, depression, and mortality after myocardial infarction in the ENRICHD trial. Med Sci Sports Exerc. 2004;746-755 doi:10.1249/01.MSS.0000125997.63493.13.
27. Wannamethee SG, Shaper AG, Walker M. Physical activity and mortality in older men with diagnosed coronary heart disease. Circulation. 2000;102:1358–63.
28. Janssen I, CJ J. Influence of physical activity on mortality in elderly with coronary artery disease. Med Sci Sports Exerc. 2006:418–23.
29. Al-Khalili F, Janszky I, Andersson A, Svane B, Schenck-Gustafsson K. Physical activity and exercise performance predict long-term prognosis in middle-aged women surviving acute coronary syndrome. J Intern Med. 2007;261:178–87.
30. Moholdt T, Wisløff U, Nilsen TIL, Slørdahl SA. Physical activity and mortality in men and women with coronary heart disease: a prospective population-based cohort study in Norway (the HUNT study). Eur J Cardiovasc Prev Rehabil. 2008;15:639–45.
31. Apullan FJ, Bourassa MG, Tardif JC, Fortier A, Gayda M, Nigam A. Usefulness of self-reported leisure-time physical activity to predict long-term survival in patients with coronary heart disease. Am J Cardiol. 2008;102:375–9.
32. Gerber Y, Myers V, Goldbourt U, Benyamini Y, Scheinowitz M, Drory Y. Long-term trajectory of leisure time physical activity and survival after first myocardial infarction: a population-based cohort study. Eur J Epidemiol. 2011;26:109–16.
33. Mons U, Hahmann H, Brenner H. A reverse J-shaped association of leisure time physical activity with prognosis in patients with stable coronary heart disease: evidence from a large cohort with repeated measurements. Heart. 2014;100:1043–9.
34. Yu C, Li LS, Ho HH, Lau C. Long-term changes in exercise capacity, quality of life, body anthropometry, and lipid profiles after a cardiac rehabilitation program in obese patients with coronary heart disease. Am J Cardiol. 2003;91:321–5.
35. Shibata Y, Hayasaka S, Yamada T, Ojima T, Ishikawa S, et al. Physical activity and risk of fatal or non-fatal cardiovascular disease among CVD survivors – the JMS cohort study. Circ J. 2011;75:1368–72.
36. Godin G, Desharnais R, Jobin J, Cook J. The impact of physical fitness and health-age appraisal upon exercise intentions and behavior. J Behav Med. 1987;10:241–50.
37. Kavanagh T, Mertens DJ, Hamm LF, Beyene J, Kennedy J, Corey P, Shephard RJ. Prediction of long-term prognosis in 12 169 men referred for cardiac rehabilitation. Circulation. 2002;106:666–71.
38. Valeur N, Clemmensen P, Saunamaki K, Grande P. The prognostic value of pre-discharge exercise testing after myocardial infarction treated with either primary PCI or fibrinolysis: a DANAMI-2 sub-study. Eur Heart J. 2005;26:119–27.
39. Lund LH, Aaronson KD, Mancini DM. Validation of peak exercise oxygen consumption and the Heart Failure Survival Score for serial risk stratification in advanced heart failure. Am J Cardiol. 2005;95:734–41.
40. O'Neill JO, Young JB, Pothier CE, Lauer MS. Peak oxygen consumption as a predictor of death in patients with heart failure receiving beta-blockers. Circulation. 2005;111:2313–8.
41. Myers J, Prakash M, Froelicher V, Do D, Partington S, Atwood JE. Exercise capacity and mortality among men referred for exercise testing. N Engl J Med. 2002;346:793–801.
42. Keteyian SJ, Brawner CA, Savage PD, Ehrman JK, Schairer J, Divine G, Aldred H, Ophaug K, Ades PA. Peak aerobic capacity predicts prognosis in patients with coronary heart disease. Am Heart J. 2008;156:292–300.
43. Martin BJ, Arena R, Haykowsky M, Hauer T, Austford LD, Knudtson M, Aggarwal S, Stone JA, for the APPROACH Investigators. Cardiovascular fitness and mortality after contemporary cardiac rehabilitation. Mayo Clin Proc. 2013;88:455–63.

44. Ades PA, Savage PD, Brawner CA, Lyon CE, Ehrman JK, Bunn JY, Keteyian SJ. Aerobic capacity in patients entering cardiac rehabilitation. Circulation. 2006;113:2706–12.
45. Karmisholt K, Gotzsche PC. Physical activity for secondary prevention of disease. Systematic reviews of randomised clinical trials. Dan Med Bull. 2005;52:90–4.
46. Rees K, Taylor RS, Singh S, Coats AJ, Ebrahim S. Exercise based rehabilitation for heart failure. Cochrane Database Syst Rev. 2004;(4):CD003331.
47. Ades PA. Cardiac rehabilitation and secondary prevention of coronary heart disease. N Engl J Med. 2001;345:892–902.
48. Wenger NK, Froelicher ES, Smith LK, Ades PA, Berra K, Blumenthal JA, Certo CM, Dattilo AM, Davis D, DeBusk RF, et al. Cardiac rehabilitation as secondary prevention. Agency for Health Care Policy and Research and National Heart, Lung, and Blood Institute. Clin Pract Guidel Quick Ref Guide Clin. 1995;17:1–23.
49. Piepoli MF, Corrà U, Adamopoulos S, Benzer W, Bjarnason-Wehrens B, et al. Secondary prevention in the clinical management of patients with cardiovascular diseases. Core components, standards and outcome measures for referral and delivery: A Policy statement from the cardiac rehabilitation section of the European Association for Cardiovascular Prevention & Rehabilitation. Endorsed by the Committee for Practice Guidelines of the European Society of Cardiology. Eur J Prev Cardiol. 2012;21:664–81.
50. Cornelissen V, Smart NA. Exercise training for blood pressure: a systematic review and meta-analysis. J Am Heart Assoc. 2013;2:e004473. doi:10.1161/JAHA.112.004473.
51. Pan XR, Li GW, Hu YH, Wang JX, Yang WY, An ZX, Hu ZX, Lin J, Xiao JZ, Cao HB, et al. Effects of diet and exercise in preventing NIDDM in people with impaired glucose tolerance. The Da Qing IGT and Diabetes Study. Diabetes Care. 1997;20(4):537–44.
52. Tuomilehto J, Lindstrom J, Eriksson JG, Valle TT, Hamalainen H, Ilanne-Parikka P, Keinanen-Kiukaanniemi S, Laakso M, Louheranta A, Rastas M, et al. Prevention of type 2 diabetes mellitus by changes in lifestyle among subjects with impaired glucose tolerance. N Engl J Med. 2001;344:1343–50.
53. Boule NG, Haddad E, Kenny GP, Wells GA, Sigal RJ. Effects of exercise on glycemic control and body mass in type 2 diabetes mellitus: a meta-analysis of controlled clinical trials. JAMA. 2001;286:1218–27.
54. Kodama S, Tanaka S, Saito K, Shu M, Sone Y, Onitake F, Suzuki E, Shimano H, Yamamoto S, Kondo K, et al. Effect of aerobic exercise training on serum levels of high-density lipoprotein cholesterol: a meta-analysis. Arch Intern Med. 2007;167:999–1008.
55. Halverstadt A, Phares DA, Wilund KR, Goldberg AP, Hagberg JM. Endurance exercise training raises high-density lipoprotein cholesterol and lowers small low-density lipoprotein and very low-density lipoprotein independent of body fat phenotypes in older men and women. Metabolism. 2007;56(4):444–50.
56. Kelley GA, Kelley KS. Aerobic exercise and HDL2-C: a meta-analysis of randomized controlled trials. Atherosclerosis. 2006;184:207–15.
57. Kelley GA, Kelley KS, Franklin B. Aerobic exercise and lipids and lipoproteins in patients with cardiovascular disease: a meta-analysis of randomized controlled trials. J Cardpulm Rehabil. 2006;26:131–9.
58. DiPietro L. Physical activity in the prevention of obesity: current evidence and research issues. Med Sci Sports Exerc. 1999;31(11 Suppl):S542–6.
59. Garrow JS, Summerbell CD. Meta-analysis: effect of exercise, with or without dieting, on the body composition of overweight subjects. Eur J Clin Nutr. 1995;49:1–10.
60. Borg G. Perceived exertion as an indicator of somatic stress. Scand J Rehabil Med. 1970;2:92–8.
61. Ilarraza H, Myers J, Kottman W, Rickli H, Dubach P. An evaluation of training responses using self-regulation in a residential rehabilitation program. J Cardpulm Rehabil. 2004;24:27–33.
62. Wassermann K, Hansen JE, Sue DY, Casaburi R, BJ W. Principles of exercise testing ind interpretation. 3rd ed. Lippincott Williams & Wikins: Baltimore; 1999.
63. Gitt AK, Wasserman K, Kilkowski C, Kleemann T, Kilkowski A, Bangert M, Schneider S, Schwarz A, Senges J. Exercise anaerobic threshold and ventilatory efficiency identify heart failure patients for high risk of early death. Circulation. 2002;106:3079–84.

64. Mezzani A, Hamm LF, Jones AM, McBride PE, Moholdt T, Stone JA, Urhausen A, Williams MA, European Association for Cardiovascular Prevention and Rehabilitation; American Association of Cardiovascular and Pulmonary Rehabilitation; Canadian Association of Cardiac Rehabilitation. Aerobic exercise intensity assessment and prescription in cardiac rehabilitation: a joint position statement of the European Association for Cardiovascular Prevention and Rehabilitation, the American Association of Cardiovascular and Pulmonary Rehabilitation, and the Canadian Association of Cardiac Rehabilitation. J Cardiopulm Rehabil Prev. 2012;32:327–50.

65. Dubach P, Sixt S, Myers J. Exercise training in chronic heart failure: why, when and how. Swiss Med Wkly. 2001;131:510–4.

66. Wen CP, Wai JPM, Tsai MK, Yang YC, Cheng TYD, Lee M, et al. Minimum amount of physical activity for reduced mortality and extended life expectancy: a prospective cohort study. Lancet. 2011;378:1244–53.

67. Pattyn N, Coeckelberghs E, Buys R, Cornelissen VA, Vanhees L. Aerobic interval training vs. moderate continous training in coronary artery disease patients: a systematic review and meta-analysis. Sports Med. 2014;44:687–700.

68. Elliott AD, Rajopadhyaya K, Bentley DJ, Beltrame JF, Aromataris EC. Interval training versus continuous exercise in patients with coronary artery disease a meta-analysis. Heart Lung Circ. 2015;24:149–57.

69. Rognmo O, Moholdt T, Bakken H, Hole T, Mølstad P, Myhr NE, Grimsmo J, Wisløff U. Cardiovascular risk of high- versus moderate-intensity aerobic exercise in coronary heart disease patients. Circulation. 2012;126:1436–40.

70. Moholdt T, Amundsen BH, Rustad LA, Løvø KT, Gullikstad LR, Bye A, Skogvoll E, Wisløff U, Slørdahl SA. Aerobic interval training versus continuous moderate exercise after coronary artery bypass surgery: a randomized study of cardiovascular effects and quality of life. Am Heart J. 2009;158:1031–7.

71. Munk PS, Butt N, Larsen AI. High-intensity interval exercise training improves heart rate variability in patients following percutaneous coronary intervention for angina pectoris. Int J Cardiol. 2009;145:312–4.

72. Rognmo O, Hetland E, Helgerud J, Hoff J, Slørdahl SA. High intensity aerobic interval exercise is superior to moderate intensity exercise for increasing aerobic capacity in patients with coronary artery disease. Eur J Cardiovasc Prev Rehabil. 2004;11:216–22.

73. Warburton DE, McKenzie DC, Haykowsky MJ, Taylor A, Shoemaker P, Ignaszewski AP, Chan SY. Effectiveness of high-intensity interval training for the rehabilitation of patients with coronary artery disease. Am J Cardiol. 2005;95:1080–4.

74. Conraads VM, Pattyn N, De Maeyer C, Beckers PJ, Coeckelberghs E, Cornelissen VA, Denollet J, Frederix G, Goetschalckx K, Hoymans VY, Possemiers N, Schepers D, Shivalkar B, Voigt JU, Van Craenenbroeck EM, Vanhees L. Aerobic interval training and continuous training equally improve aerobic exercise capacity in patients with coronary artery disease; The SAINTEX-CAD study. Int J Cardiol. 2015;179:203–10.

75. Hofmann R, Gogol C, Karoff M Bjarnason-Wehrens B. Impact of continuous exercise intensity versus high intensity interval exercise training on endurance capacity in coronary artery disease patients with preserved left ventricular function. Abstract P181, EuroPRevent 2014, Amsterdam.

76. Nechwatal RM, Duck C, Gruber G. Physical training as interval or continuous training in chronic heart failure for improving functional capacity, hemodynamics and quality of life – a controlled study. Z Kardiol. 2002;91:328–37.

77. Wisloff U, Stoylen A, Loennechen JP, Bruvold M, Rognmo O, Haram PM, Tjonna AE, Helgerud J, Slordahl SA, Lee SJ, et al. Superior cardiovascular effect of aerobic interval training versus moderate continuous training in heart failure patients: a randomized study. Circulation. 2007;115:3086–94.

78. Smart NA, Dieberg G, Giallauria F. Intermittent versus continuous exercise training in chronic heart failure: a meta-analysis. Int J Cardiol. 2013;186:352–8.

79. Haykowsky MJ, Timmons MP, Kruger C, McNeely M, Taylor DA, Clark AM. Meta-analysis of aerobic interval training on exercise capacity and systolic function in patients with heart failure and reduced ejection fractions. Am J Cardiol. 2013;111:1466–9.

80. Ismail H, McFarlane JR, Nojoumian AH, Dieberg G, Smart NA. Clinical outcomes and cardiovascular responses to different exercise training intensities in patients with heart failure. J Am Coll Cardiol Heart Fail. 2013;1:514–22.

81. Pattyn N, Vanhees L, Cornelissen VA, Coeckelberghs E, De Maeyer C, Goetschalckx K, Possemiers N, Wuyts K, Van Craenenbroeck EM, PJ B. The long-term effects of a randomized trial comparing aerobic interval versus continuous training in coronary artery disease patients: 1-year data from the SAINTEX-CAD study. Eur J Prev Cardiol. 2016;23:1154–64. doi:10.1177/2047487316631200.

82. Meyer K, Samek L, Schwaibold M, Westbrook S, Hajric R, Beneke R, Lehmann M, Roskamm H. Interval training in patients with severe chronic heart failure: analysis and recommendations for exercise procedures. Med Sci Sports Exerc. 1997;29(3):306–12.

83. Kelley GA, Kelley KS, Tran ZV. Walking and resting blood pressure in adults: a meta-analysis. Prev Med. 2001;33:120–7.

84. Kelley GA, Kelley KS, Tran ZV. Walking and non-HDL-C in adults: a meta-analysis of randomized controlled trials. Prev Cardiol. 2005;8:102–7.

85. Murphy MH, Nevill AM, Murtagh EM, Holder RL. The effect of walking on fitness, fatness and resting blood pressure: a meta-analysis of randomised, controlled trials. Prev Med. 2007;44:377–85.

86. Church TS, Earnest CP, Morss GM. Field testing of physiological responses associated with Nordic Walking. Res Q Exerc Sport. 2002;73:296–300.

87. Willson J, Torry MR, Decker MJ, Kernozek T, Steadman JR. Effects of walking poles on lower extremity gait mechanics. Med Sci Sports Exerc. 2001;33:142–7.

88. Schwameder H, Roithner R, Muller E, Niessen W, Raschner C. Knee joint forces during downhill walking with hiking poles. J Sports Sci. 1999;17:969–78.

89. Kraemer WJ, Ratamess NA, French DN. Resistance training for health and performance. Curr Sports Med Rep. 2002;1:165–71.

90. Kraemer WJ, Ratamess NA, Fry AC, French DN. Strength testing: development and evaluation of methodology. In: Maud PJ, Foster C, editors. Physiological assessment of human fitness. 2nd ed. Champaign: Human Kinetics; 2006. p. 119–50.

91. Narici MV, Reeves ND, Morse CI, Maganaris CN. Muscular adaptations to resistance exercise in the elderly. J Musculoskelet Neuronal Interact. 2004;4:161–4.

92. Latham NK, Bennett DA, Stretton CM, Anderson CS. Systematic review of progressive resistance strength training in older adults. J Gerontol A Biol Sci Med Sci. 2004;59:48–61.

93. Latham N, Anderson C, Bennett D, Stretton C. Progressive resistance strength training for physical disability in older people. Cochrane Database Syst Rev. 2003;(2):CD002759.

94. Pu CT, Johnson MT, Forman DE, Hausdorff JM, Roubenoff R, Foldvari M, Fielding RA, Singh MA. Randomized trial of progressive resistance training to counteract the myopathy of chronic heart failure. J Appl Physiol. 2001;90:2341–50.

95. Williams AD, Carey MF, Selig S, Hayes A, Krum H, Patterson J, Toia D, Hare DL. Circuit resistance training in chronic heart failure improves skeletal muscle mitochondrial ATP production rate – a randomized controlled trial. J Card Fail. 2007;13:79–85.

96. Braith RW, Magyari PM, Pierce GL, Edwards DG, Hill JA, White LJ, Aranda Jr JM. Effect of resistance exercise on skeletal muscle myopathy in heart transplant recipients. Am J Cardiol. 2005;95:1192–8.

97. Braith RW, Magyari PM, Fulton MN, Aranda J, Walker T, Hill JA. Resistance exercise training and alendronate reverse glucocorticoid-induced osteoporosis in heart transplant recipients. J Heart Lung Transplant. 2003;22:1082–90.

98. Gillespie LD, Gillespie WJ, Robertson MC, Lamb SE, Cumming RG, Rowe BH. Interventions for preventing falls in elderly people. Cochrane Database Syst Rev. 2003;(4):CD000340.

99. Marzolini Oh PI, Brooks D. Effect of combined aerobic and resistance training versus aerobic training alone in individuals with coronary artery disease: a meta-analysis. Eur J Prev Cardiol. 2012;19:81–94.

100. Hwang CL, Chien CL, Wu YT. Resistance training increases 6-minute walk distance in people with chronic heart failure: a systematic review. J Physiother. 2010;56:87–96.

101. Hunter GR, Treuth MS, Weinsier RL, Kekes-Szabo T, Kell SH, Roth DL, Nicholson C. The effects of strength conditioning on older women's ability to perform daily tasks. J Am Geriatr Soc. 1995;43:756–60.
102. Hunter GR, Wetzstein CJ, Fields DA, Brown A, Bamman MM. Resistance training increases total energy expenditure and free-living physical activity in older adults. J Appl Physiol. 2000;89:977–84.
103. Banz WJ, Maher AM, Thompson WG, Bassett DR, Moore W, Ashraf M, Keefer DJ, Zemel MB. Effects of resistance versus aerobic training on coronary artery disease risk factors. Exp Biol Med. 2003;228:434–40.
104. Brooks N, Layne JE, Gordon PL, Roubenoff R, Nelson ME, Castaneda-Sceppa C. Strength training improves muscle quality and insulin sensitivity in Hispanic older adults with type 2 diabetes. Int J Med Sci. 2007;4:19–27.
105. Kim HJ, Lee JS, Kim CK. Effect of exercise training on muscle glucose transporter 4 protein and intramuscular lipid content in elderly men with impaired glucose tolerance. Eur J Appl Physiol. 2004;93:353–8.
106. Holten MK, Zacho M, Gaster M, Juel C, Wojtaszewski JF, Dela F. Strength training increases insulin-mediated glucose uptake, GLUT4 content, and insulin signaling in skeletal muscle in patients with type 2 diabetes. Diabetes. 2004;53:294–305.
107. Castaneda C, Layne JE, Munoz-Orians L, Gordon PL, Walsmith J, Foldvari M, Roubenoff R, Tucker KL, Nelson ME. A randomized controlled trial of resistance exercise training to improve glycemic control in older adults with type 2 diabetes. Diabetes Care. 2002;25:2335–41.
108. Fiatarone MA, Marks EC, Ryan ND, Meredith CN, Lipsitz LA, Evans WJ. High-intensity strength training in nonagenarians. Effects on skeletal muscle. JAMA. 1990;263:3029–34.
109. King PA, Savage P, Ades PA. Home resistance training in an elderly woman with coronary heart disease. J Cardpulm Rehabil. 2000;20:126–9.
110. Brochu M, Savage P, Lee M, Dee J, Cress ME, Poehlman ET, Tischler M, Ades PA. Effects of resistance training on physical function in older disabled women with coronary heart disease. J Appl Physiol. 2002;92:672–8.
111. Ades PA, Savage PD, Brochu M, Tischler MD, Lee NM, Poehlman ET. Resistance training increases total daily energy expenditure in disabled older women with coronary heart disease. J Appl Physiol. 2005;98:1280–5.
112. Ades PA, Savage PD, Cress ME, Brochu M, Lee NM, Poehlman ET. Resistance training on physical performance in disabled older female cardiac patients. Med Sci Sports Exerc. 2003;35:1265–70.
113. Lee IM, Hsieh CC, Paffenbarger Jr RS. Exercise intensity and longevity in men. The Harvard Alumni Health Study. JAMA. 1995;273:1179–84.
114. Volaklis KA, Tokmakidis SP. Resistance exercise training in patients with heart failure. Sports Med. 2005;35:1085–103.
115. Benton MJ. Safety and efficacy of resistance training in patients with chronic heart failure: research-based evidence. Prog Cardiovasc Nurs. 2005;20:17–23.
116. Bartlo P. Evidence-based application of aerobic and resistance training in patients with congestive heart failure. J Cardiopulm Rehabil Prev. 2007;27:368–75.
117. Piepoli MF, Conraads V, Corrà U, Dickstein K, Francis DP, Jaarsm T, McMurray J, Pieske B, Piotrowicz E, Schmid JP, Anker SD, Solal AC, Filippatos GS, Hoes AW, Gielen S, Giannuzzi P, Ponikowsk PP. Exercise training in heart failure: from theory to practice. A consensus document of the Heart Failure Association and the European Association for Cardiovascular Prevention and Rehabilitation. Eur J Heart Fail. 2011;13:347–57.
118. Braith RW, Stewart KJ. Resistance exercise training: its role in the prevention of cardiovascular disease. Circulation. 2006;113:2642–50.
119. Lind AR, McNicol GW. Muscular factors which determine the cardiovascular responses to sustained and rhythmic exercise. Can Med Assoc J. 1967;96:706–15.
120. Sale DG, Moroz DE, McKelvie RS, MacDougall JD, McCartney N. Comparison of blood pressure response to isokinetic and weight-lifting exercise. Eur J Appl Physiol Occup Physiol. 1993;67:115–20.

121. Mitchell JH, Payne FC, Saltin B, Schibye B. The role of muscle mass in the cardiovascular response to static contractions. J Physiol. 1980;309:45–54.
122. Lamotte M, Fleury F, Pirard M, Jamon A, de Borne P v. Acute cardiovascular response to resistance training during cardiac rehabilitation: effect of repetition speed and rest periods. Eur J Cardiovasc Prev Rehabil. 2010;17:329–36.
123. Fleck S, Falkel J, Harman E. Cardiovascular responses during resistance training. Med Sci Sports Excerc. 1989;21:114.
124. Williams MA, Haskell WL, Ades PA, Amsterdam EA, Bittner V, Franklin BA, Gulanick M, Laing ST, Stewart KJ. Resistance exercise in individuals with and without cardiovascular disease: 2007 update: a scientific statement from the American Heart Association Council on Clinical Cardiology and Council on Nutrition, Physical Activity, and Metabolism. Circulation. 2007;116:572–84.
125. Graf C, Rost R. Herz und Sport. Balingen: Spitta Verlag; 2001.
126. Schmid JP, Anderegg M, Romanens M, Morger C, Noveanu M, Hellige G, Saner H. Combined endurance/resistance training early on, after a first myocardial infarction, does not induce negative left ventricular remodeling. Eur J Cardiovasc Prev Rehabil. 2008;15:341–6.
127. Arthur HM, Gunn E, Thorpe KE, Ginis KM, Mataseje L, McCartney N, McKelvie RS, Ginis KM, Mataseje L, McCartney N, McKelvie RS. Effect of aerobic versus combined aerobic-strength training on 1-year, post-cardiac rehabilitation outcomes in woman after a cardiac event. J Rehabil Med. 2007;39:730–5.
128. Karlsdottir AE, Foster C, Porcari JP, Palmer-McLean K, White-Kube R, Backes RC. Hemodynamic responses during aerobic and resistance exercise. J Cardpulm Rehabil. 2002;22:170–7.
129. Bjarnason-Wehrens B, Mayer-Berger W, Meister ER, Baum K, Hambrecht R, Gielen S. Recommendations for resistance exercise in cardiac rehabilitation. Recommendations of the German Federation for Cardiovascular Prevention and Rehabilitation. Eur J Cardiovasc Prev Rehabil. 2004;11:352–61.
130. Braith RW, Graves JE, Pollock ML, Leggett SL, Carpenter DM, Colvin AB. Comparison of 2 vs 3 days/week of variable resistance training during 10- and 18- week programmes. Int J Sports Med. 1989;10:450–4.
131. Rhea MR, Alvar BA, Burkett LN, Ball SD. A meta-analysis to determine the dose response for strength development. Med Sci Sports Exerc. 2003;35:456–64.
132. Feiereisen P, Vaillant M, Eischen D, Delagardelle C. Isokinetic versus one-repetition maximum strength assessment in chronic heart failure. Med Sci Sports Exerc. 2010;42:2156–63.
133. Levinger I, Goodman C, Hare DL, Jerums G, Toia D, Selig S. The reliability of the 1RM strength test for untrained middle-aged individuals. J Sci Med Sport. 2009;12:310–6.
134. Barnard KL, Adams KJ, Swank AM, Mann E, Denny DM. Injuries and muscle soreness during the one repetition maximum assessment in a cardiac rehabilitation population. J Cardpulm Rehabil. 1999;19:52–8.
135. Schroeder ET, Wang Y, Castaneda-Sceppa C, Cloutier G, Vallejo AF, Kawakubo M, Jensky NE, Coomber S, Azen SP, Sattler FR. Reliability of maximal voluntary muscle strength and power testing in older men. J Gerontol A Biol Sci Med Sci. 2007;62:543–9.
136. Brzycki M. Strength testing-Prediction a one-rep max from reps-to-fatigue. JOPERD. 1993;68:88–90.

Angina Pectoris

5

Dumitru Zdrenghea and Dana Pop

Currently, the majority of patients diagnosed with stable angina receive drug therapy, provided that the European clinical practice guidelines only recommend percutaneous myocardial revascularization (after coronary angiography) in patients continuing to present symptoms caused by ischemic heart disease despite optimal medical therapy [1].

As an example, we report the case of a 62-year-old female that was referred to the cardiac rehabilitation unit in the cardiology department.

The patient is an already retired women and nonsmoker, with menopause at 54 years and, after this, with slightly increased blood pressure (150/95 mmHg), not treated by drugs.

She presented for 3 months retrosternal burning pain, which appeared during walking and climbing stairs, especially at the beginning of the effort and in case of cold weather.

The rest-ECG was normal, but during the cycle ergometer exercise stress test, it was registered a maximal ST segment depression of 1.25 mm in leads V4–V6, associated with chest pain (Fig. 5.1). The peak exercise level was 100 W (seven METs), the peak heart rate 130/min, and the double product (SBP × HR) 23,000, corresponding to the ischemic threshold of the patient (Fig. 5.2).

A 24-h ambulatory ECG monitoring was also performed, during which a painful ischemic episode (ST segment depression 1.5 mm) and five painless ischemic episodes (ST segment depression 1 mm) were registered, with a total ischemic burden of 70 min/24 h.

Coronary angiography showed a single-vessel coronary artery disease (75 % stenosis in the circumflex artery). The echo-Doppler examination revealed a normal systolic and diastolic ventricular function and a small, grade I, mitral regurgitation

D. Zdrenghea (✉) • D. Pop
University of Medicine and Pharmacy "Iuliu Haţieganu" Rehabilitation Hospital,
Cluj-Napoca, Romania
e-mail: dzdrenghea@yahoo.com

© Springer International Publishing AG 2017
J. Niebauer (ed.), *Cardiac Rehabilitation Manual*,
DOI 10.1007/978-3-319-47738-1_5

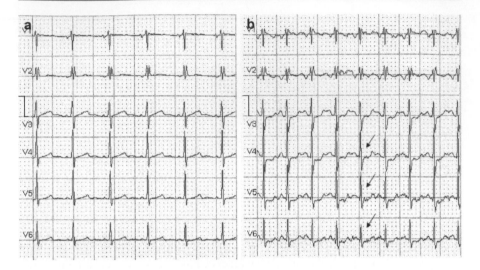

Fig. 5.1 (**a**) Rest ECG – normal; (**b**) Stress ECG (125 W) – RS, HR = 130/min, horizontal ST segment depression 1.25 mm V4–V6 associated with chest pain

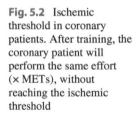

Fig. 5.2 Ischemic threshold in coronary patients. After training, the coronary patient will perform the same effort (× METs), without reaching the ischemic threshold

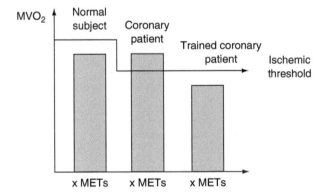

through calcification of the posterior mitral annulus. Intravascular ultrasound (IVUS), which was performed during coronarography, showed no unstable plaques; the stenotic lesion was fibrotic.

The laboratory data showed the following values: total cholesterol (TC) of 220 mg/dl, LDL cholesterol (LDL) of 135 mg/dl, HDL cholesterol (HDL) of 40 mg/dl, triglyceride (TG) of 260 mg/dl, and a fasting blood glucose level of 98 mg/dl. The body mass index (BMI) was 28 kg/m², and the waist circumference 86 cm.

Thus, the patient was diagnosed as suffering from chronic coronary artery disease and stable effort angina, CCS (Canadian Cardiovascular Society) class II, hypertension grade I with very high added risk and metabolic syndrome.

The patient was advised to follow a hypocaloric Mediterranean diet to lose weight; a drug treatment regimen consisting of aspirin 75 mg/day, bisoprolol 10 mg/day, rosuvastatin 10 mg/day, and perindopril 5 mg/day was initiated.

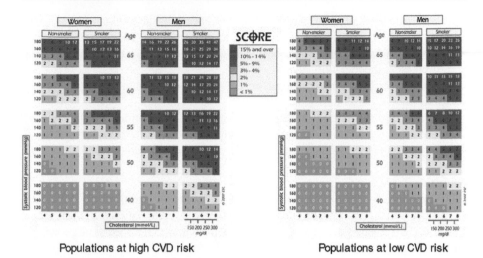

Populations at high CVD risk   Populations at low CVD risk

Fig. 5.3 SCORE chart: 10-year risk of fatal CVD in high and low risk regions of Europe (The European Society of Cardiology)

The blood pressure value returned to normal (130/80 mmHg), and angina pectoris attacks during daily activities disappeared.

The patient was then addressed to the ambulatory rehabilitation unit and submitted to an 8-week, five times per week, 1-h duration, physical rehabilitation program, consisting of dynamic but also resistance training. It was recommended, in the other 2 days, to perform physical exercises and walking for at least 30 min/day at home. After 8 weeks, a new maximal exercise stress test was performed, proving an increase of exercise capacity with 25 W, but with the same maximal ST depression.

After this, the patient was addressed to a community-based training program, with the recommendation to be followed for 6–12 months. After 12 months, the patient was recommended to perform a daily moderate or vigorous activity of 30–60-min duration, on an individual non-supervised basis, consisting of physical exercises, walking, games, and swimming.

Question 1

What is the cardiovascular risk of the patient according to the SCORE cardiovascular risk chart?

The SCORE chart (Fig. 5.3) is used only in primary prevention to evaluate the risk of cardiovascular death for the next 10 years, a value more than 5 % being considered high and imposing special prevention measures [2].

The present patient already presents an ischemic heart disease as stable angina pectoris. In this case, the risk is already considered very high, imposing secondary prevention measures, and the use of SCORE chart is no longer indicated [2].

Question 2

Does the patient present a metabolic syndrome?

The principal feature of the metabolic syndrome is abdominal obesity. Our patient presents overweight, but according to the American Diabetes Association (ADA) criteria for abdominal obesity (>88 cm in women, >102 cm in men), she doesn't present the metabolic syndrome [3].

In turn, according to the European criteria (abdominal circumference >80 cm in women and >94 cm in men), the patient presents the metabolic syndrome because other criteria are still present (hypertension, low HDL, and increased TG). This will increase the cardiovascular risk because of atherogenic dyslipidemia (increased TG, low HDL, small dense LDL particles) and because of increased risk of diabetes [2].

Question 3

What categories of treatment are recommended for angina pectoris?

Lifestyle changes are recommended in all cardiovascular patients or with cardiovascular risk factors. For patients with metabolic syndrome, a special target will be to lose weight [2].

Drug treatment is recommended according to current guidelines: antiplatelets, beta-blockers, and statins; in some cases, but not ours, calcium channel blockers (CCBs) may be added [1]. Also, for second-line treatment, it is recommended to add long-acting nitrates, ivabradine, nicorandil, or ranolazine, according to heart rate, blood pressure, and tolerance [1, 4].

Myocardial revascularization is a good opportunity to decrease myocardial ischemia and to treat angina, but it is not recommended in this patient: the angina is not only stable, but the ischemic threshold, evaluated through double product (DP), is high (23,000) [1]. The maximum ST segment depression is less than 2 mm, and it appears at a high level of effort (100 W) and of heart rate (87 % of maximum heart rate). The patient presents a moderate single-vessel disease (Fig. 5.4a, b); revascularization is recommended for severe one or for multivessel or left main disease. In addition, IVUS confirmed a stable atherosclerotic plaque (Fig. 5.5). The total ischemic burden is more than 60 min (limit to indicate angiography and revascularization), but other criteria for revascularization are not fulfilled [1].

Question 4

Which components of the cardiac rehabilitation are indicated for the patient?

The treatment of risk factors (dyslipidemia, overweight, and hypertension) is indicated, but it is not specific for angina. The targets are those recommended by current guidelines [1].

Physical activity as the main component of cardiac rehabilitation is strongly recommended because it was demonstrated that physical activity and training can increase the quality of life and chances of survival for cardiovascular patients [1, 5].

There are two components of physical activity: physical training represents the organized and supervised form of physical activity [6–8]. For itself, physical training is not strongly recommended in this patient, whose exercise capacity is normal (seven METs). Still, there are at least two reasons to apply it. The first is represented by the direct and especially indirect effects on cardiovascular risk factors [9, 10]. The patient presents hypercholesterolemia, hypertriglyceridemia, and high blood pressure, which can be favorably influenced by physical training [7, 9]. Even more important, patients

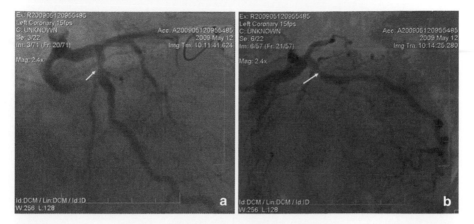

Fig. 5.4 Coronary angiography in RAO (**a**) and LAO (**b**) projection, respectively with caudal angulation. 75% stenosis of the circumflex artery (*arrow*) (Courtesy of Associate Professor A. Iancu)

Fig. 5.5 IVUS. Atherosclerotic plaque (*arrow*). Calcification suggests a fibrotic, stable plaque (Courtesy of Associate Professor A. Iancu)

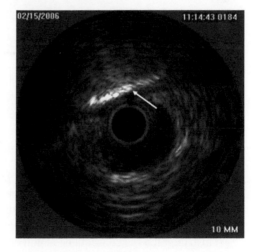

included in cardiac rehabilitation programs are more adherent to the secondary prevention measures, particularly in this case, when the patient presents, according to European criteria, a metabolic syndrome [2, 11–13]. The second reason is represented by the effect of physical training, beyond the increasing of exercise capacity. It was demonstrated that physical training, especially the high-intensity one, has antiatherogenic, anti-inflammatory, and antithrombotic properties, decreasing the progression of atherosclerotic plaque and its complications [12–15] (Fig. 5.6). Last but not least, to increase the patient's quality of life, it is recommended to obtain the maximal exercise capacity permitted by the underlying disease [16, 17].

Physical counseling, to perform a daily physical activity of 30–60 min every day, 5 days, or minimum 3 days/week, is also recommended for our patient because of the abovementioned benefices [1, 9]. On the days when physical training is performed, individual physical activity is still recommended, but not compulsory [7].

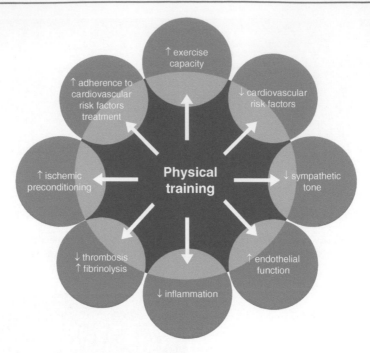

Fig. 5.6 The most important benefits of physical training in cardiovascular patients, including angina patients

Question 5

Which are the objectives of physical training for a patient with stable effort angina?

As for all cardiovascular patients, the increase of exercise capacity is a very important target for cardiac rehabilitation programs [11]. It was demonstrated that after phase II rehabilitation programs, the exercise capacity VO_2 increases with 20–25 % without a significant increase of the ischemic threshold but with much less increase of MVO_2 for the same level of exercise (Fig. 5.2).

It also targeted the consequence upon cardiovascular risk factors through a direct effect, but also by increasing the adherence to the specific measures applied to control them (e.g.,, quit smoking) [12, 16–18].

The pleiotropic effects upon atherogenic mechanisms are also very important, being demonstrated during clinical studies [15, 16].

Question 6

Which are the recommended cardiac rehabilitation modalities?

Inpatient cardiac rehabilitation is indicated only during the acute phase of the disease (phase I rehabilitation) or in complicated patients during phase II [7, 16, 19, 20].

Outpatient cardiac rehabilitation. For our patient, already asymptomatic under drug treatment, outpatient rehabilitation is the only indicated method. It is possible to be performed in a cardiac rehabilitation unit or even in a community center because the cardiovascular risk of the patient is moderate (class B), and tight medical supervision of physical training is not compulsory [7, 21–24].

Table 5.1 The comparative effects of aerobic and resistance training

Variable	Aerobic exercise	Resistance exercise	
VO2max	↑↑	↑0	
Muscle strength	0	↑↑	
Hemodynamic effect			
Systolic blood pressure (rest)		0	0
Diastolic blood pressure (rest)		0	0
Double product during submaximal exercise (MVO₂)		↓↓	↓
Stroke volume, *resting and maximal*		↑↑	0
Mx CO		↑↑	0
Heart rate (rest)		↓↓	0
Metabolic effect			
HDL		↑0	↑0
LDL		↓0	↓0
Insulin sensitivity		↑↑	↑↑
% fat		↓↓	↓

↑ increase, ↓ decrease, 0 unchanged, *HDL* high-density lipoprotein cholesterol, *LDL* low-density lipoprotein cholesterol

Home cardiac rehabilitation can be recommended if supervised physical training is not possible [15, 25]. Because the exercise capacity of our patient is high, in this case, the physical training will consist of physical exercises, rapid walking, or domestic activities (30–60 min/day), with the recommendation to avoid the appearance of pain (effort under the ischemic threshold) [26–29].

Question 7

Which training modalities and what frequency of training sessions are recommended for our patient?

Physical training can use three types of exercise:

Stretching exercises are used to maintain the joint mobility and flexibility. It has no effect on exercise capacity [16]. It can be used as a part of physical training program, but not to assure the training effect [30].

Aerobic training. It represents the main type of exercise, recommended in all cardiovascular patients, including stable angina patients [31–33]. It associates the abovementioned effect upon exercise capacity, mainly through peripheral but also through central mechanisms [34, 35]. In patients with stable effort angina, not only an increase of ischemic threshold (angina threshold) and a decrease in number and intensity of anginal attacks but also an increase in survival were registered [35–37]. It has the best hemodynamic cardiovascular effects (Table 5.1), and because it does not increase, but in fact decreases peripheral resistance during exercise, it increases systolic output, maximal cardiac output, and VO₂ max; at the same time, it is well tolerated even by patients with depressed LV systolic performance [38].

Resistance training. The isometric component of exercise cannot be avoided during daily life, and, consequently, resistance exercises have to be used during training sessions, especially in patients with normal LV performance, as is our patient. It was demonstrated (Table 5.1) that under survey and at an intensity of 20–30 % of MCV (maximal voluntary contraction), its hemodynamic effect is not detrimental (but at the same time not beneficial) upon LV performance, because of increasing afterload

[17, 32]. In time, they can increase moderately the exercise capacity of the patients and decrease the double product, improving the quality of life and having neutral or favorable metabolic effects. The muscular strength is even more increased as during aerobic training (Table 5.1). They will be used in association with aerobic training in some of the training sessions (2–3 times per week).

The recommended training frequency in cardiovascular patients, including stable angina pectoris, was initially two to three times per week, but it was demonstrated that the best results are obtained by using five training sessions per week [16, 39]. The minimum training session to obtain a significant training effect is three times per week. It is ideal to perform seven sessions per week, however is not possible for practical reasons [2, 8]. That's why the patients are encouraged to exercise by themselves, 30 min/day, using physical exercises and walking, in other days than those with supervised physical training [2, 8].

It is to mention that in physical training recommendations, we must consider the particularities of women. Thus, long-term exercise training sessions must be diversified; exercise must be conducted in intervals rather than continuously or in small groups.

They should also provide support for women emotionally, socially, and psychologically. There are recommended "open discussions" on secondary prevention measures (particularly weight loss, quitting smoking, and prescription of medication with cardioprotective effects) and on the role of physical training [6].

Question 8

Which is the recommended intensity and duration of training sessions and what types of exercise are recommended?

The duration of training sessions is generally recommended to be 50–60 min; lesser duration is recommended only in heart failure patients [16, 18]. For our patient, with stable coronary artery disease, the duration is maximal – 60 min [30, 31, 40].

The intensity of the performed exercise can be assessed using the Borg scale of perceived exertion. This scale can be used by the patient himself to determine optimal training intensity. From 3 to 4, it represents a moderate activity, accounting for 40–60 % of the maximum capacity (VO2 max). From 5 to 6, the activity is considered difficult, accounting for 60–85 % of the maximum exercise capacity, this level being recommended in stable ischemic heart disease, as in our case.

The intensity can be low, moderate, and high (Table 5.2).

Low-intensity physical training: 20–40 % of peak tVO2 (maximal VO2 realized during maximal exercise stress testing, before including the patients in training programs) and 40–50 % of peak heart rate. The intensity is too low to increase the exercise capacity and to result in pleiotropic effects. This low intensity is sometimes recommended in heart failure patients to avoid further physical deconditioning [13, 37, 41, 42].

Moderate-intensity training (50–60 % MxVO2, 60–70 % MxHR) increases the exercise capacity, but only by 15–20 %, and the pleiotropic cardiovascular effects are modest or even absent. That's why moderate training is recommended only to physically deconditioned patients or patients with LV dysfunction, arrhythmias, etc. It can also be realized during home rehabilitation, when the training cannot be

Table 5.2 The effects of physical training in relationship with effort intensity

	VO2	Cardiovascular risk factors control	Pleiotropic effects
Low	0	0	0
Moderate	↑	↓	↑
High	↑↑	↓↓	↑↑
Very high	Contraindicated		

supervised. It is not recommended in our patient, with high exercise capacity and without LV dysfunction [13, 37, 41, 42].

High-intensity physical training (60–75 % of peak VO2, 70–85 % of max HR at peak effort) assures the maximal (25–35 %) increase of VO_2 and, in angina, of ischemic threshold. It has maximal effect upon the quality of life and survival. It assures also the maximal pleiotropic effects of exercise, some of them registered [37, 41] only after intense physical training. It was demonstrated that in stable angina patients, high-intensity physical training results in outcomes as good as or even better than those obtained through interventional myocardial revascularization [15]. Our patient belongs to a moderate-risk class, has already a near-normal exercise capacity, and was recommended to perform physical training on an outpatient basis. Therefore, high-intensity training can be applied to obtain a maximum and optimal result. However, in patients with stable angina pectoris, it is recommended that training heart rate remains below the ischemic threshold, determined during maximal exercise stress test. In our patient, it occurred at 130/min, which means that a training heart rate about 115–120/min (10 beats/min under the angina threshold) for 30–40 min/training session would be suitable, of course preceded and followed by 10-min warm-up and 10-min cooldown exercises [13, 42].

Very high-intensity training (80–90 % of peak VO_2, 90–100 % of max HR at peak effort) will result in ischemia and probably angina, which have to be avoided during training sessions; hence, this is not recommended even in our stable effort angina patient. Moreover, this high-intensity training is not at all recommended in cardiovascular patients [13, 16, 37, 41, 42].

Question 9
How long is practicing physical training and physical activity recommended for our patient?

As for other cardiovascular patients, physical training is recommended for a limited period of time, but physical activity for a lifetime, this representing the last, phase III, of cardiovascular rehabilitation [16]. Physical training itself, representing the phase II rehabilitation, is recommended to be of 6–8 weeks duration and about 36 training sessions. A shorter period of training (2–4 weeks) is not enough to obtain the training effect, respectively, the increase in the exercise capacity and the appearance of the pleiotropic effects [43–46]. Classically, the objective of phase II cardiac rehabilitation is to increase exercise capacity at seven METs. The patient about whom we already discussed has this exercise capacity. Consequently, the objective of physical training will be to more increase the exercise capacity, but mainly the appearance of pleiotropic effects, and a good adherence to lifestyle changes and later physical activity. Unfortunately, after such a short period, long-term compliance to lifestyle changes is poor. That is why, whenever possible, it is recommended to continue institutional (supervised) physical training another 8–12 months. Some authors consider this period as phase III rehabilitation, but we prefer to call it "extended phase II rehabilitation" to avoid confusion in understanding the sequential phases of cardiac rehabilitation [43–46]. After the period of 6–8 weeks or 8–12 months, the patient will continue physical exercise on an individual basis, as a lifestyle, for the whole life. This is necessary, because the training effects (the benefits of physical activity) will disappear after 3–6 weeks of sedentary life [43–47].

Question 10

Does late ischemic preconditioning intervene to assure the increase of exercise capacity during physical training?

Ischemic preconditioning refers to the finding, experimental at first and then clinical, that short episodes of myocardial ischemia protect the myocardium from unwanted effects of subsequent ischemic events. The protective effect occurs a few minutes after the initial preconditioning episode and lasts 1–2 h, representing the so-called early window of ischemic preconditioning or early ischemic preconditioning. After 24 h, the protective effect reappears even in the absence of other ischemic episodes, the protective effect being weaker but longer, up to 72 h, achieving the second window of preconditioning or late preconditioning [48].

Both types of ischemic preconditioning (early and late) have clinical, electric, arrhythmic, hemodynamic, and metabolic consequences. Ischemic preconditioning correlates with mitochondrial protection, thus preserving mitochondrial activity and energy production, which increases cell survival [48].

The mechanisms of both early and late preconditioning are complex (Fig. 5.7), early preconditioning being assured , mainly through adenosine and $K+$ ATP channels and late preconditioning mainly through iNOS and nitric oxide (Fig. 5.8) [49]. It was demonstrated that after moderate-to-intense physical training for a few weeks, ST depression was delayed, maximal depression was lower, and the ischemic threshold was raised during exercise test performed at the end of the rehabilitation program (ET2), compared with the one (ET1) from the beginning of the program (Table 5.3) [50]. Because late preconditioning disappears after 72 h, it is not permitted to stop the physical activity more than 2 days to preserve the training effect, also through this mechanism [48].

Question 11

For long-term secondary prevention, are some categories of drugs useful or lifestyle changes and physical activity enough?

To obtain the very high targets for dyslipidemia and hypertension, in many cases, lifestyle changes are not enough and drugs are also necessary to control these risk factors. Even more, some drugs are useful not only to control the cardiovascular risk factors but they also have direct antiatherogenic effects or preventive effects upon

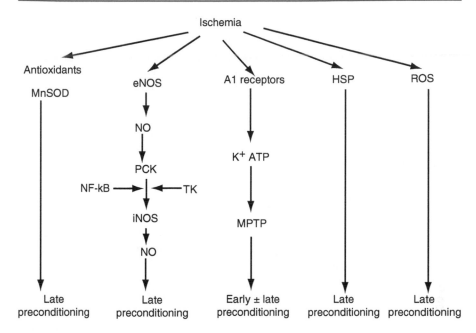

Fig. 5.7 Main mechanisms of ischemic preconditioning (*HSP* heat shock proteins, *eNOS* endothelial nitric oxide synthase, *iNOS* inducible nitric oxide synthase, *Mn-SOD* Manganese Superoxide Dismutase, *ROS* Reactive oxygen species, *NO* nitric oxide, *MPTP* mitochondrial permeability transition pore, *PKC* protein kinase C, *NF-kB* necrosis factor kB, *TK* tyrosine kinase)

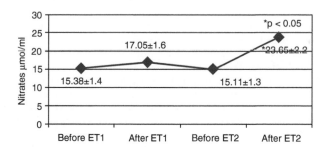

Fig. 5.8 The role of NO in late ischemic preconditioning. Nitrates blood level before and after ET_1 and ET_2 performed at 24-h interval in 22 coronary patients with positive exercise stress testing. Nitrates level rises insignificantly after ET_1 but rises significantly after ET_2, suggesting that NO is involved in late ischemic preconditioning

Table 5.3 Exercise testing data during ET_1 and ET_2 performed at 4 weeks interval in trained group A and untrained group B stable effort angina patients

	Group A		Group B	
	ET_1	ET_2	ET_1	ET_2
Peak effort (W·s)	80.3 ± 7.2	$93.4 \pm 8.3^*$	65.2 ± 5.8	72.9 ± 6.5
Double product (mmHg · b/min)	$21,573 \pm 3122$	$24,168 \pm 3423$	$23,551 \pm 3100$	$21,000 \pm 2752$
Maximal ST depression (mm)	1.52 ± 0.23	$0.74 \pm 0.12^*$	1.46 ± 0.32	1.17 ± 0.21

$^*p < 0.05$

atherosclerotic complications (thrombosis, arrhythmias, etc.). They are considered as secondary preventive drugs. Statins, antiplatelet drugs, and ACE inhibitors or ARBs are included in this category [1, 2]. They are recommended in any patient with ischemic heart disease, including stable effort angina, even if the patient is asymptomatic [1]. For the statins, the indication is reinforced and becomes compulsory in the presence of dyslipidemia – high total and LDL cholesterol. On the other hand, not all drugs used in ischemic patients, for angina or for other reasons, offer protection against atherosclerosis and its complications [1, 2, 8, 51]. As an example, nitrates are excellent for the prevention and control of anginal pain, but do not improve the prognosis of ischemic patients [1]. Calcium channel blockers are excellent antianginal drugs, and in some experimental research, they proved to have anti-atherosclerotic effects [1]. In turn, there are not enough clinical data to support their usefulness for secondary prevention. For fibrates, recommended to treat hypertriglyceridemia, there is also some experimental support of antiatherogenic effect, but clinical data are lacking, and until now, they are not recommended as preventive therapy in ischemic patients [52–54].

References

1. Task Force Members, Montalescot G, Sechtem U, Achenbach S, Andreotti F, Arden C, Budaj A, Bugiardini R, Crea F, Cuisset T, Di Mario C, Ferreira JR, Gersh BJ, Gitt AK, Hulot JS, Marx N, Opie LH, Pfisterer M, Prescott E, Ruschitzka F, Sabaté M, Senior R, Taggart DP, van der Wall EE, Vrints CJ, ESC Committee for Practice Guidelines, Zamorano JL, Achenbach S, Baumgartner H, Bax JJ, Bueno H, Dean V, Deaton C, Erol C, Fagard R, Ferrari R, Hasdai D, Hoes AW, Kirchhof P, Knuuti J, Kolh P, Lancellotti P, Linhart A, Nihoyannopoulos P, Piepoli MF, Ponikowski P, Sirnes PA, Tamargo JL, Tendera M, Torbicki A, Wijns W, Windecker S, Reviewers D, Knuuti J, Valgimigli M, Bueno H, Claeys MJ, Donner-Banzhoff N, Erol C, Frank H, Funck-Brentano C, Gaemperli O, Gonzalez-Juanatey JR, Hamilos M, Hasdai D, Husted S, James SK, Kervinen K, Kolh P, Kristensen SD, Lancellotti P, Maggioni AP, Piepoli MF, Pries AR, Romeo F, Rydén L, Simoons ML, Sirnes PA, Steg PG, Timmis A, Wijns W, Windecker S, Yildirir A, Zamorano JL. 2013 ESC guidelines on the management of stable coronary artery disease: the Task Force on the management of stable coronary artery disease of the European Society of Cardiology. Eur Heart J. 2013;34(38):2949–3003.
2. Perk J, De Backer G, Gohlke H, Graham I, Reiner Z, WM V, Albus C, Benlian P, Boysen G, Cifkova R, Deaton C, Ebrahim S, Fisher M, Germano G, Hobbs R, Hoes A, Karadeniz S, Mezzani A, Prescott E, Ryden L, Scherer M, Syvänne M, Op Reimer WJ S, Vrints C, Wood D, JL Z, Zannad F, Fifth Joint Task Force of the European Society of Cardiology and Other Societies on Cardiovascular Disease Prevention in Clinical Practice; European Association for Cardiovascular Prevention and Rehabilitation. European Guidelines on cardiovascular disease prevention in clinical practice (version 2012): the Fifth Joint Task Force of the European Society of Cardiology and Other Societies on Cardiovascular Disease Prevention in Clinical Practice (constituted by representatives of nine societies and by invited experts). Eur J Prev Cardiol. 2012;19(4):585–667.
3. Grundy SM, Hansen B, Smith Jr SC, Cleeman JI, Kahn RA, American Heart Association; National Heart, Lung, and Blood Institute; American Diabetes Association. Clinical management of metabolic syndrome: report of the American Heart Association/National Heart, Lung, and Blood Institute/American Diabetes Association conference on scientific issues related to management. Circulation. 2004;109:551–6.

4. Henri C, O'Meara E, De Denus S, Elzir L, Tardif JC. Ivabradine for the treatment of chronic heart failure. Expert Rev Cardiovasc Ther. 2016;14(5):553–61.
5. Anderson L, Oldridge N, Thompson DR, Zwisler AD, Rees K, Martin N, Taylor RS. Exercise-based cardiac rehabilitation for coronary heart disease: cochrane systematic review and meta-analysis. J Am Coll Cardiol. 2016;67(1):1–12.
6. Reed JL, Prince SA, Cole CA, Nerenberg KA, Hiremath S, Tulloch HE, Fodor JG, Szczotka A, McDonnell LA, Mullen KA, Pipe AL, Reid RD. E-Health physical activity interventions and moderate-to-vigorous intensity physical activity levels among working-age women: a systematic review protocol. Syst Rev. 2015;4:3. doi:10.1186/2046-4053-4-3.
7. Wenger NK. Current status of cardiac rehabilitation. J Am Coll Cardiol. 2008;51(17): 1619–31.
8. Balady GJ, Williams MA, Ades PA, Bittner V, Comoss P, Foody JAM, Franklin B, Sanderson B, Southard D. Core components of cardiac rehabilitation/secondary prevention programs: 2007 update: a scientific statement from the American Heart Association Exercise, Cardiac Rehabilitation, and Prevention Committee, the Council on Clinical Cardiology; the Councils on Cardiovascular Nursing, Epidemiology and Prevention, and Nutrition, Physical Activity, and Metabolism; and the American Association of Cardiovascular and Pulmonary Rehabilitation. Circulation. 2007;115:2675–82.
9. Lavie CJ, Morshedi-Meibodi A, Milani RV. Impact of cardiac rehabilitation on coronary risk factors, inflammation, and the metabolic syndrome in obese coronary patients. J Cardiometab Syndr. 2008;3(3):136–40.
10. Warner Jr JG, Brubaker PH, Zhu Y, et al. Long-term (5-year) changes in HDL cholesterol in cardiac rehabilitation patients. Do sex differences exist? Circulation. 1995;92:773–7.
11. Woodgate J, Brawley LR. Self-efficacy for exercise in cardiac rehabilitation: review and recommendations. J Health Psychol. 2008;13(3):366–87. Review
12. Hambrecht R. The molecular base of exercise. In: Perk J et al., editors. Cardiovascular prevention and rehabilitation. London: Springer; 2007. p. 67–76.
13. Gohlke H. Exercise training in coronary heart disease. In: Perk J et al., editors. Cardiovascular prevention and rehabilitation. London: Springer; 2007. p. 125–37.
14. Wang JS. Exercise prescription and thrombogenesis. J Biomed Sci. 2006;13(6):753–61.
15. Hambrecht R, Wolf A, Gielen S, et al. Effect of exercise on coronary endothelial function in patients with coronary artery disease. N Engl J Med. 2000;342:454–60.
16. Zdrenghea D. Recuperare și prevenție cardiovasculară. Cluj-Napoca: Ed. Clusium; 2008.
17. Williams MA, Haskell WL, Ades PA, Amsterdam EA, Bittner V, Franklin BA, Gulanick M, Laing ST, Stewart KJ. Comparison of effects of aerobic endurance training with strength training. Resistance exercise in individuals with and without cardiovascular disease:2007 update; a scientific statement from the American Heart Association Council on Clinical Cardiology and Council on Nutrition, Physical Activity, and Metabolism. Circulation. 2007;116: 572–84.
18. Gianuzzi P. Rehabilitation modalities. In: Perk J et al., editors. Cardiovascular prevention and rehabilitation. London: Springer; 2007. p. 454–9.
19. AACVPR. Guidelines for Cardiac Rehabilitation and Secondary Prevention Programs. 4th ed. Champaign: Human Kinetics; 2004.
20. Lloyd GW. Preventive cardiology and cardiac rehabilitation programmes in women. Maturitas. 2009;63(1):28–33.
21. Lavie CJ, Thomas RJ, Squires RW, Allison TG, Milani RV. Exercise training and cardiac rehabilitation in primary and secondary prevention of coronary heart disease. Mayo Clin Proc. 2009;84(4):373–83.
22. Fuchs AR, Meneghelo RS, Stefanini E, De Paola AV, Smanio PE, Mastrocolla LE, Ferraz AS, Buglia S, Piegas LS, Carvalho AA. Exercise may cause myocardial ischemia at the anaerobic threshold in cardiac rehabilitation programs. Braz J Med Biol Res. 2009;42(3):272–8.
23. Beckie TM, Mendonca MA, Fletcher GF, Schocken DD, Evans ME, Banks SM. Examining the challenges of recruiting women into a cardiac rehabilitation clinical trial. J Cardiopulm Rehabil Prev. 2009;29(1):13–21.

24. Jeger RV, Rickenbacher P, Pfisterer ME, Hoffmann A. Outpatient rehabilitation in patients with coronary artery and peripheral arterial occlusive disease. Arch Phys Med Rehabil. 2008;89(4):618–21.
25. Oliveira J, Ribeiro F, Gomes H. Effects of a home-based cardiac rehabilitation program on the physical activity levels of patients with coronary artery disease. J Cardiopulm Rehabil Prev. 2008;28(6):392–6.
26. Higginson R. Women and cardiac rehab: overcoming the barriers. Br J Nurs. 2008;17(22): 1380–1.
27. O'Keefe-McCarthy S. Women's experiences of cardiac pain: a review of the literature. Can J Cardiovasc Nurs. 2008;18(3):18–25. Review
28. Grace SL, Gravely-Witte S, Brual J, Suskin N, Higginson L, Alter D, Stewart DE. Contribution of patient and physician factors to cardiac rehabilitation referral: a prospective multilevel study. Nat Clin Pract Cardiovasc Med. 2008;5(10):653–62.
29. Blanchard C. Understanding exercise behaviour during home-based cardiac rehabilitation: a theory of planned behaviour perspective. Can J Physiol Pharmacol. 2008;86(1–2):8–15.
30. Squires RW, Montero-Gomez A, Allison TG, Thomas RJ. Long-term disease management of patients with coronary disease by cardiac rehabilitation program staff. J Cardiopulm Rehabil Prev. 2008;28(3):180–6.
31. Koutroumpi M, Pitsavos C, Stefanadis C. The role of exercise in cardiovascular rehabilitation: a review. Acta Cardiol. 2008;63(1):73–9. Review
32. Amundsen BH, Rognmo Ø, Hatlen-Rebhan G, Slørdahl SA. High-intensity aerobic exercise improves diastolic function in coronary artery disease. Scand Cardiovasc J. 2008;42(2): 110–7.
33. Brochu M, Poehlman ET, Savage P, Fragnoli-Munn K, Ross S, Ades PA. Modest effects of exercise training alone on coronary risk factors and body composition in coronary patients. J Cardpulm Rehabil. 2000;20:180–8.
34. Iellamo F, Pagani M, Volterrani M. Cardiac rehabilitation and prevention of cardiovascular disease a role for autonomic cardiovascular regulation. J Am Coll Cardiol. 2008;52(13):1105.
35. Schachinger V, Britten MB, Zeiher AM. Prognostic impact of coronary vasodilator dysfunction on adverse long-term outcome of coronary heart disease. Circulation. 2000;101: 1899–906.
36. Fox KF, Nuttall M, Wood DA, Wright M, Arora B, Dawson E, Devane P, Stock K, Sutcliffe SJ, Brown K. A cardiac prevention and rehabilitation programme for all patients at first presentation with coronary artery disease. Heart. 2001;85:533–8.
37. Thompson PD. Exercise prescription and proscription for patients with coronary artery disease. Circulation. 2005;112:2354–63.
38. Chursina TV, Shcherbatykh SI, Tarasov KM, Molchanov AV. Physical rehabilitation of in patients with ischemic heart disease. Klin Med (Mosk). 2008;86(7):31–5.
39. Tanasescu M, Leitzmann MF, Rimm EB, Willett WC, Stampfer MJ, Hu FB. Exercise type and intensity in relation to coronary heart disease in men. JAMA. 2002;288:1994–2000.
40. Balady GJ, Fletcher BJ, Froelicher EF, et al. Cardiac rehabilitation programs: a statement for healthcare professionals from the American Heart Association. Circulation. 1994;90: 1602–10.
41. AHA Scientific Statement. Exercise standards for testing and training. Circulation. 2001;104:1694.
42. Gielen S, Brutsaert D, Saner H, Hambrecht R. Cardiac rehabilitation. In: Camm AJ, Lüscher TF, Serruys PW, et al., editors. ESC textbook of cardiovascular medicine. Malden: Blackwell Publishing; 2006. p. 783–806.
43. DA M, Gersch BJ. Chronic coronary artery disease. In: Libby P, Bonow RO, Mann DL, Zipes DP, editors. Braunwald's heart disease. Philadelphia: W.B. Saunders Company; 2007. p. 1353–418.
44. Papadakis S, Reid RD, Coyle D, Beaton L, Angus D, Oldridge N. Cost-effectiveness of cardiac rehabilitation program delivery models in patients at varying cardiac risk, reason for referral, and sex. Eur J Cardiovasc Prev Rehabil. 2008;15(3):347–53.

45. Womack L. Cardiac rehabilitation secondary prevention programs. Clin Sports Med. 2003;22(1):135–60.
46. Mendes MF. Long term maintenance programs. In: Perk J et al., editors. Cardiovascular prevention and rehabilitation. London: Springer; 2007. p. 347–51.
47. Migam A, JC T. The place of exercise in the patient with chronic stable angina. Heart Metab. 2008;38:37.
48. Zdrenghea D, Poantă L, Pop D, Zdrenghea V, Zdrenghea M. Physical training – beyond increasing exercise capacity. Rom J Intern Med. 2008;46(1):17–27.
49. Zdrenghea D, Bódizs G, Ober MC, Ilea M. Ischemic preconditioning by repeated exercise tests involves nitric oxide up-regulation. Rom J Intern Med. 2003;41(2):137–44.
50. Zdrenghea D, Potâng E, Timiş D, Bogdan E. Does ischemic preconditioning occur during rehabilitation of ischemic patients? Rom J Intern Med. 1999;37(3):201–6.
51. McSweeney JC, Rosenfeld AG, Abel WM, Braun LT, Burke LE, Daugherty SL, Fletcher GF, Gulati M, Mehta LS, Pettey C, Reckelhoff JF, American Heart Association Council on Cardiovascular and Stroke Nursing, Council on Clinical Cardiology, Council on Epidemiology and Prevention, Council on Hypertension, Council on Lifestyle and Cardiometabolic Health, and Council on Quality of Care and Outcomes Research. Preventing and experiencing ischemic heart disease as a woman: state of the science: a scientific statement from the American Heart Association. Circulation. 2016;133(13):1302–31.
52. Stone NJ, Robinson JG, Lichtenstein AH, Bairey Merz CN, Blum CB, Eckel RH, Goldberg AC, Gordon D, Levy D, Lloyd-Jones DM, McBride P, Schwartz JS, Shero ST, Smith Jr SC, Watson K, Wilson PW, American College of Cardiology/American Heart Association Task Force on Practice Guidelines. 2013 ACC/AHA guideline on the treatment of blood cholesterol to reduce atherosclerotic cardiovascular risk in adults: a report of the American College of Cardiology/American Heart Association Task Force on practice guidelines. J Am Coll Cardiol. 2014;63(25 Pt B):2889–934.
53. Miller M, Stone NJ, Ballantyne C, Bittner V, Criqui MH, Ginsberg HN, Goldberg AC, Howard WJ, Jacobson MS, Kris-Etherton PM, Lennie TA, Levi M, Mazzone T, Pennathur S, American Heart Association Clinical Lipidology, Thrombosis, and Prevention Committee of the Council on Nutrition, Physical Activity, and Metabolism; Council on Arteriosclerosis, Thrombosis and Vascular Biology; Council on Cardiovascular Nursing; Council on the Kidney in Cardiovascular Disease. Triglycerides and cardiovascular disease: a scientific statement from the American Heart Association. Circulation. 2011;123(20):2292–333.
54. Lloyd-Jones DM, Morris PB, Ballantyne CM, Birtcher KK, Daly DD Jr, DePalma SM, Minissian MB, Orringer CE, Smith SC Jr. 2016 ACC Expert consensus decision pathway on the role of non-statin therapies for LDL-cholesterol lowering in the management of atherosclerotic cardiovascular disease risk: a report of the American College of Cardiology Task Force on clinical expert consensus documents. J Am Coll Cardiol 2016. pii: S0735-1097(16)32398-1. 10.1016/j.jacc.2016.03.519. [Epub ahead of print].

Diabetes Mellitus Type 2 and Cardiovascular Disease

6

David Niederseer, Gernot Diem, and Josef Niebauer

6.1 Clinical Information

A 54-year-old man presents at the Institute of Sports Medicine, Prevention and Rehabilitation for an assessment of his physical fitness. His wife gave him a voucher for a physical fitness check as a birthday present since he has never had an assessment of his physical fitness before. He is a carpenter and reports to be healthy and free of symptoms. Two years ago, he had a non-ST-elevation myocardial infarction of the anterior wall. The left descending artery had been treated with a drug-eluting stent in the local cardiology department. On presentation, he reports no angina or other cardiac disorders. The patient smokes one pack of cigarettes per day (30 pack years). Both of his parents are still alive, his father is 76 years old and suffers from type 2 diabetes and chronic obstructive pulmonary disease, whereas his 75-year-old mother has no known disorders. Neither his two brothers nor his sister has any cardiovascular diseases, and his two sons who are 27 and 30 years old are also healthy. He reports 30–45 min of jogging once a week, and his present medication includes 100 mg of acetylsalicylic acid, a beta-blocker (metoprolol 50 mg 1/2-0-0), an

D. Niederseer, MD, PhD, BSc
Department of Cardiology, University Heart Center, University Hospital Zurich, Zurich, Switzerland

Institute of Sports Medicine, Prevention and Rehabilitation, Paracelsus Medical University, Institute of Sports Medicine of the State of Salzburg, Sports Medicine of the Olympic Center Salzburg-Rif, Lindhofstraße 20, 5020 Salzburg, Austria

G. Diem, MD
Clinical Center Bad Hall for Cardiac and Neurological Rehabilitation, Bad Hall, Austria

J. Niebauer, MD, PhD, MBA (✉)
Institute of Sports Medicine, Prevention and Rehabilitation, Paracelsus Medical University, Institute of Sports Medicine of the State of Salzburg, Sports Medicine of the Olympic Center Salzburg-Rif, Lindhofstraße 20, 5020 Salzburg, Austria
e-mail: j.niebauer@salk.at

© Springer International Publishing AG 2017
J. Niebauer (ed.), *Cardiac Rehabilitation Manual*,
DOI 10.1007/978-3-319-47738-1_6

Fig. 6.1 Lung function test. *FVC* functional vital capacity, *FEV1* forced expiratory volume in first second, *PEF* peak expiratory flow, *NHANES III* third national health and nutrition examination survey, *l* liters, *s* seconds

Parameter	Unit	Value measured	Value in % of predicted value (NHANES III)
FVC	l	5.44	93%
FEV1	l	4.3	94%
FEV1/FVC		0.79	101%
PEF	l/s	10.61	97%

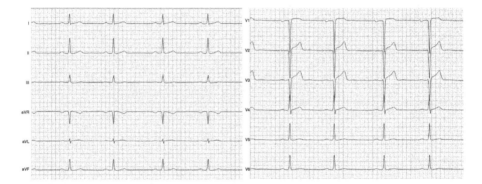

Fig. 6.2 ECG with left ventricular hypertrophy

angiotensin-converting enzyme (ACE) inhibitor (ramipril 2.5 mg 1-0-0), and a statin (simvastatin 40 mg 0-0-1).

On physical examination, body mass index (BMI; 31.1 kg/m², i.e., 94.3 kg; 1.74 m), waist circumference (105 cm), and blood pressure (145/95 mmHg) were elevated. Auscultation of the heart and lungs revealed no pathologic findings and no signs of heart failure were noted. Lung function parameters (Fig. 6.1) were within normal limits. The ECG (Fig. 6.2) revealed signs of left ventricular hypertrophy (Sokolow-Lyon Index, 4.8 mV).

A maximal exercise stress test was performed on a cycle ergometer (Fig. 6.3) starting with a workload of 50 watts (W) which was increased by 25 W every 2 minutes (min). The patient had to terminate the test due to exhaustion at 150 W. His heart rate at rest was 56/min and 152/min on exhaustion. Throughout the stress test and the recovery period, the patient was free of symptoms, and there were no signs of ischemia or arrhythmia on the ECG. The only pathologic finding was an increased blood pressure at peak exercise of 230/120 mmHg. Due to the elevated blood pressure and the positive Sokolow-Lyon Index, echocardiography (Fig. 6.4) was performed. A concentric left ventricular hypertrophy (end-diastolic diameter of the intraventricular septum [IVSd] in M-mode in the parasternal long axis view of 13 mm) and a mildly reduced left ventricular function with an ejection fraction of 49 % and hypokinesia of the anterior and anterolateral midventricular to apical segments were noted.

Stage	Workload	Time min:sec	Heart rate [1/min]	Blood pressure [mmHg]	Rate pressure product	RPE
0	rest	0	56	145/95	10440	8
1	50	2	108	160/100	17280	10
2	75	4	124	180/100	22320	13
3	100	6	130	210/110	27300	15
4	125	8	147	220/115	32340	18
5	150	9:32	152	230/120	34960	20
post	recovery 1 min	1	134	215/110	28810	17
post	recovery 3 min	3	112	190/100	21280	13
post	recovery 5 min	5	89	175/90	15575	11

Fig. 6.3 Data of cycle ergometer. *RPE* rate of perceived exertion

Fig. 6.4 Left ventricular hypertrophy (LVH)

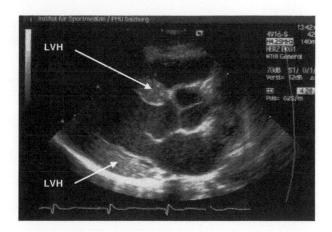

Blood tests (Fig. 6.5) showed a fasting plasma glucose of 6.6 mmol/L (119 mg/dL), HbA1c of 6.4 %, and dyslipidemia. Although treated with a statin, total cholesterol was 7.0 mmol/L (270 mg/dL), low-density lipoprotein (LDL) cholesterol was 4.0 mmol/L (155 mg/dL), high-density lipoprotein (HDL) cholesterol was 2.2 mmol/L (85 mg/dL), and triglycerides were 1.7 mmol/L (148 mg/dL).

Urine analysis (Fig. 6.6) showed microalbuminuria and glucosuria.

6.2   Risk Stratification

In order to raise the patient's awareness and understanding for essential and mandatory lifestyle changes, it is very useful to assess his risk for future vascular events. The following questions arise:

Parameter	Unit	Value	Flag
potassium	mmol/l	3.8	
sodium	mmol/l	140	
urea	mg/dl	21	
kreatinin	mg/dl	0.9	
calcium	mmol/l	2.44	
total proteine	g/dl	7.8	
glucose	mmol/l; mg/dl	6.6; 119	high
c-reactive proteine	mg/dl	<0.6	
hsCRP	mg/dl	0.3	high
uric acid	mg/dl	6.2	
HbA1c	%	6.4	high
total bilirubin	mg/dl	1.1	
cholesterol	mmol/l; mg/dl	7.0; 270	high
triglycerides	mmol/l; mg/dl	1.7; 148	
HDL-cholesterol	mmol/l; mg/dl	2.2; 85	high
LDL-cholesterin	mmol/l; mg/dl	4.0; 155	high
creatinkinase	U/l	151	
CK-MB	U/l	11	
PTT	seconds	32	
fibrinogen	mg/dl	317	
erythrocytes	T/L.	4.6	
hemoglobin	g/dl	13.8	
hematocrit	%	40.0	
leukocytes	G/L.	3.59	
thrombocytes	G/L.	170	
albumin	g/dl	4.9	
homocystein	µmol/l	12.00	

Fig. 6.5 Blood parameters. *hsCRP* high-sensitivity C-reactive protein, *HDL* high-density lipoprotein, *LDL* low-density lipoprotein, *CK-MB* creatine kinase muscle-brain type, *PTT* partial thromboplastin time

Fig. 6.6 Urinary analysis. *Neg* negative finding, *kg* kilogram, *m* meter, *pH* pondus hydrogenii, *mg* milligram, *dl* deciliter

weight density	kg/m³	1.015
pH		6
leucocytes	-	neg
nitrite	-	neg
proteine	-	neg
glucose	++	100 mg/dl
keton bodies	-	neg
urobilinogen	-	neg
bilirubin	-	neg
erythrocytes	-	neg
microalbumin	++	50 mg/dl

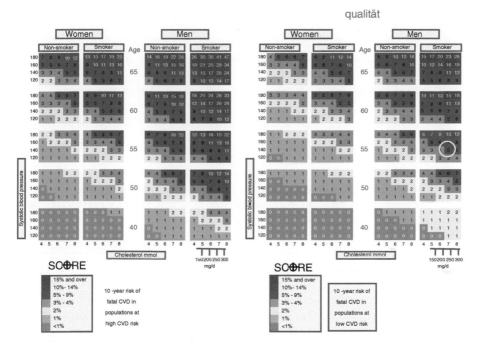

Fig. 6.7 Score charts for high- and low-risk countries

1. Which variables do you need to predict the 10-year risk of heart attack and stroke according to HeartScore® in this patient?

Age, gender, smoking status, systolic blood pressure, total cholesterol, and country of residence [1] (see Fig. 6.7) are mandatory to calculate the 10-year risk for cardiovascular death according to HeartScore®. The inclusion of BMI into HeartScore® has been tested several times and BMI has been proven to be a very weak risk factor for CVD. As a result, the addition of BMI does not improve the predictive power of HeartScore® [1, 2]. According to the European Guidelines on CVD Prevention, patients with diabetes are considered at high risk and should

Table 6.1 Score charts for high and low risk countries

European low risk	Andorra, Austria, Belgium*, Cyprus, Denmark, Finland, France, Germany, Greece*, Iceland, Ireland, Israel, Italy, Luxembourg, Malta, Monaco, the Netherlands*, Norway, Portugal, San Marino, Slovenia, Spain*, Sweden*, Switzerland, and the United Kingdom
European high risk	All other European countries
Very high risk	Armenia, Azerbaijan, Belarus, Bulgaria, Georgia, Kazakhstan, Kyrgyzstan, Latvia, Lithuania, Macedonia, FYR, Moldova, Russia, Ukraine, and Uzbekistan
National versions are available for*	Belgium, Germany, Greece, the Netherlands, Spain, Sweden, and Poland

therefore be treated with maximum intensity. Therefore, the inclusion of diabetes is not useful, since patients are being classified as high risk already.

2. There are two models, high risk and low risk, which of them do you use?

The model has to be chosen according to the country of residence of the patient (see Table 6.1).

For Austria, the low-risk model has to be chosen and calculates a 10-year risk of 5 % (age, 54 years; smoker; systolic blood pressure, 145 mmHg; total cholesterol, 7.0 mmol/L).

In our patient, risk estimation alone indicates an urgent need for preventive intervention to avoid a second cardiovascular event.

6.3   Diagnosis of Diabetes

Because of an elevated fasting plasma glucose level of 6.6 mmol/L (119 mg/dL), an elevated HbA1c of 6.4 % (46 mmol/mol), microalbuminuria, and glucosuria, it is mandatory to test for diabetes mellitus.

How do you efficiently and accurately diagnose diabetes in cardiac patients?

According to the most recent ESC Guidelines on diabetes, pre-diabetes, and cardiovascular diseases [2], it is recommended that the diagnosis of diabetes is based on HbA1c (if >6.5 % or > 48 mmol/mol) and fasting glucose (if >7.0 mmol/L or 126 mg/dL) combined or on an oral glucose tolerance test (OGTT, 2 h glucose > 11.1 mmol/L or >200 mg/dL) if still in doubt. (I, B) Since 2010, HbA1c may also be used to diagnose diabetes. Furthermore, HbA1c helps to assess the success of anti-glycemic therapy. HbA1c testing is highly specific compared with a 2 h OGTT or a fasting plasma glucose test. However, because HbA1c testing is not sensitive enough to rule out diabetes if levels are normal, the test should not be used for excluding diabetes [2]. Lower than expected levels of HbA1c can be seen in people with shortened red blood cell life span, as seen in glucose-6-phosphate dehydrogenase deficiency, sickle-cell disease, or any other condition causing premature red

Fig. 6.8 How to perform an oral glucose tolerance test

- fasting (except water) for the previous 8 -14 hours
- oral glucose tolerance test 7:00 -8:00 am
- baseline blood sample
- ingestion of standardized glucose solution (1.75 grams of glucose per kilogram of body weight, to a maximum dose of 75 grams) within 5 minutes
- blood draw after 2 hours

Diagnose / measurement	WHO 2006/2011	ADA 2003 and 2012
Diabetes		
HbA1c	**Can be used** If measured ≥6.5 % (48 mmol/mol)	**Recommended** ≥6.5% (48 mmol/mol)
FPG	Recommended ≥7.0 mmol/L (≥126 mg/dL)	≥7.0 mmol/L (≥126 mg/dL)
2hPG	Or ≥11.1 mmol/L (≥200 mg/dL)	Or ≥11.1 mmol/L (≥200 mg/dL)
IGT		
FPG	<7.0 mmol/l (<126 mg/dL)	<7.0 mmol/l (<126 mg/dL)
2hPG	≥7.8-<11.1 mmol/L (≥ 140-200 mg/dL)	**Not required** If measured 7.8-11.0 mmol/L (140-198 mg/dL)
IFG		
FPG	6.1-6.9 mmol/L (110-125 mg/dL)	5.6-6.9 mmol/L (100-125 mg/dL)
2hPG	**If measured** <7.8 mmol/l (<140 mg/dL)	--

Fig. 6.9 Comparison of 2006 World Health Organization (WHO) and 2003/2011 and 2012 American Diabetes Association (ADA) diagnostic criteria for impaired fasting glucose, impaired glucose tolerance, and diabetes

blood cell death. Conversely, higher than expected levels can be seen in people with a longer red blood cell life span, as in patients with vitamin B12 or folate deficiency. Elevated HbA1c levels represent poor glucose control. However, normal HbA1c levels still conform with a history of recent hypoglycemia or with spikes of hyperglycemia. Furthermore, HbA1c measures are not reliable, if the patient went on a diet or medical therapy within the last 6 weeks. In addition, patients with recent blood loss or hemolytic anemia are not suitable for this test [2].

Performing an OGTT is the method of choice to diagnose diabetes mellitus in this patient. Early stages of hyperglycemia and asymptomatic type 2 diabetes are best diagnosed by an OGTT (Fig. 6.8 [2] and 6.9) with an intake of 75 mg of glucose dissolved in 250–300 mL water within 5 min (body weight × 1.75 = mg of glucose for test; in this patient: 93.4 × 1.75 = 163.45 mg; but intake should not exceed 75 mg). In this patient the 2 h post-load glucose level was 12.2 mmol/L (220 mg/dL), which is diagnostic for diabetes (>11.1 mmol/L or 200 mg/dL). On a side note, his HbA1c was 6.4 % (48 mmol/mol) and fasting glucose was 6.6 mmol/L or 119 mg/dL, and consequently without an OGTT, the diagnosis of diabetes would have been missed.

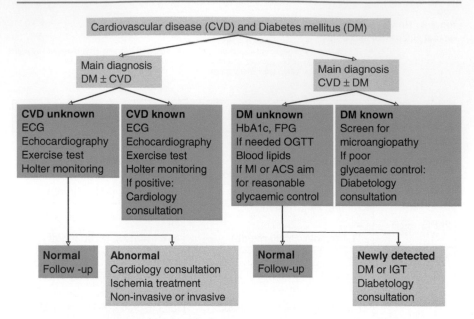

Fig. 6.10 Algorithm for patients with coronary artery disease and diabetes mellitus. *CAD* coronary arterial disease, *DM* diabetes mellitus, *HbA1C* hemoglobin A1c, *MI* myocardial infarction, *ECG* electrocardiogram, *ACS* acute coronary syndrome, *PFG* plasma fasting glucose, *IGT* impaired glucose tolerance

Besides the diagnosis of diabetes, also impaired fasting glucose (IFG) and impaired glucose tolerance (IGT) may be diagnosed using fasting glucose and OGTT.

An early diagnosis of diabetes is of utmost importance, since diabetes mellitus is associated with a more than twofold increase of cardiac mortality. Whereas patients with a previous myocardial infarction do have an increased risk of 4.0, the addition of the risk factor diabetes mellitus leads to a further increase, accumulating to 6.4 [2]. Figure 6.10 [2] presents a diagnostic algorithm of an efficient and practical diagnostic decision-making pathway for patients with diabetes mellitus (DM) or coronary artery disease (CAD). The presence of diabetes sets the patient at the highest possible risk regardless of other comorbidities. In a subsample of the Euro Heart Survey more than one-third of the patients with CAD who underwent an OGTT had an impaired glucose tolerance. Implementation of this simple, effective, and inexpensive test into clinical routine of patients with CAD would help diagnose diabetes mellitus and thus grant these high-risk patients access to an optimal medical, interventional, and surgical therapy [3].

Generally, metformin is recommended as the first-line therapy in newly diagnosed diabetes following evaluation of renal function. An estimated glomerular filtration rate (eGFR) of >50 ml/min is regarded as a cutoff value for metformin. If a target HbA1c of <7 % (53 mmol/mol) is not reached after a repeated measurement of HbA1c, the dosage of metformin may be increased up to 3000 mg, or, alternatively, a second agent may be added. In selected patients, such as our patient, a more stringent glucose control (HbA1c 6.0–6.5 % – 42–48 mmol/mol) might be considered if it can be achieved without hypoglycemia or other adverse events [2]. In concordance with the current guidelines, we started with metformin 500 mg 1-0-1 in our patient, as his eGFR is 74 mL/min.

6.4   Improving the Risk Factor Profile

The patient's risk profile includes arterial hypertension, physical inactivity, smoking, obesity, dyslipidemia, and diabetes mellitus. Treatment goals for cardiovascular risk factors are depicted in Fig. 6.11.

Blood pressure was 145/95 mmHg at rest and 230/120 mmHg at maximal exercise. Blood testing shown in Fig. 6.5 revealed a fasting plasma glucose of 6.6 mmol/L (119 mg/dL) and dyslipidemia although treated with a statin with total cholesterol of 7.0 mmol/L (270 mg/dL), LDL cholesterol of 4.0 mmol/L (155 mg/dL), HDL cholesterol of 2.2 mmol/L (85 mg/dL), and triglycerides of 1.7 mmol/L (148 mg/dL).

The patient's medication already included 100 mg of acetylsalicylic acid, a beta-blocker (metoprolol 50 mg 1/2-0-0), an ACE inhibitor (ramipril 2.5 mg 1-0-0), and a statin (simvastatin 40 mg 0-0-1).

To improve the risk factor profile in this patient, it is necessary to expand drug therapy immediately and instruct the patient on how to make lifestyle changes at the same time. Starting a structured program for lifestyle changes now and considering additional drug therapy some time later would not be enough to improve the risk factor profile in this patient. Additional pharmaceutical therapy is warranted. By not starting an intervention, the patient would continue to remain at a high cardiac risk. The history of this patient does not allow any more time for therapeutic nihilism.

The patient's blood pressure is not treated adequately. A blood pressure of 145/90 mmHg at rest and 230/120 mmHg at maximal exercise is still too high. Also, in cardiac patients with a reduced LVEF, a heart rate at rest of $\geq$70/min is associated with increased mortality (Fig. 6.10) [4, 5]. Thus, the beta-blocker ought to be increased to the highest tolerable dosage. As a result, an additional If-channel blocker most likely will not be needed. It is mandatory to increase the dose of the ACE inhibitor and beta-blocker to sufficiently treat hypertension in this patient. If a third agent is needed, a thiazide diuretic like hydrochlorothiazide may be added. According to the SPRINT study [6], the target blood pressure in a patient like ours could be <120/80 mmHg; however, the guidelines have not yet included this trial.

Hypertension	< 140/85 mmHg
LDL -Cholesterol	<1.8 mmol/l (< 70 mg/dl)
Fasting glucose:	4.4–6.1 mmol/l (80–110 mg/dl)
HbA1c:	< 6,5 %(48 mmol/mol)
BMI:	< 25 kg/m²
Waist circumference:	< 102 cm
Physical activity:	30-60 minutes on 3-7 days/week (>150 min/week) moderate to vigorous moderate-intensity aerobic physical activity (as walking, cycling, etc.) with 50–70% of maximum heart rate.

Fig. 6.11 Goals for risk reduction. *HbA1C* hemoglobin A1c

To reach the goals of risk reduction, a structured program for lifestyle changes like a comprehensive cardiac rehabilitation program has to be started immediately in order to implement all non-pharmacological treatment options.

Dyslipidemia is not sufficiently treated in this patient. According to the current guidelines on diabetes, pre-diabetes, and cardiovascular disease, a statin therapy is recommended in patients with diabetes and very high risk (i.e., if combined with documented cardiovascular disease, severe chronic kidney disease, or with one or more cardiovascular risk factors and/or target organ damage) with an LDL cholesterol of <1.8 mmol/L (<70 mg/dL) or at least a >50 % reduction of LDL cholesterol if this target goal cannot be reached [2]. Consequently, we changed simvastatin to a more potent statin, namely, rosuvastatin 20 mg 1-0-0. It is still under investigation what role PCSK-9 inhibitors (proprotein convertase subtilisin/kexin type 9 inhibitor) will play in such a patient [7].

With respect to obesity and physical inactivity, at least 150 min/week of moderate to vigorous aerobic physical activity (e.g., walking, jogging, cycling) with initially 50 % but then 70 % of his maximum heart rate has to be initiated and ideally ought to be performed for 30–60 min per day on 3–7 days a week. On a side note, maximal heart rate is not calculated or derived from tables but assessed during maximal ergometry, which is terminated either by exhaustion, symptoms, or ECG changes. Exercise training has a major beneficial impact on most cardiovascular risk factors. Effects include a decrease in glucose and triglycerides, increase in HDL cholesterol, and reduction of weight and blood pressure levels [2]. While some of the positive effects of exercise training can be achieved by pharmaceutical agents as well, effects on endothelial dysfunction and exercise capacity are more strongly conveyed by exercise training [8, 9].

Besides physical exercise, a dietary approach is warranted. Daily caloric intake should be reduced to 1500 kcal and the fat intake to 30–35 % of the daily total energy uptake [2, 10].

Smoking cessation is key to improve the cardiovascular risk profile in this patient. Smoking cessation programs help smokers to quit smoking [10].

In the chronic phase (>12 months) after myocardial infarction, daily 100 mg of acetylsalicylic acid is recommended for secondary prevention [7].

The goals for risk reduction according to current guidelines [2, 10] are listed in Fig. 6.11. Participation in a comprehensive cardiac rehabilitation program helps the patient to reach the goals of risk reduction and reduces the overall mortality by 26–31 % [10].

6.5   Exercise Prescription

The patient reports physical activity of 30–45 min of jogging once a week at the most.

Which additional exercise prescription is recommended for this patient?

According to current literature, 150 min/week of moderate to vigorous moderate-intensity aerobic physical activity (e.g., walking, cycling, etc.) has to be performed with 50–70 % of maximum heart rate at least five times a week. Alternatively, high-intensity

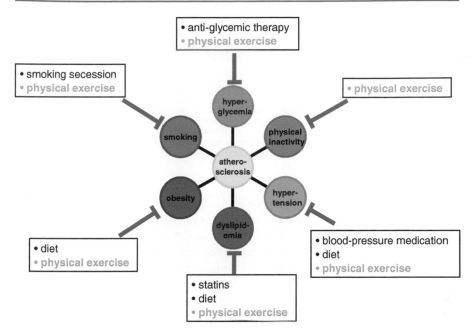

Fig. 6.12 Therapeutic options to treat modifiable risk factors

interval training may also be performed, which has been shown to be rather equipotent [11]. Patients who follow such exercise programs can expect to experience a beneficial effect on glycemic control, which is not primarily mediated by weight loss. Even though there is less evidence for resistance training, an increase in muscle bulk will lead to improved insulin sensitivity and reduced levels of glucose. In addition, the patient should perform resistance training three times a week, targeted at all major muscle groups, progressing to three sets of either 10–12 repetitions at 70 % of the one-repetition maximum (1-RM) or 25–30 repetitions at 40 % 1-RM [12, 13] (Fig. 6.12).

Two weeks after assessment of his physical fitness, our patient agreed to participate in an outpatient rehabilitation program at the Institute of Sports Medicine, Prevention and Rehabilitation. This rehabilitation program lasted 12 months and consisted of three training sessions during the first 6 weeks followed by training session per week per the rest of the year. A training session included endurance training, resistance training, and training of proprioception and flexibility. Furthermore, patients received psycho-cardiological advice and nutritional support, participated in a smoking cessation program, and were encouraged to also exercise at home [14]. Long-term but not short-term multifactorial intervention with focus on exercise training improves coronary endothelial dysfunction in diabetes mellitus type 2 and CAD, as previously reported [15].

Sessions are held in small groups of three to ten patients. Training sessions last 60 min and consist of 5 min warm-up, 50 min endurance and resistance training, and 5 min cool-down. Before each training session blood glucose is measured in each diabetic subject.

Fig. 6.13 Hypoglycemia
manifestations

Adrenergic manifestations
anxiety, nervousness, tremor, palpitations, tachycardia, sweating, feeling of
warmth, pallor, coldness, mydriasis, parasthaesia in the fingers

Glucagon manifestations
hunger, nausea, vomiting, abdominal discomfort, headache

Neuroglycopenic manifestations
impaired judgment, anxiety, moodiness, depression, crying, negativism,
irritability, rage, personality change, emotional lability, fatigue, weakness,
apathy, lethargy, daydreaming, sleep, confusion, amnesia, dizziness, blurred
vision, double vision, automatic behavior, difficulty speaking, incoordination,
paralysis, hemiparesis, paresthesia, headache, stupor, coma, abnormal
breathing, generalized or focal seizures.

In addition calisthenics, stretching exercises, and exercises on unstable surfaces are performed. Endurance training is carried out on a cycle ergometer with ECG monitoring throughout the session. The first session is started with a heart rate equivalent to 50 % of VO_2 peak as measured during ergospirometry. The cycle ergometer automatically adjusts the workload so that the heart rate always lies in the previously defined range. During the following sessions, the workload is increased up to 70–80 % of VO_2 peak. If possible, patients are asked to exercise continuously for 30 min with the aim to train for 60 min per session. Two additional sessions per week are resistance training. The first sessions are used to familiarize the patients with weight lifting equipment. During the following weeks resistance training is increased up to three sets of eight to ten repetitions at 75–85 % of the one-repetition maximum (1-RM) in six to eight muscle groups.

While our patient was well into the program, a serious incident occurred. Since routine presession blood glucose measurement showed 11.2 mmol/L (200 mg/dL), which compared well to his previous presession measurements, he started to train. After 10 min of ergometer training, his heart rate started to rise although his workload was constantly decreasing from 75 to 45 W. The patient also reported to feel dizziness and experienced a dry mouth. A closer look at the ECG revealed several ventricular premature beats. What is the most likely cause of the patient's symptoms? Hypoglycemia manifestations are summarized in Fig. 6.13.

Immediate blood glucose measurement showed a blood glucose concentration of 19.4 mmol/L (350 mg/dL), indicating hyperglycemia in this patient.

Usual hyperglycemic symptoms are polyphagia; polydipsia; polyuria; blurred vision; fatigue; weight loss; poor wound healing; dry mouth; dry or itchy skin; impotence (male); recurrent infections such as vaginal yeast infections; groin rash; external ear infections (swimmer's ear); Kussmaul hyperventilation: deep, rapid breathing; cardiac arrhythmia; stupor; and coma.

After some minutes of rest the patient recovered well, but blood glucose remained elevated at 19.4 mmol/L (342 mg/dL) after a third measurement 15 min later. The patient reported to have had a demanding week at his job and furthermore some domestic problems. He therefore suffered from sleeplessness during the last week. To find relief from stress, he exercised on his cycle ergometer for a home-based training session 2 h before the scheduled training session at our institute. Once measurements were obtained and it became obvious that he had hyperglycemia, he was instructed not to

Fig. 6.14 Blood glucose measurements and urinary tests after serious incident

When?	Blood glucose [mmol/l] ([mg/dl])	Keton bodies in urine
before training	11.2 (200)	not assessed
immediately after incident	19.4 (350)	++ (50 mg/dl)
15 minutes after incident	19.0 (342)	not assessed
next day	9.6 (174)	neg.

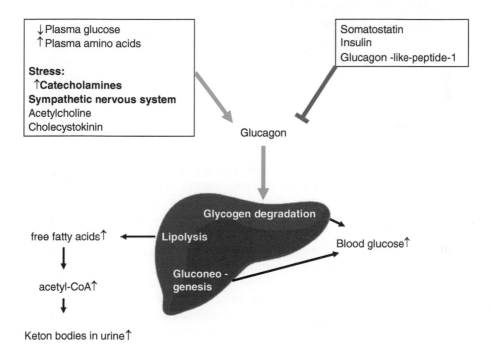

Fig. 6.15 Role of glucagon in diabetes mellitus

perform any exercise for the rest of the day and to continuously measure blood glucose levels every 15 min. Furthermore, a urinary analysis was performed and revealed ketone bodies in his urine. The next day the patient's urine was checked again and all parameters were within normal limits. His blood glucose level was 9.6 mmol (174 mg/dL) and the patient reported a complete recovery after a day of rest. His blood glucose measurements and urinary tests are depicted in Fig. 6.14. Exhaustion causes glucose production in the liver (glycogenesis and glycogenolysis) plus enhanced free fatty acid release by adipose tissue and reduced muscle uptake of glucose (Fig. 6.15).

Value	unit	pre	post	trend
Weight	kg	94.3	92.8	↓
BMI	kg/m²	31.1	30.7	↓
Pmax	W	150/1:32	200/1:06	↑
Hfrest	beats/min	72	66	↓
Hfmax	beats/min	152	163	↑
BPrest	mmHg	145/95	125/90	↓
BPmax	mmHg	230/120	215/110	↓
HbA1c	%	6.9	6.2	↓
Glucose	mmol/l; mg/dl	6.6; 119	6.5; 117	↓
LDL-Cholesterol	mmol/l; mg/dl	4.0; 155	2.1; 81	↓
total Cholesterol	mmol/l; mg/dl	7.0; 270	3.5; 135	↓
HDL-Cholesterol	mmol/l; mg/dl	2.2; 85	2.2; 84	=
Triglycerides	mmol/l; mg/dl	1.7; 148	1.3; 111	↓

Fig. 6.16 Pre- and post-measurements

No such event happened in the following months and the patient completed 52 weeks of training with an attendance rate of 95 %. Importantly, the continuous smoking cessation counseling in this patient resulted in a gradual decrease of the number of cigarettes he smoked. At the end of the 48th week of the rehabilitation program, he proudly announced that he had managed to quit smoking. Pre- and post-intervention measurements are shown in Fig. 6.16. Besides weight, body composition, and exercise capacity, his glucose metabolism, lipid profile, and his blood pressure profile also improved due to a combined approach of medication and lifestyle intervention. A follow-up echocardiography revealed a normalization of the left ventricular hypertrophy (IVSd,d 11 mm). The quality of life questionnaire demonstrated a significant improvement in seven out of eight tested domains: vitality, physical functioning, general health, perceptions physical role, functioning emotional role, functioning social role, and functioning mental health. No improvement was observed in the domain entitled "bodily pain." These results were in keeping with those of other patients in other outpatient cardiac rehabilitation programs [16, 14].

Conclusion

This 54-year-old man presents at the Institute of Sports Medicine, Prevention and Rehabilitation for an assessment of his physical fitness with a history of non-ST-elevation myocardial infarction of the anterior wall 2 years ago. Due to multiple modifiable cardiac risk factors, he has to change his lifestyle immediately. It is important that he enrolls in a comprehensive cardiac rehabilitation program. Exercise training should be performed three to five times a week at an intensity of 50 % of his maximum heart rate increasing to 150 min/week of moderate to vigorous aerobic physical activity (e.g., walking, jogging, cycling, etc.) with then 70 % of his maximum heart rate, ideally performed every day of the week. Exercise training is important, since it has a major beneficial impact on most risk factors. Effects include a decrease in triglycerides, increase in HDL cholesterol, and reduction of weight and blood pressure levels [12]. In addition, it is recommended to perform resistance training three times a week, targeted at all major muscle groups, progressing to three sets of eight to ten repetitions at a weight that cannot be lifted more than eight to ten times (8–10 RM) [12].

All lifestyle changes have to be supported by treating the risk factors appropriately with drugs for arterial hypertension, dyslipidemia, and diabetes. Furthermore, daily caloric intake should be reduced to 1500 kcal and the fat intake to 30–35 % of the daily total energy uptake [2, 10]. Smoking cessation should be encouraged by utilization of special programs. Also, antiplatelet therapy with aspirin or other antiplatelet drugs, if aspirin is contraindicated, has to be initiated and maintained [7].

To guide such patients in a reasonable way is a time-consuming and lifelong task, to which there is no alternative.

References

1. Conroy RM, Pyorala K, Fitzgerald AP, Sans S, Menotti A, De Backer G, De Bacquer D, Ducimetiere P, Jousilahti P, Keil U, Njolstad I, Oganov RG, Thomsen T, Tunstall-Pedoe H, Tverdal A, Wedel H, Whincup P, Wilhelmsen L, Graham IM, group Sp. Estimation of ten-year risk of fatal cardiovascular disease in Europe: the SCORE project. Eur Heart J. 2003;24(11):987–1003.
2. Authors/Task Force M, Ryden L, Grant PJ, Anker SD, Berne C, Cosentino F, Danchin N, Deaton C, Escaned J, Hammes HP, Huikuri H, Marre M, Marx N, Mellbin L, Ostergren J, Patrono C, Seferovic P, Uva MS, Taskinen MR, Tendera M, Tuomilehto J, Valensi P, Zamorano JL, Guidelines ESCCfP, Zamorano JL, Achenbach S, Baumgartner H, Bax JJ, Bueno H, Dean V, Deaton C, Erol C, Fagard R, Ferrari R, Hasdai D, Hoes AW, Kirchhof P, Knuuti J, Kolh P, Lancellotti P, Linhart A, Nihoyannopoulos P, Piepoli MF, Ponikowski P, Sirnes PA, Tamargo JL, Tendera M, Torbicki A, Wijns W, Windecker S, Document R, De Backer G, Sirnes PA, Ezquerra EA, Avogaro A, Badimon L, Baranova E, Baumgartner H, Betteridge J, Ceriello A, Fagard R, Funck-Brentano C, Gulba DC, Hasdai D, Hoes AW, Kjekshus JK, Knuuti J, Kolh P, Lev E, Mueller C, Neyses L, Nilsson PM, Perk J, Ponikowski P, Reiner Z, Sattar N, Schachinger V, Scheen A, Schirmer H, Stromberg A, Sudzhaeva S, Tamargo JL, Viigimaa M, Vlachopoulos C, Xuereb RG. ESC guidelines on diabetes, pre-diabetes, and cardiovascular diseases developed in collaboration with the EASD: the Task Force on diabetes, pre-diabetes, and cardiovascular diseases of the European Society of Cardiology (ESC) and developed in collaboration with the European Association for the Study of Diabetes (EASD). Eur Heart J. 2013;34(39):3035–87. doi:10.1093/eurheartj/eht108.
3. Drechsler K, Fikenzer S, Sechtem U, Blank E, Breithardt G, Zeymer U, Niebauer J. The Euro Heart Survey – Germany: diabetes mellitus remains unrecognized in patients with coronary artery disease. Clin Res Cardiol Off J German Cardiac Soc. 2008;97(6):364–70. doi:10.1007/s00392-008-0643-z.
4. McMurray JJ, Adamopoulos S, Anker SD, Auricchio A, Bohm M, Dickstein K, Falk V, Filippatos G, Fonseca C, Gomez-Sanchez MA, Jaarsma T, Kober L, Lip GY, Maggioni AP, Parkhomenko A, Pieske BM, Popescu BA, Ronnevik PK, Rutten FH, Schwitter J, Seferovic P, Stepinska J, Trindade PT, Voors AA, Zannad F, Zeiher A, Guidelines ESCCfP. ESC guidelines for the diagnosis and treatment of acute and chronic heart failure 2012: the Task Force for the Diagnosis and Treatment of Acute and Chronic Heart Failure 2012 of the European Society of Cardiology. Developed in collaboration with the Heart Failure Association (HFA) of the ESC. Eur Heart J. 2012;33(14):1787–847. doi:10.1093/eurheartj/ehs104.

5. Fox K, Ford I, Steg PG, Tendera M, Robertson M, Ferrari R. Heart rate as a prognostic risk factor in patients with coronary artery disease and left-ventricular systolic dysfunction (BEAUTIFUL): a subgroup analysis of a randomised controlled trial. Lancet. 2008;372(9641):817–21. doi:10.1016/s0140-6736(08)61171-x.
6. Group TSR. A randomized trial of intensive versus standard blood-pressure control. N Engl J Med. 2015;373(22):2103–16. doi:10.1056/NEJMoa1511939.
7. Latimer J, Batty JA, Neely DD, Kunadian V. PCSK9 inhibitors in the prevention of cardiovascular disease. J Thromb Thrombolysis. 2016; doi:10.1007/s11239-016-1364-1.
8. Sixt S, Rastan A, Desch S, Sonnabend M, Schmidt A, Schuler G, Niebauer J. Exercise training but not rosiglitazone improves endothelial function in prediabetic patients with coronary disease. Eur J Cardiovasc Prev Rehabil. 2008;15(4):473–8. doi:10.1097/HJR.0b013e3283002733.
9. Niebauer J. Treatment after coronary artery bypass surgery remains incomplete without rehabilitation. Circulation. 2016;133(24):2529–37.
10. Perk J, De Backer G, Gohlke H, Graham I, Reiner Z, Verschuren M, Albus C, Benlian P, Boysen G, Cifkova R, Deaton C, Ebrahim S, Fisher M, Germano G, Hobbs R, Hoes A, Karadeniz S, Mezzani A, Prescott E, Ryden L, Scherer M, Syvanne M, Scholte op Reimer WJ, Vrints C, Wood D, JL Z, Zannad F. European guidelines on cardiovascular disease prevention in clinical practice (version 2012). The Fifth Joint Task Force of the European Society of Cardiology and Other Societies on Cardiovascular Disease Prevention in Clinical Practice (constituted by representatives of nine societies and by invited experts). Eur Heart J. 2012;33(13):1635–701. doi:10.1093/eurheartj/ehs092.
11. Tschentscher M, Eichinger J, Egger A, Droese S, Schonfelder M, Niebauer J. High-intensity interval training is not superior to other forms of endurance training during cardiac rehabilitation. Eur J Prev Cardiol. 2016;23(1):14–20. doi:10.1177/2047487314560100.
12. Sigal RJ, Kenny GP, Wasserman DH, Castaneda-Sceppa C, White RD. Physical activity/exercise and type 2 diabetes: a consensus statement from the American Diabetes Association. Diabetes Care. 2006;29(6):1433–8. doi:10.2337/dc06-9910.
13. Egger A, Niederseer D, Diem G, Finkenzeller T, Ledl-Kurkowski E, Forstner R, Pirich C, Patsch W, Weitgasser R, Niebauer J. Different types of resistance training in type 2 diabetes mellitus: effects on glycaemic control, muscle mass and strength. Eur J Prev Cardiol. 2013;20(6):1051–60. doi:10.1177/2047487312450132.
14. Niebauer J, Mayr K, Tschentscher M, Pokan R, Benzer W. Outpatient cardiac rehabilitation: the Austrian model. Eur J Prev Cardiol. 2013;20(3):468–79. doi:10.1177/2047487312446137.
15. Sixt S, Beer S, Bluher M, Korff N, Peschel T, Sonnabend M, Teupser D, Thiery J, Adams V, Schuler G, Niebauer J. Long- but not short-term multifactorial intervention with focus on exercise training improves coronary endothelial dysfunction in diabetes mellitus type 2 and coronary artery disease. Eur Heart J. 2010;31(1):112–9. doi:10.1093/eurheartj/ehp398.
16. Niebauer J, Mayr K, Harpf H, Hofmann P, Muller E, Wonisch M, Pokan R, Benzer W. Long-term effects of outpatient cardiac rehabilitation in Austria: a nationwide registry. Wien Klin Wochenschr. 2014;126(5–6):148–55. doi:10.1007/s00508-014-0527-3.

Cardiac Rehabilitation After Acute Myocardial Infarction: The Influence of Psychosocial Disorders

7

Werner Benzer

A 52-year-old gentleman developed intensive chest pain at six o'clock in the morning. He went to the emergency room of his community hospital. After 12-lead ECG registration, an acute posterior wall ST-elevation myocardial infarction (STEMI) was diagnosed (1). ECG was tele-transmitted to the percutaneous coronary intervention (PCI) centre. Diagnosis was confirmed by interventional cardiologists, and the logistics of care were immediately initiated. The patient was monitored. ASS, prasugrel and unfractionated heparin were given. Following current guidelines the patient was transferred to the PCI centre for emergency cardiac catheterization [1]. The delay from the first medical contact to the start of the cath lab procedure lasted approximately 80 min. Coronary angiography demonstrated a subtotal occlusion in the mid right coronary artery caused by acute plaque rupture (Fig. 7.1). PCI was performed using balloon dilatation of the plaque burden ruptured. The procedure could be finalized with drug-eluting stent implantation.

Did the emergency logistics care of this case meet the current guidelines?
The 2012 ESC guidelines for the management of acute myocardial infarction [1] defines current prehospital and in-hospital management and reperfusion strategies within 24 h of first medical contact. These guidelines result to primary PCI within a time window preferably <90 min after first medical contact (Fig. 7.2).

Following these guidelines for patients with the clinical presentation of STEMI within 24 h after symptom onset and with persistent ST-segment elevation or new or presumed new left bundle branch block, PCI should be performed as early as possible, but within 90 min after first medical contact (Fig. 7.2).

Primary PCI is defined as angioplasty and/or stenting without prior or concomitant fibrinolytic therapy and is the preferred therapeutic option when performed by

W. Benzer, MD, FESC
Outpatient Cardiac Rehabilitation Centre, Cardiac Disease Management Centre,
Grenzweg 10, 6800 Feldkirch, Austria
e-mail: wbenzer@cable.vol.at

© Springer International Publishing AG 2017
J. Niebauer (ed.), *Cardiac Rehabilitation Manual*,
DOI 10.1007/978-3-319-47738-1_7

Fig. 7.1 ECG
tele-transmission
showed posterior wall
STEMI

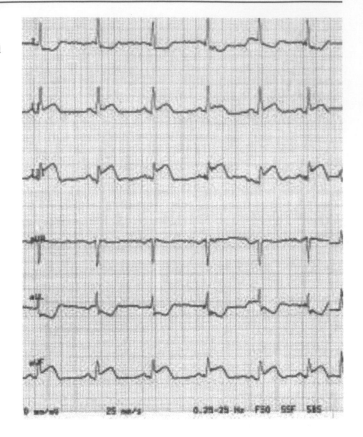

experienced team. Primary PCI is effective in securing and maintaining coronary artery patency and avoids some of the bleeding risks of fibrinolysis. Randomized clinical trials comparing timely performed primary PCI with in-hospital fibrinolytic therapy in high-volume, experienced centres have shown more effective restoration of patency, less reocclusion, improved residual left ventricular function and better clinical outcome with primary PCI [2]. Routine coronary stent implantation in patients with STEMI decreases the need for target vessel revascularization but is not associated with significant reductions in death or re-infarction rates.

After successful percutaneous coronary intervention (Fig. 7.3), the patient was transferred to the coronary care unit of the PCI centre and was further monitored for 24 h. Then he was sent back to the community hospital, where he experienced the rest of his hospital stay without any complications.

Primary PCI during the early hours of myocardial infarction has become the preferred therapeutic option, if it can be performed within 90 min after the first medical contact. In contrast to fibrinolytic therapy followed by delayed PCI practised in former times, after primary PCI and stenting, in uncomplicated cases,

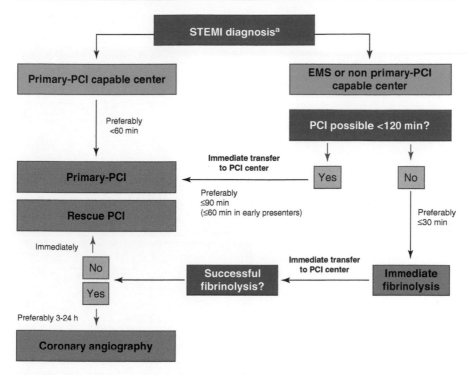

Fig. 7.2 Prehospital and in-hospital management and reperfusion strategies within 24 h of first medical contact [1]. *a*The time point the diagnosis is confirmed with patient history and ECG ideally within 10 min from the first medical contact (FMC). All delays are related to FMC (first medical contact). *Cath* catheterization laboratory, *EMS* emergency medical system, *FMC* first medical contact, *PCI* percutaneous coronary intervention, *STEMI* ST-segment elevation myocardial infarction

phase I cardiac rehabilitation can start the next day, and such patients can be walking around the flat and walking upstairs within a few days. Patients with larger myocardial damage and heart failure, shock or serious arrhythmias should be kept bedridden, and their physical activity increased slowly, dependent upon their symptoms and the extent of myocardial damage. After primary PCI, patients who experience an uncomplicated course of the event can be discharged after a hospital stay of 2–3 days. Exercise-based rehabilitation is recommended in all patients after acute myocardial infarction (Class I; Evidence Level A) [1, 3].

At day of discharge an interview was performed to detect patient's risk factors. Except an occupational distress during many years, no acquired cardiovascular risk factors could be detected (Table 7.1). Nevertheless cardiac rehabilitation was strongly recommended to the patient because of the current cardiovascular event. After financial agreement of his health insurance 2 weeks after hospital discharge, the patient could be admitted to an outpatient rehabilitation centre.

Fig. 7.3 (**a**) Coronary angiography demonstrated plaque rupture in the mid right coronary artery; (**b**) primary PCI was performed immediately and (**c**) resulted in open vessel with TIMI 3 flow

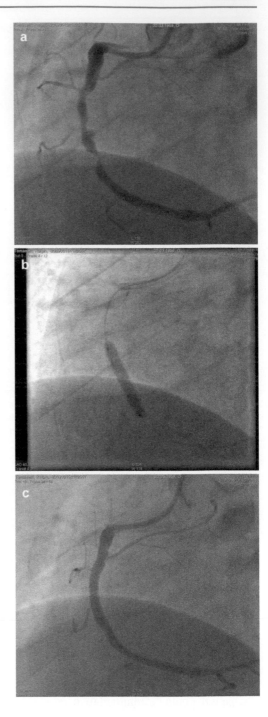

Table 7.1 Cardiovascular risk factors of the patient presented

Male	Yes	Family history CV disease	Yes
Height (cm)	176	Creatinine (mg/dl)	1.0
Weight (kg)	78	Cholesterol (mg/dl)	189
Blood pressure (mmHg)	125/80	LDL-C (mg/dl)	105
Smoker	No	HDL-C (mg/dl)	58
Physically active	Regular	Triglycerides	167
Distress	Yes	Fasting blood sugar (mg/dl)	95

Did the rest of the hospital course meet the current guidelines?

Patients without significant LV damage can sit out of bed late on the first day, be allowed to use a commode and undertake self-care and self-feeding. Ambulation can start the next day, and such patients can be walking up to 200 m on the flat and walking upstairs within a few days. Those who have experienced heart failure, shock or serious arrhythmias should be kept in bed longer, and their physical activity increased slowly, dependent upon their symptoms and the extent of myocardial damage.

Following routine clinical practice of the hospital, where this patient was clinically managed after primary PCI, he was discharged with prescription of aspirin, prasugrel, nebivolol, candesartan and atorvastatin.

What is the evidence of optimal pharmacological treatment after STEMI?

The ESC guidelines for the management of acute myocardial infarction in patients presenting with ST-segment elevation recommend in its 2012 version [1].

- In the acute phase of coronary artery syndromes and for the following 12 months, dual antiplatelet therapy with a P2Y12 inhibitor (ticagrelor or prasugrel) added to aspirin is recommended unless contraindicated due to such as excessive risk of bleeding. In patients who cannot receive ticagrelor or prasugrel, clopidogrel (600 mg loading dose, 75 mg daily dose) is recommended (Class I; Evidence Level A).
- It is recommended to initiate or continue highdose statins early after admission in all STEMI patients without contraindication or history of intolerance, regardless of initial cholesterol values (Class I; Evidence Level A).
- ACE inhibitors should be considered in all patients in the absence of contraindications (Class IIa; Evidence Level A).
- Oral treatment with beta-blockers should be considered during hospital stay and continued thereafter in all STEMI patients without contraindications (Class IIa; Evidence Level A).

After acute myocardial infarction, risk assessment is important to identify patients at high risk of further events. When primary PCI has been performed successfully in the acute phase, early risk assessment is less important since it can be assumed that the infarct-related coronary lesion has been treated and stabilized. After hospital discharge, phase II cardiac rehabilitation should start as early as possible. The aim is to restore the patient to as full a life as possible, including return to work. Dependent upon local facilities, in-hospital cardiac rehabilitation for 4 weeks can be useful in patients with severe left ventricular dysfunction or relevant co-morbidity. All other patients can start with outpatient cardiac rehabilitation immediately after hospital discharge and should be continued the succeeding weeks and months but at least reach rehabilitation targets. Outpatient stress testing within 2 weeks in combination with ECG or imaging techniques would be appropriate in these patients.

A bicycle stress test was performed before starting phase II cardiac rehabilitation. Patient could perform only 75 W of 150 W expected by age and gender. He was not limited by symptoms of angina or dyspnoea. He only reported fatigue as he also felt during the weeks before his event.

Guidelines of bicycle stress test after acute coronary syndrome [4]

Acute coronary syndrome (unstable angina or acute myocardial infarction) represents an acute phase in the life cycle of the patient with chronic coronary disease. Thus, the role and timing of exercise testing in ACS relates to this acute and convalescent period. Only limited evidence available supports the use of exercise testing in patients with STEMI with appropriate indications as soon as the patient has stabilized clinically. Only three studies investigated a symptom-limited pre-discharge (3–7 days) exercise test in patients with unstable angina or non-Q-wave infarction. The major independent predictors of 1-year infarction-free survival in multivariable regression analysis were the number of leads with ischemic ST-segment depression and peak exercise workload achieved [5]. Because of the extraordinary fatigue and mood disturbance of the patient presented without clinical meaningful test results, psychological aspects were focused in the initial phase of cardiac rehabilitation.

Anxiety is almost inevitable, in both patients and their associates, so that reassurance and explanation of the nature of the illness are of great importance and must be handled sensitively. It is also necessary to warn of the frequent occurrence of depression and irritability that more frequently occurs after returning home. It must also be recognized that denial is common; while this may have a protective effect in the acute stage, it may make subsequent acceptance of the diagnosis more difficult. Large studies suggest a role for psychosocial factors as prognostic factors in cardiovascular disease with the strongest evidence for depression as a negative factor in post-infarction patients [6]. However, whether depression is an independent risk (after adjustment for conventional risk factors) is still unclear, and there is, so far, little evidence that any intervention targeting these factors improves prognosis.

In the early 1980s and early 1990s, studies reported that life stress, psychological distress, depressive symptoms and hostility or anger were all linked to poor outcomes after STEMI. Depression has been associated with an increased risk of coronary heart disease in both men and women. In the INTERHEART study, the authors showed that feeling sad, blue or depressed for 2 weeks or more in a row was associated with acute myocardial infarction across different populations and across groups of people with different ethnic origins [7].

After administration of the Hospital Anxiety and Depression Scale (HADS), which was routinely performed in this particular outpatient cardiac rehabilitation centre where the patient was admitted, he presented no anxiety but clinical meaningful depression score.

Is the HADS the right instrument to detect anxiety and depression in patients after an acute cardiac event?

A number of instruments have been used by various studies and trials to identify and monitor post-MI patients with depression. Unfortunately, very little information exists on the operating characteristics of these instruments in this population [8]. The Hospital Anxiety and Depression Scale (HADS) has been extensively used in clinical trials, gives clinically meaningful results as a psychological screening test and is responsive to changes in the course of disease and with interventions. We used the validated German version of the HADS to assess anxiety and depression in this study [9].

With the result of the HADS, patient was sent to short-term psychotherapy. At the same time exercise-based cardiac rehabilitation was started. Three sessions of 1 h each per week was prescribed for 3 months.

Did exercise prescription in this case follow the current guidelines?

Patients recovering from acute myocardial infarction should be admitted to an exercise-based cardiac rehabilitation programme. Exercise training should start at a more moderate intensity, shorter duration and lower frequency than the ultimate goal. A moderate activity is in the range of 40–60 % of maximal O_2 uptake or 55–70 % of the age-adjusted maximal heart rate [10]. Most patients will be on a beta-blocker, which tends to decrease the heart range in a variable manner. Success should be assessed and reinforcement provided regularly. Gradual increases in activity are not only safer for sedentary patients with coronary artery disease but short-term successes may increase the patient's self-efficacy for being physically active. The guidelines for secondary prevention of coronary disease for patients in a chronic and stable phase suggest that physical activities of moderate intensity 4–5 times per week for 30–45 min are desirable. This adds up to an exercise volume of 2 h to almost 4 h with a kcal expenditure between 900 and 1700 kcal per week. Endurance activities like walking, jogging or bicycling are preferable. The intensity of the endurance activity should be in the moderate range. It is important to consider the age-adjusted exercise capacity and heart rate to avoid overexertion and not to endanger persons who have been rather inactive for long periods of time.

Three months later, patient's mood circumstances presented much better. Repeated HADS test showed values near normal. The physical performance of the patient also has improved in the meantime to150 W without any symptoms. At the end of the rehabilitation programme, the cardiac rehabilitation team stated in his medical report that in this patient, the comprehensive programme including short-term psychotherapy did meet the rehabilitation goals.

As demonstrated in this case, anxiety and depression are almost inevitable and must be handled sensitively. It is also necessary to warn of the request occurrence of depression and irritability that more frequently occur after returning home. Large studies suggest a role for psychosocial factors as prognostic factors in cardiovascular disease with the strongest evidence for depression as a negative factor in post-infarction patients [11]. Therefore management of psychological risk factor and behavioural interventions is important. Observational studies indicate that psychological factors strongly influence the course of coronary artery disease. Management approaches include routinely screening for psychosocial risk factors, referring patients with severe psychological distress to behavioural specialists and directly treating patients with milder forms of psychological distress with brief targeted interventions. A number of behavioural interventions have been evaluated for their ability to reduce adverse cardiac events among patients presenting with psychosocial risk factors. Although the efficacy of stand-alone psychosocial interventions remains unclear, both exercise and comprehensive cardiac rehabilitation with psychosocial interventions have demonstrated a reduction in cardiac events [12]. Furthermore, recent data suggest that psychopharmacologic interventions may also be effective [13]. However, whether depression is an independent risk is still unclear, and there is, so far, little evidence that any intervention targeting these factors improves prognosis [14].

Only the ENRICHD and MIND-IT studies were designed to assess cardiovascular outcomes in depressive disorders, although the MIND-IT study had very low statistical power [13, 15, 16]. Neither found evidence that depression treatment affects cardiac outcomes. Among patients with depression and history of myocardial infarction in the ENRICHD clinical trial, there was no difference in event-free survival between participants treated with cognitive behavioural therapy supplemented by an antidepressant vs. usual care (75.5 % vs. 74.7 %) [15]. Cardiac event-free survival in the MIND-IT trial was 86.2 % for patients in the treatment group and 87.3 % for patients in the control group [13].

Depression treatment with medication or cognitive behavioural therapy in patients with cardiovascular disease is associated with modest improvement in depressive symptoms but no improvement in cardiac outcomes. No clinical trials have assessed whether screening for depression improves depressive symptoms or cardiac outcomes in patients with cardiovascular disease [8].

Current guidelines for the detection and management of post-myocardial infarction depression

The American Academy of Family Physicians (AAFP) Commission on Science convened a panel to review the evidence on the effect of depression on persons after myocardial infarction [17].

This guideline pertains directly only to patients who have sustained STEMI. For guideline recommendations, see Table 7.2.

Evidence question 1: What is the prevalence of depression during initial hospitalization for myocardial infarction?

The updated evidence review continued to show a wide range of prevalence (7.2–41.2 %) depending on the method used to assess depression. Structured interviews tended to produce lower prevalence estimates, and rating scales, such as the BDI,

Table 7.2 Post-myocardial infarction depression clinical practice guidelines [17]

Recommendation		Level of evidence
1	Patients having a myocardial infarction should be screened for depression using a standardized depression symptom checklist at regular intervals during the post-myocardial infarction	A
2	Post-MI patients with a diagnosis of depression should be treated to improve their depression symptoms, with systems in place to ensure regular follow-up	A
3	Selective serotonin reuptake inhibitors (SSRIs) are preferred to tricyclic antidepressants for treatment of depression in post-MI patients	A
4	Psychotherapy may be beneficial for treatment of depression in post-MI patients. The existing evidence base does not establish what form of psychotherapy is preferred	B

produced higher prevalence estimates. In general, across the studies, about one of every five patients with myocardial infarction have depression during an initial hospitalization.

Evidence question 2: What is the independent association of measures of depression with post-myocardial infarction outcome?

All studies support the association between post-MI depression and cardiac-related mortality, with a direct relation between severity of depression symptoms and probability of death. Six independent studies meet inclusion criteria that reported cardiac event rates among depressed patients. One study found that the association between cardiac events and depression disappeared with adjustment for fatigue symptoms, and two others found the same when adjusting for a measure of anxiety. Studies of similar methodological quality have shown relations between post-MI depression symptoms and hospital readmission and nonfatal cardiac events or symptoms.

Five randomized clinical trials that specifically evaluated antidepressant medication treatment (typically with selective serotonin reuptake inhibitors (SSRIs)) could be identified. A trend towards improved cardiac outcomes in the largest and best designed of the medication studies did not reach statistical significance. Three additional publications have addressed medication treatment. A post-hoc subgroup analysis of the ENRICHD trial [15] found a 43 % reduction in death, nonfatal MI and all-cause mortality among those patients taking SSRIs. SSRIs appear to be safe from a cardiac standpoint and effective in reducing depression symptoms. SSRIs are preferred over tricyclic antidepressants because of the heart rate and conduction effects of tricyclic antidepressants.

The effects of psychotherapy are difficult to interpret because of the heterogeneity of the modalities used; however, at least cognitive behavioural therapy appears to improve depression symptoms. Subgroup analyses of several studies suggest that benefit accrues to patients with pre-existing depression or previous episodes of depression, whereas patients whose initial symptoms appear after myocardial infarction have a very high placebo response rate and generally improve regardless of therapy.

Following recent recommendations from the Cardiac Rehabilitation Section of the European Association of Cardiovascular Prevention and Rehabilitation of the European Society of Cardiology, a multimodal behavioural intervention, integrating counselling for PSRFs and coping with illness, should be included within comprehensive CR. Patients with psychosocial disorders after acute myocardial infarction should be referred for psychological counselling or psychologically focused interventions and/or psychopharmacological treatment. To conclude, the success of CR may critically depend on the interdependence of the body and mind, and this interaction needs to be reflected through the assessment and management of PSRFs in line with robust scientific evidence, by trained staff, integrated within the core CR team [18].

Learning objectives of this case:

- How to manage a patient with STEMI from the first medical contact
- How to initiate cardiac rehabilitation after STEMI and primary percutaneous coronary intervention
- Prevalence of depression after STEMI
- Detection and management of post-STEMI depression

References

1. Steg PG, James SK, Atar D, for The Task Force on the management of ST-segment elevation acute myocardial infarction of the European Society of Cardiology, et al. ESC guidelines for the management of acute myocardial infarction in patients presenting with ST-segment elevation. Eur Heart J. 2012;33:2569–619.
2. Keeley EC, Boura JA, Grines CL, et al. Primary angioplasty vs. intravenous thrombolytic therapy for acute myocardial infarction: a quantitative review of 23 randomised trials. Lancet. 2003;361:13–20.
3. Perk J, De Backer G, Gohlke H, for The Fifth Joint Task Force of the European Society of Cardiology and Other Societies on Cardiovascular Disease Prevention in Clinical Practice, et al. European guidelines on cardiovascular disease prevention in clinical practice (version 2012). Eur Heart J. 2012;33:1635–701.
4. Fletcher GF, Ades PA, Kligfield P, For The American Heart Association Exercise, Cardiac Rehabilitation, and Prevention Committee of the Council on Clinical Cardiology, Council on Nutrition, Physical Activity and Metabolism, Council on Cardiovascular and Stroke Nursing, and Council on Epidemiology and Prevention, et al. Exercise standards for testing and training: a scientific statement from the American Heart Association. Circulation. 2013;128: 873–934.
5. Nyman I, Larsson H, Areskog M, for the RISC Study Group, et al. The predictive value of silent ischemia at an exercise test before discharge after an episode of unstable coronary artery disease. Am Heart J. 1992;123:324–31.

6. Wells KB, Stewart A, Hays RD, Burnam MA, et al. The functioning and well-being of depressed patients. Results from the Medical Outcomes Study. JAMA. 1989;262:914–9.
7. Rosengren A, Hawken S, Ounpuu S, for the INTERHEART investigators, et al. Association of psychosocial risk factors with risk of acute myocardial infarction in 11119 cases and 13648 controls from 52 countries (the INTERHEART study). Lancet. 2004;364:953–62.
8. Thombs BD, de Jonge P, Coyne JC, et al. Depression screening and patient outcomes in cardiovascular care: a systematic review. JAMA. 2008;300:2161–271.
9. Bjelland I, Dahl AA, Haug TT, et al. The validity of the hospital anxiety and depression scale. An updated literature review. J Psychosom Res. 2002;52:69–77.
10. Fletcher FG, Balady GJ, Ezra A, et al. Exercise standards for testing and training: a statement for healthcare professionals from the American Heart Association. Circulation. 2013;104: 1694–740.
11. Rozanski A, Blumenthal JA, Davidson KW, et al. The epidemiology, pathophysiology, and management of psychosocial risk factors in cardiac practice: the emerging field of behavioural cardiology. J Am Coll Cardiol. 2005;45:637–51.
12. Rees K, Bennett P, West R, et al. Psychological interventions for coronary heart disease. Cochrane Database Syst Rev. 2004;2:CD002902.
13. Honig A, Kuyper AM, Schene AH, for the MIND-IT investigators, et al. Treatment of post-myocardial infarction depressive disorder: a randomized, placebo-controlled trial with mirtazapine. Psychosom Med. 2007;69:606–13.
14. Nicholson A, Kuper H, Hemingway H, et al. Depression as an aetiologic and prognostic factor in coronary heart disease: a meta-analysis of 6362 events among 146 538 participants in 54 observational studies. Eur Heart J. 2006;27:2763–74.
15. Berkman LF, Blumenthal J, Burg M, et al. Effects of treating depression and low perceived social support on clinical events after myocardial infarction: the Enhancing Recovery in Coronary Heart Disease patients (ENRICHD) randomized trial. JAMA. 2003;289:3106–16.
16. Van Melle JP, de Jonge P, Honig A, et al. Effects of antidepressant treatment following myocardial infarction. Br J Psychiatry. 2009;190:460–6.
17. Green LA. Post-myocardial infarction depression clinical practice guideline panel. Ann Fam Med. 2009;7:71–9.
18. Pogosova N, Saner H, Pedersen SS, for the Cardiac Rehabilitation Section of the European Association of Cardiovascular Prevention and Rehabilitation of the European Society of Cardiology, et al. Psychosocial aspects in cardiac rehabilitation: from theory to practice. A position paper from the Cardiac Rehabilitation Section of the European Association of Cardiovascular Prevention and Rehabilitation of the European Society of Cardiology. Eur J Prev Cardiol. 2015;10:1290–306.

Stable Coronary Artery Disease: Exercise-Based Cardiac Rehabilitation Reduces the Risk of Recurrent Angina After PCI in the Case of Arterial Hypertension

8

Werner Benzer

A 70-year-old lady presented with hypertension and angina to the general practitioner. He sent her to the cardiologist for exercise stress testing. The result was inconclusive. During exercise, angina could be reproduced, but no ECG abnormalities were recorded. The cardiologist decided to send the patient to his concurrent invasive cardiology department for coronary angiography. An intermediate stenosis of the circumflex artery could be detected (Fig. 8.1). After coronary flow reserve measurement with pressure wire, the fractional flow reserve showed 0.85 (Fig. 8.2). Regarding the angina symptoms of the patient, the interventional cardiologist decided to dilate the lesion. He ended up with uncomplicated drug-eluting stent implantation (Fig. 8.3). A day after the procedure, the patient could be discharged from the hospital. ASS and clopidogrel was administered for 4 weeks. At the time of discharge, systolic blood pressure was 170/100 mmHg.

The guidelines of the European Society of Cardiology strongly support the use of PCI in clinically stable patients with coronary artery disease and angina [1]. But in patients with chronic stable conditions and in the absence of a recent myocardial infarction, PCI does not offer any benefit in terms of death, myocardial infarction or the need for subsequent revascularization compared with conservative medical treatment [2]. Patients with stable coronary artery disease and angina were included in the recently published COURAGE Trial [3]. Patients were randomly assigned to undergo PCI and optimal medical therapy or optimal medical therapy alone. This study showed very clearly, that, as an initial management strategy in patients with stable coronary artery disease and angina, PCI did not reduce the risk of death, myocardial infarction or other major cardiovascular events when added to optimal

W. Benzer, MD, FESC
Outpatient Cardiac Rehabilitation Centre, Cardiac Disease Management Centre,
Grenzweg 10, 6800, Feldkirch, Austria
e-mail: wbenzer@cable.vol.at

© Springer International Publishing AG 2017
J. Niebauer (ed.), *Cardiac Rehabilitation Manual*,
DOI 10.1007/978-3-319-47738-1_8

Fig. 8.1 Intermediate stenosis of the left circumflex artery

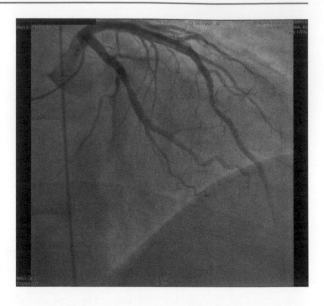

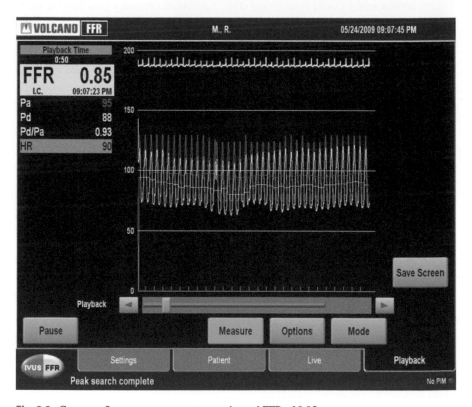

Fig. 8.2 Coronary flow reserve measurement showed FFR of 0.85

Fig. 8.3 Left circumflex
artery after PCI and stent
implantation

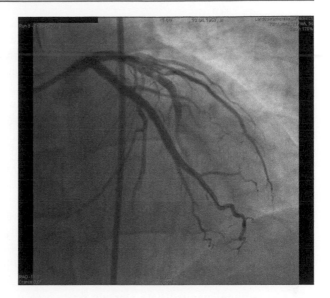

medical therapy. However, exercise-based cardiac rehabilitation is associated with a
25 % reduction in overall mortality and mortality from cardiovascular causes at 3
years [4].

*Indications for revascularization in patients with stable angina or silent isch-
aemia* [1]:

- Left main disease with stenosis > 50 % (Class I; Evidence Level A)
- Any proximal LAD stenosis > 50 % (Class I; Evidence Level A)
- Two-vessel or three-vessel disease with stenosis > 50 % with impaired LV func-
  tion = LVEF < 40 % (Class I; Evidence Level A)
- Large area of ischaemia (> 10 % LV) (Class I; Evidence Level B)
- Single remaining patent coronary artery with stenosis > 50 % (Class I; Evidence
  Level C)
- For symptoms in any coronary stenosis > 50 % and in the presence of limiting
  angina or angina equivalent, unresponsive to medical therapy (Class I; Evidence
  Level A)

In general PCI is effective at reducing angina in patients with symptomatic coronary artery disease. But in stable patients PCI fails to reduce further cardiac events
beyond intensive medical therapy. This should be taken in account, when decision
to intervention is made.

Decision-making for PCI is important to optimize the success rate, to safe costs
and to prevent complications during the procedure. It is generally accepted that
revascularization of a coronary stenosis responsible for reversible ischaemia is justi-
fied as it relieves angina complaints and in some situations improves patient outcome [1]. In today's interventional practice, however, a stenosis not clearly

responsible for symptoms is often treated, even if ischaemia cannot be attributed to the lesion and even if it is only of mild or moderate severity. This applies to either a single intermediate stenosis or to an intermediate stenosis found incidentally in a patient undergoing stenting because of a more severe stenosis elsewhere in the coronary arteries.

This approach not evidence based, and it is unnecessarily expensive. It might even be harmful because the risk of peri-procedural myocardial infarction or late stent thrombosis is not negligible, even when drug-eluting stents are used [5]. It is unlikely that stenting a haemodynamically non-significant stenosis will improve complaints, and there is no data suggesting that it will improve patient prognosis. Defining the haemodynamic significance of a stenosis from the angiogram is difficult.

Fractional flow reserve (FFR) is an accurate invasive index to determine in the catheterization laboratory whether an angiographically equivocal stenosis is of functional significance (i.e. responsible for reversible ischaemia) [6]. FFR can be simply and rapidly determined just before the planned intervention or during routine diagnostic catheterization. FFR expresses maximum achievable blood flow to the myocardium supplied by a stenotic artery as a fraction of normal maximum flow. Its normal value is 1.0, and a value of 0.75 identifies stenosis associated with inducible ischaemia with a high diagnostic accuracy. A recent study has suggested that FFR-based decision-making about revascularization of an intermediate coronary stenosis results in an excellent long-term outcome [7].

Antihypertensive medication was continued as administered previously. The pharmacological treatment combination contents candesartan and a thiazide diureticum. Because of drug-eluting stent implantation, dual platelet inhibition with aspirin and clopidogrel was started and continued for a minimum of 12 months. No further recommendation for risk factor modification was given by the interventional cardiologist.

Question

Did the interventional cardiologist follow the current guidelines for management of patients with stable coronary artery disease and hypertension?

In practice, classification of hypertension and risk assessment should continue to be based on systolic and diastolic blood pressure (Table 8.1). This should be definitely the case for decision concerning the blood pressure threshold and goal for treatment (Fig. 8.4).

For a long time, hypertension guidelines focused on blood pressure values as the only variable determining the need and the type of treatment. The 2013 ESH-ESC Guidelines emphasized that diagnosis and management of hypertension should be related to quantification of global cardiovascular risk [8]. This concept is based on the fact that only a small fraction of the hypertensive population has an elevation of blood pressure alone, with the great majority exhibiting additional cardiovascular risk factors, with a relationship between the severity of the blood pressure elevation and that of alterations in glucose and lipid metabolism. Furthermore, when

Table 8.1   Definitions and classification of blood pressure levels (mmHg) (8)

Category	Systolic		Diastolic
Optimal	< 120	and	< 80
Normal	120–129	and/or	80–84
High normal	130–139	and/or	5–89
Grade 1 hypertension	140–159	and/or	90–99
Grade 2 hypertension	160–179	and/or	100–109
Grade 3 hypertension	≥ 180	and/or	≥ 110
Isolated systolic hypertension	≥ 140	and	< 90

Other risk factors, asymptomatic organ damage or disease	Blood Pressure (mmHg)			
	High normal SBP 130-139 or DBP 85-89	Grade I HT SBP 140-159 or DBP 90-99	Grade 2 HT SBP 160-179 or DBP 100-109	Grade 3 HT SBP ≥180 or DBP ≥110
No other RF		Low risk	Moderate risk	High risk
1-2 RF	Low risk	Μοδερατε ρισκ	Moderate to high risk	High risk
≥3RF	Low to Moderate risk	Moderate to high risk	High Risk	High risk
OD, CKD stage 3 diabetes	Moderate to high risk	High risk	High risk	High to very high risk
Symptomatic CVD, CKD stage ≥4 or diabetes with OD/ RFs	Very high risk		Very high risk	Very high risk

BP = blood pressure; CKD- chronic kidney disease; CV= cardiovascular; CVD= cardiovascular disease; DBP = diastolic blood pressure; HT = hypertension; OD = organ damage; RF = risk factor; SBP = systolic blood pressure.

Fig. 8.4 Stratification of total cardiovascular risk in categories of low, moderate, high and very high risk according to systolic blood pressure and diastolic blood pressure and prevalence of risk factors, asymptomatic organ damage, diabetes, chronic kidney disease stage or symptomatic cardiovascular disease. Subjects with a high normal office but a raised out-of-office blood pressure (masked hypertension) have a cardiovascular risk in the hypertension range. Subjects with a high office blood pressure but normal out-of-office blood pressure (white coat hypertension), particularly if there is no diabetes, organic disease, cardiovascular disease or chronic kidney disease, have lower risk than sustained hypertension for the same office blood pressure (8)

concomitantly present, blood pressure and metabolic risk factors potentate each other, leading to a total cardiovascular risk that is greater than the sum of its individual components [9]. Finally, evidence is available that in high-risk individuals (Fig. 8.4) thresholds and goals for antihypertensive treatment, as well as other treatment strategies, should be different from those to be implemented in lower- or higher-risk individuals (Fig. 8.5a, b). In order to maximize cost-efficacy of the management of hypertension, the intensity of the therapeutic approach should be graded as a function of total cardiovascular risk.

Total cardiovascular disease risk can easily be derived from printed SCORE charts (see illustrations in Fig. 8.5a, b) or additionally from the web where the SCORE system will provide physicians and patients with information on how total risk can be reduced by interventions (both lifestyles and drugs) that have been proven to be efficacious and safe in descriptive cohort studies and/or in randomized controlled trials [9]. The SCORE system also allows the estimation of total cardiovascular disease risk to be projected to age 60 which may be of particular importance for guiding young adults at low absolute risk at the age of 20 or 30 but already with an unhealthy risk profile which will put them at much higher risk when they grow older. Furthermore, both systems allow the use of relative risk estimates that could be of interest in particular cases [9].

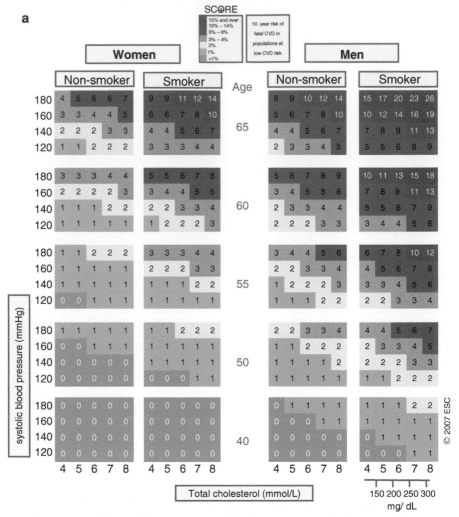

Fig. 8.5 (**a**) SCORE chart: 10-year risk of fatal cardiovascular disease in countries at low cardiovascular disease risk based on the following risk factors: age, sex, smoking, systolic blood pressure and total cholesterol. Note that the risk of total (fatal + nonfatal) cardiovascular disease events will be approximately three times higher than the figures given (9). (**b**) SCORE chart: 10-year risk of fatal cardiovascular disease in countries at high cardiovascular disease risk based on the following risk factors: age, sex, smoking, systolic blood pressure and total cholesterol (9)

b

SC❋RE

15% and over
10% – 14%
5% – 9%
3% – 4%
2%
1%
<1%

10 -year risk of fatal CVD in populations at high CVD risk

Women

| | Non-smoker | Smoker | Age | Men Non-smoker | Smoker |

Women – Non-smoker / Smoker; Age 65

	Non-smoker	Smoker		Non-smoker	Smoker
180	7 8 9 10 12	13 15 17 19 22		14 16 19 22 26	26 30 35 41 47
160	5 5 6 7 8	9 10 12 13 16		9 11 13 15 16	18 21 25 29 34
140	3 3 4 5 6	6 7 8 9 11	65	6 8 9 11 13	13 15 17 20 24
120	2 2 3 3 4	4 5 5 6 7		4 5 6 7 9	9 10 12 14 17

180	4 4 5 6 7	8 9 10 11 13		9 11 13 15 18	18 21 24 28 33
160	3 3 3 4 5	5 6 7 8 9		6 7 9 10 12	12 14 17 20 24
140	2 2 2 3 3	3 4 5 5 6	60	4 5 6 7 9	8 10 12 14 17
120	1 1 2 2 2	2 3 3 4 4		3 3 4 5 6	6 7 8 10 12

180	2 2 3 3 4	4 5 5 6 7		6 7 8 10 12	12 13 16 19 22
160	1 2 2 2 3	3 3 4 4 5		4 5 6 7 8	8 9 11 13 16
140	1 1 1 1 2	2 2 2 3 3	55	3 3 4 5 6	5 6 8 9 11
120	1 1 1 1 1	1 1 2 2 2		2 2 3 3 4	4 4 5 6 8

180	1 1 1 2 2	2 2 3 3 4		4 4 5 6 7	7 8 10 12 14
160	1 1 1 1 1	1 2 2 2 3		2 3 3 4 5	5 6 7 8 10
140	0 1 1 1 1	1 1 1 1 2	50	2 2 2 3 3	3 4 5 6 7
120	0 0 1 1 1	1 1 1 1 1		1 2 2 2	2 3 3 4 5

180	0 0 0 0 0	0 0 0 1 1		1 1 1 2 2	2 2 3 3 4
160	0 0 0 0 0	0 0 0 0 0		1 1 1 1 1	1 2 2 2 3
140	0 0 0 0 0	0 0 0 0 0	40	0 1 1 1 1	1 1 1 2 2
120	0 0 0 0 0	0 0 0 0 0		0 0 1 1 1	1 1 1 1 1

systolic blood pressure (mmHg)

| 4 5 6 7 8 | 4 5 6 7 8 | | 4 5 6 7 8 | 4 5 6 7 8 |

© 2007 ESC

Total cholesterol (mmol/L)

150 200 250 300 mg/ dL

High CVD risk countries are all those not listed under the low risk chart (figure 4). Of these, some are at very high rish and the high riskv chart may underestimate resk in these. These countries are Armenia, Azerbaijan, Belgium, Bulgaria, Georgia, Kazakhstan, Kyrgystan, Latvia, Lithuania, Macedonia FYR, MOdova, Russia, UKraine, and Uzbekistan.

Fig. 8.5 (continued)

Blood pressure is characterized by large spontaneous variations both during the day and between days, months and seasons. Therefore the diagnosis of hypertension should be based on multiple blood pressure measurements, taken on separate occasions over a period of time. If blood pressure is only slightly elevated, repeated measurements should be obtained over a period of several months to define the patients 'usual' blood pressure as accurately as possible. On the other hand, if the patient has a more marked blood pressure elevation, evidence of hypertension-related organ damage or a high- or very-high cardiovascular risk profile, repeated measurements should be obtained over shorter periods of time (weeks or days). In general, the diagnosis of hypertension should be based on at least two blood pressure measurements per visit and at least 2–3 visits although in particularly severe cases the diagnosis can be based on measurements taken at a single visit. 24-h ambulatory blood pressure monitoring is recommended if blood pressure is not acceptable after first treatment.

Treatment can start with a single drug, which should initially be administered at low dose. If blood pressure is not controlled, either a full dose of the initial agent can be given or patients can be switched to an agent of a different class (which should also be administered, first at low and then at full dose). Switching to an agent from a different class is mandatory in case the first agent had no blood pressure lowering or induced important side effects. This 'sequential monotherapy' approach may allow to find the drug to which any individual patient best responds both in terms of efficacy and tolerability. However, although the so-called responder rate (systolic and diastolic blood pressure reduction ≥ 20 and 10 mmHg, respectively) to any agent in monotherapy is approximately 50 %, the ability of any agent used alone to achieve target blood pressure values ($< 140/90$ mmHg) does not exceed 20–30 % of the overall hypertensive population except in subjects with grade 1 hypertension. Furthermore the procedure is laborious and frustrating for both doctors and patients, leading to low compliance and unduly delaying urgent control of blood pressure in high-risk hypertensive patients. Hopes are placed on pharmacogenomics, which in the future may succeed in identifying the drugs having the best chance of being effective and beneficial in individual patients [8, 9].

Antihypertensive drugs of different classes can be combined if (1) they have different and complementary mechanisms of action, (2) there is evidence that the antihypertensive effect of the combination is greater than that of either combination component and (3) the combination may have a favourable tolerance profile, the complementary mechanisms of action of the components minimizing their individual side effects. The following two-drug combinations have been found to be effective and well tolerated and have been favourably used in randomized efficacy trials.

- Thiazide diuretics and ACE inhibitors
- Thiazide diuretics and angiotensin receptor antagonists
- Calcium antagonists and ACE inhibitors
- Calcium antagonists and angiotensin receptor antagonists
- Calcium antagonists and thiazide diuretics
- Beta-blockers and calcium antagonists (e.g. dihydropyridine)

Antihypertensive treatment is also beneficial in hypertensive patients with chronic coronary heart disease. The benefit can be obtained with different drugs and drug combinations (including calcium antagonists) and appears to be related to the degree of blood pressure reduction. A beneficial effect has been demonstrated also when initial blood pressure is $< 140/90$ mmHg and for achieved blood pressure around 130/80 mmHg or less.

In the case of the old lady presenting to other general practitioner with persistent angina after PCI, he did not change the pharmacological treatment prescribed by the interventional cardiologist. But he offered the patient to be admitted to a cardiac rehabilitation programme. She was not sure to agree, because the interventional cardiologist did not recommend such activities to her. Because of persistent symptoms of angina, the lady went back to the general practitioner 6 week later and asked now for participation in an outpatient cardiac rehabilitation programme.

How can an outpatient cardiac rehabilitation programme add to the interventional treatment of angina? First of all antihypertensive medication of this patient was adapted following current guidelines of the management of arterial hypertension. Exercise training within days after PCI is safe. Therefore it is recommended that subjects begin or resume exercise training as soon as possible after the procedure. Care must be taken to assure that angina symptoms are recorded and properly evaluated and that catheterization access sites are healed and stable. Exercise testing may be of considerable value in assessing new or different symptoms or in patients with incomplete revascularization (i.e. those in whom not all stenotic lesions have been dilated) [10].

Exercise is also recommended as a component of the initial treatment of hypertension for as long as 12 months in patients with stage 1 hypertension (140–99 mmHg) with no other coronary risk factors and no evidence of cardiovascular disease and for as long as 6 months in those with one other risk factor, not including diabetes. For patients with diabetes or cardiovascular disease or those with stage 2 or 3 hypertension (160/100 mmHg), drug therapy should be initiated concurrently with exercise and other lifestyle modification programmes [8].

A slight increase in systolic pressure may precede exercise training sessions due to anticipation and is generally not a cause for concern. Incremental increases in systolic blood pressure during exercise are normal, although unusually high blood pressures (> 190 mmHg systolic), particularly during low-level activity, may warrant adjustment in medical therapy. A 10–15 mmHg fall in blood pressure from resting levels during exercise is a cause for concern. Exercise must be discontinued in such instances, and the patient should be further evaluated before returning to training sessions.

After 3 months of exercise training three times a week, the old lady experienced that angina symptoms improved. With a two-drug combination of calcium antagonist and a thiazide diuretic, blood pressure was now 140/90 mmHg. Antihypertensive medication was still maintained.

Regular physical exercise in patients with stable coronary artery disease and angina has been shown to improve myocardial perfusion and to retard disease progression. A randomized study in patients with stable coronary artery disease and angina comparing the effects of exercise training versus standard PCI with stenting showed that exercise training resulted in superior event-free survival and better exercise capacity, notably owing to reduced rehospitalizations and repeat revascularization [11]. This study also adds an important piece of evidence to the rationale for exercise-based cardiac rehabilitation also in patients with stable coronary artery disease and angina. It documents very clearly that an optimized medical therapy together with exercise training as a lifestyle intervention can be an alternative approach to an interventional strategy in selected motivated patients with stable coronary artery disease.

Nevertheless, in most symptomatic patients with stable coronary artery disease and angina, PCI will remain the therapy of choice but should be combined with a more aggressive lifestyle intervention, initiated by exercise-based cardiac rehabilitation. In this sense, PCI not followed by cardiac rehabilitation should be viewed as a suboptimal therapeutic strategy.

Learning objectives of this case:

- Decision-making of PCI in clinically stable patients with coronary artery disease
- Treatment of hypertension
- How to assess cardiovascular risk in patients with hypertension
- Medical treatment of hypertension
- Cardiac rehabilitation in patients with hypertension

References

1. Windecker S, Kolh P, Alfonso F, et al. The task force on myocardial revascularization of the European Society of Cardiology (ESC) and the European Association for Cardio-Thoracic Surgery (EACTS). 2014 ESC/EACTS Guidelines on myocardial revascularization. Eur Heart J. 2014;35:2541–261.
2. Katritsis DG, Ioannidis JP. Percutaneous coronary intervention versus conservative therapy in nonacute coronary artery disease: a meta-analysis. Circulation. 2005;111:2906–12.
3. Boden WE, O'Rourke RA, Teo KK, et al. Optimal medical therapy with or without PCI for stable coronary disease. N Engl J Med. 2007;356:1503–15164.
4. Ades PA. Cardiac rehabilitation and secondary prevention of coronary heart disease. N Engl J Med. 2001;345:892–902.
5. Kastrati A, Dibra S, Eberle A, et al. A sirolimus-eluting stents vs paclitaxel-eluting stents in patients with coronary artery disease: meta-analysis of randomized trials. JAMA. 2005;294:819–25.
6. De Bruyne B, Fearon WF, Pijls NH et al. for the FAME 2 Trial Investigators. Fractional flow reserve-guided PCI for stable coronary artery disease. N Engl J Med. 2014;371(13):1208–1217.
7. Van Nunen LX, Zimmermann FM, Tonino PA et al. for the FAME Study Investigators. Fractional flow reserve versus angiography for guidance of PCI in patients with multivessel coronary artery disease (FAME): 5-year follow-up of a randomised controlled trial. Lancet. 2015;386:1853–1860.
8. Mancia G, Fagard R, Narkiewicz K, et al. For The task Force for the management of arterial hypertension of the European Society of Hypertension (ESH) and of the European Society of Cardiology (ESC). 2013 ESH/ESC guidelines for the management of arterial hypertension. Eur Heart J. 2013;34(28):2159–219.
9. Perk J, De Backer G, Gohlke H, et al. for The Fifth Joint Task Force of the European Society of Cardiology and Other Societies on Cardiovascular Disease Prevention in Clinical Practice. European Guidelines on cardiovascular disease prevention in clinical practice (version 2012). Eur Heart J. 2012;33:1635–701.

10. Fletcher GF, Balady GJ, Ezra A et al. for The American Heart Association Exercise, cardiac rehabilitation, and prevention committee of the council on clinical cardiology, council on nutrition, physical activity and metabolism, council on cardiovascular and stroke nursing, and council on epidemiology and prevention. Exercise standards for testing and training: a scientific statement from the American Heart Association Circulation. 2013;128:873–934.
11. Hambrecht R, Walther C, Möbius-Winkler S, et al. Percutaneous coronary angioplasty compared with exercise training in patients with stable coronary artery disease: a randomized trial. Circulation. 2004;109:1371–8.

Rehabilitation of Patients After CABG/Sternotomy

9

Paul Dendale and Ines Frederix

9.1 Case: Coronary Artery Bypass Surgery

A 64-year old poorly controlled type 2 diabetic patient (HbA1c 10.4 %) is admitted for exercise-induced angina pectoris. He is known with a history of COPD GOLD II (Tiffeneau index 61 %, FEV1 55 % predicted) and still smokes 10–15 cigarettes/day. His cholesterol is 270 mg/dl, he weighs 117 kg for 1.69 m (BMI, 41 kg/m²) and his blood pressure is 165/95 mmHg. He suffers from chronic kidney disease stage IIIa (GFR, 50 ml/min/1.73 m²).

He is currently treated with metformin 850 mg bd and bisoprolol 5 mg od. On admission, troponines remain normal, and a coronary angiography shows multivessel coronary artery disease including (1) a proximal complex LAD lesion and (2) a 90 % stenosis of the RCA. Echocardiography shows a moderate LV hypertrophy (IVS 1.5 cm, PW 1.4 cm, LV mass index 118 g/m², relative wall thickness (RWT) 0.45) with a preserved systolic function (EF, 60 %; biplane Simpson's method).

P. Dendale (✉)
Faculty of Medicine and Life Sciences, Hasselt University, Hasselt, Belgium
Department of Cardiology, Jessa Hospital, Hasselt, Belgium
e-mail: paul.dendale@jessazh.be

I. Frederix
Faculty of Medicine and Life Sciences, Hasselt University, Hasselt, Belgium
Department of Cardiology, Jessa Hospital, Hasselt, Belgium
Faculty of Medicine and Health Sciences, Antwerp University, Antwerp, Belgium

© Springer International Publishing AG 2017
J. Niebauer (ed.), *Cardiac Rehabilitation Manual*,
DOI 10.1007/978-3-319-47738-1_9

Classical coronary artery bypass surgery was the initially suggested option, based on the coronary angiography findings.

Question

Which risk factors for pulmonary complications are present in this patient, and how can they be modified by the rehabilitation team?

Answer

1. Current smoking: Several trials have shown that patients who continue to smoke in the immediate preoperative period have a significant increase in pulmonary complications, wound healing problems and a longer stay in the intensive care unit. An intervention study in orthopaedic patients showed that a six-week period of smoking cessation significantly reduces these risks. The rehabilitation team should stress the importance of smoking cessation and propose treatment with bupropion or vareniclin. An individual support increases the chances of successful abstinence. As the patient is stable, the surgery can safely be postponed for several weeks.

2. The presence of reduced pulmonary function: As the median sternotomy which is typically used in bypass surgery is known to reduce the vital capacity in the first weeks after surgery, patients with a reduced pulmonary function are at risk of respiratory insufficiency in the postoperative period. Optimal treatment by betamimetic inhalation and if necessary inhaled corticoid or an oral course of corticosteroids is advised. Preoperative testing of inspiratory muscle strength can be useful to detect those patients who might have benefit of preoperative inspiratory muscle strength training exercises. Studies [1–4] have shown that a six-week training program for the inspiratory muscles decreases postoperative complications.

3. Obesity: Vital capacity is further reduced by obesity, which increases the risk of pulmonary complications. Obesity is known as one of the risk factors for perioperative complications, and preoperative weight reduction has been shown to result in better postoperative recovery [5]. Therefore if the surgery can be postponed safely for weeks, an individual preoperative follow-up by a dietician may be useful. Using a short course of a protein diet, 5–10 kg of weight loss can be obtained.

4. Insufficiently treated diabetes: In long-standing diabetes, the risks of slow or incomplete healing of the sternotomy are a typical complication in case of bilateral mammary artery bypass grafting. The devascularisation of the sternum increases the risk of sternum dehiscence in the postoperative period, compromising pulmonary function even further. Optimal treatment of diabetes for several weeks by weight loss, low-intensity physical activity and adapted medical treatment are necessary for several weeks before surgery. Mechanical support systems (e.g. SternaSafe) are promoted as means to decrease this risk further in the first days after the operation.

Case Part 2

The patient is referred to ambulatory cardiac rehabilitation 5 days after a 3-week stay in the hospital for two vessel bypass operations. The postoperative phase was complicated by respiratory distress necessitating reintubation and ventilation for 7 days. He still feels weak and is out of breath when walking from the parking lot to the rehabilitation centre. When speaking, he needs to stop regularly to breathe. He also mentions paresthesias left of the sternotomy scar, an intermittent "rocking" sensation in his chest and pain between the shoulder blades. Clinical examination shows a heart rate of 115/min (irregular pulse), reduced breathing sounds over the left lung and swelling of both ankles. The scars all are healing well, but on palpitation, crepitations are felt next to the sternotomy scar. An ECG before discharge shows atrial fibrillation, diffuse repolarisation abnormalities and no signs of infarction; an echocardiography reveals a slightly reduced systolic function (EF, 50 %; biplane Simpson's method) and no pericardial fluid.

Question

Which is a possible reason for the dyspnoea in this patient?

1. Pleural fluid accumulation: Pleural effusions are common after sternotomy (up to 60 % of patients show some signs of pleural effusion in the first postoperative week) [6]. They can occur during hospitalisation, but sometimes also occur or increase during the ambulatory cardiac rehabilitation programme. Pleural effusions after sternotomy most often occur in the left pleura. The aetiology can be diverse: pleurotomy (for harvesting of the mammary artery), topical cooling with ice, inflammation (post-pericardiotomy syndrome, often occurring several weeks after the operation and accompanied by signs of inflammation, pain and fever) or heart failure (in this case, pleural fluid accumulates more symmetrically on both sides).
2. Reduced pulmonary function: Sternotomy has been shown to cause an important acute reduction in pulmonary function [7]. A mean reduction in vital capacity and expiratory flows of approximately 30 % in the first weeks after the operation is described in the literature. The spontaneous evolution after 3 months is not always towards a complete resolution. In some patients, the reduced pulmonary function persists at one-year follow-up. Possible causes for this reduction are a change in breathing pattern (more upper thoracic breathing instead of abdominal breathing) [8], lack of coordination of the rib cage movement [9], pleural effusion, paralysis or paresis of a haemidiaphragm due to injury to the phrenic nerve (often in case of ice cooling of the heart of mammary artery harvesting; can be diagnosed with an EMG of the phrenic nerve). Studies have shown that postoperative reduction of pulmonary function is more frequent after mammary artery surgery [10], possibly due to the use of the internal mammary artery retractor. In severe cases, sternal instability is a cause of persistently reduced pulmonary function [11, 12]

Table 9.1 Results from
initial CPET

Load max	194 Watt	
VO$_2$ max	20 ml/min/kg	78 % pred
HR max	102 bpm	62 % pred
RER max	1.21	
VE max	94 L/min	110 % pred
VE/VCO$_2$ slope	42	
πO$_2$	21.2 ml	107 % pred
FEV1	2.18 L	55 % pred
FVC	3.02 L	60 % pred
Tiffeneau index	58 %	

VO$_2$ oxygen uptake, *HR* heart rate, *RER* respiratory
exchange ratio, *VE* minute ventilation, *πO$_2$* oxygen pulse,
FEV1 forced expiratory volume in 1 second, *FVC* forced
vital capacity

Fig. 9.1 Chest X-ray
illustrating evident blunting
of the left costodiaphrag-
matic sinus, typical for a
pleural effusion

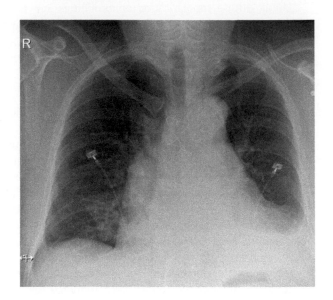

Question

An initial cardiopulmonary exercise test (CPET) was conducted, the results of
which are shown in Table 9.1. What can we learn from this CPET?

When interpreting the CPET results, we can conclude that it was a maximal
exercise test (RER max, 1.21; HR max, 62 % pred; VR = VE max/MVV = 108 %)
with ventilatory, rather than cardiovascular limitation and a reduced aerobic capacity (VO$_2$ max, 78 % pred).

Cardiovascular parameters confirmed a normal blood pressure evolution during the
CPET (not shown), a normal oxygen pulse and therapy-induced chronotropic incompetence. Ventilatory parameters revealed a mixed restrictive-obstructive lung function, an abnormally elevated VE/VCO2 slope and ventilatory exercise test limitation.

Based on these findings there was a high suspicion for a pleural effusion, which
was later confirmed by RxTx (Fig. 9.1).

Question

What can be done in the rehabilitation setting?

Diagnosis: Heightened suspicion for common complications is needed in the first weeks of ambulatory rehabilitation. Clinical examination in patients complaining of persistent dyspnoea or showing a lack of normal progression in the exercise load will easily exclude significant pleural effusion, severe paralysis of a haemidiaphragm or obstructive lung disease. An ergospirometry performed in the first weeks after the start of ambulatory rehabilitation will very often show 30–40 % reduction in the maximal tidal volume during exercise, but this tends to normalise during the program. A control ergospirometry in patients showing lack of progress will allow to differentiate between pulmonary and other causes. Further examinations can be done as needed (Rx Thorax, pleurocentesis, echocardiography, pulmonary function tests EMG of the phrenic nerve).

Rehabilitative therapy: It is not yet well known which physiotherapy techniques significantly influence the natural course of the pulmonary function after sternotomy [13, 14]. Most pleural effusions tend to disappear spontaneously or after a short course of anti-inflammatory drugs; in some cases, recurrent pleurocenteses or even pleurodesis is necessary. Hemidiaphragm paralysis due to phrenic nerve injury recovers spontaneously in 70–90 % of patients [15]. In severe cases, surgical intervention with plicage of the diaphragm is proposed [15]. Preoperative inspiratory muscle training [3, 4] can be a good technique to reduce the risk of postoperative pulmonary complications in patients with a compromised pulmonary function. If there is a place for postoperative respiratory muscle training remains to be determined. In some cases of reduced pulmonary function due to persistent respiration-dependent pain, a consultation with an osteopath can be of help to some patients [16].

Case (Part 3)

Which are the other rehabilitation problems that need attention in the first weeks after the start of the rehab program in this patient?

1. Sternal wound healing: Externally, the wounds seem to heal well, but the sensation of movement at the sternal level, especially when provoked by changing position in bed, could point to incomplete healing of the bone. Crepitations felt during palpation next to the sternal wound are a clinical sign suggesting delayed healing. Delayed healing of the sternum is more frequent in patients after bilateral mammary artery operations and diabetics. In cases where sternal instability is suspected, all (asymmetrical) exercises with the upper limbs should be avoided until complete healing. In some cases, some instability persists; in severe cases, a refixation can be planned. The pain between the shoulder blades are a typical complication of sternotomy: the costovertebral joints are stressed importantly, with local bleeding, partial dislocation and an inflammatory process as a consequence of the opening of the chest during the operation. Painkillers may be required to

allow the patient to sleep normally in the first weeks. Studies in our lab have shown that after a classical rehabilitation programme, some pain and reduced mobility persist in up to one third of the patients even 15 months after the operation. This may be related to the presence of a pleural drain and/or the exposure of the internal mammary artery. Up to now, it is not known which is the optimal therapy for these low-grade persistent pain problems: mobilisation exercises may have a place in the treatment, but definitive studies are lacking. In our rehabilitation centre, patients with persistent thoracic cage or spine problems are referred for advice by an osteopath.

2. Heart rate: The heart rate suggests recurrence of atrial fibrillation (AF), which is very common after cardiac surgery [17, 18]. Up to 60 % of patients experience an often self-limiting episode of AF in the first days after operation, but during the ambulatory rehabilitation, it is much less frequent. Patients presenting in the rehabilitation unit with AF should be treated by anticoagulation and antiarrhythmic drugs or cardioversion. The rehabilitation setting is a very good place to detect these recurrences. Some categories of patients are more prone to recurrences and need to be checked regularly: mitral valve operations, COPD, obese patients, reduced systolic function, elderly patients, patients not treated with beta-blockers, etc.

3. Obesity: After complicated surgery, it is not the ideal moment to immediately start a calorie-restricted diet. Also, more and more evidence is accumulating regarding the different roles of overweight and/or obesity in primary versus secondary prevention for cardiovascular disease (the so-called obesity paradigm) [19, 20]. In secondary prevention the optimum body weight is shifting to a higher BMI range, to appreciate the association of higher body weight and outcome in cardiovascular disease. Lifestyle recommendations for patients who are overweight/obese should be made, with more careful consideration of the often catabolic condition of chronic cardiovascular disease and may be more focused on encouraging exercise and a healthy diet that may not necessarily include caloric restriction.

4. Swollen ankles: Swelling of the ankles is a frequent phenomenon after exposure of veins for bypass surgery. Normally, the swelling disappears spontaneously after 6–12 weeks, even without intervention. Diuretics are not advised, as they can cause disturbances of electrolytes and renal function and may reduce the blood pressure, which is often low in the first 4–6 weeks after CABG. Support stockings reduce traction on the scars in the legs and are advised to be used during daytime until swelling disappears

5. Hypotension: Patients after coronary bypass surgery often show a reduced blood pressure in the first weeks after rehabilitation. This reduction in blood pressure is multifactorial (bed rest, reduced food and fluid intake, blood pressure-lowering treatment, etc.). This can give rise to orthostatic reactions if the preoperative antihypertensive therapy is not (temporarily)

reduced. In most cases, the blood pressure returns to its preoperative value 6–8 weeks after surgery, and the antihypertensive therapy will therefore often be reduced in the beginning of the rehabilitation program, while increasing treatment is needed at the end of the programme. In the meantime, advice concerning low-salt food should be given.

6. Postoperative peripheral neuropathies [21–23]: The majority of neuropathies occur as a consequence of entrapment or elongation of a part of the root of the plexus brachialis (nervus ulnaris) or of the peroneal nerve and are apparent only in the postoperative stage (often seen only in ambulatory rehabilitation):

(a) Brachial plexus palsy: With an incidence of 5 and 24 %, it is mainly caused by the positioning of the arm (or both arms) in abduction (90°) and external rotation (30°) during surgery [13, 16, 24]. This combination puts the plexus in a maximal stretch situation. The retraction of the sternum and possible fractures of the first rib are also described as causal factors [16]. The plexus stretch can be further accentuated by turning the head of the patient into the contralateral direction. Exposure of the internal mammary artery, necessitating a greater retraction of the chest wall, has also been mentioned as a causal factor. In most patients especially, the lower roots (giving rise to the ulnar nerve) are injured and general pain is the primary complaint. Medical assessment is by electromyographic evaluation of the brachial plexus region. The majority of the patients also need to be included in an extensive physiotherapeutical treatment. Nevertheless the functional recovery process of the injured nerve is often complete after an average convalescence period between 3 weeks and maximum 1 year.

(b) Peroneal nerve injury [24]: The prevalence of this postoperative nerve lesion is rare: literature sources mention an incidence of 0.30 % [13] up to 6 % [24]. In most cases the problem is attributed to excessive external rotation of the leg(s) and/or the hip(s) during surgery. Considering the superficial location of the peroneal nerve(s) compression around the head of the fibula can be expected. In most of the cases, the injury is unilateral (59 %) [13], and the patient experiences reduced dorsal flexion of the ankle as well as impairments of skin sensitivity and pain. Electromyographic evaluation is recommended, but as the first signs of nerve denervation are visible at earliest 10 up to 14 days after the first occurrence of the peripheral nerve lesion, the examination needs to be postponed to the third postoperative week. In spite of the fact that the prognosis of this problem is good in most cases, some cases with a long-term impairment of the nerve function are reported. For both neurological disorders, some comorbidity problems such as diabetes, older age, subnormal body weight and the duration of the operation can have a significant negative influence [13, 14, 16, 24].

Case (Part 4)

The patient suffered from several postoperative problems. Are there novel treatment options that could prevent some of these?

Minimally invasive coronary artery bypass grafting has become an interesting alternative to conventional coronary artery bypass grafting [25–29], not necessitating the midline sternotomy. The endoscopic atraumatic coronary artery bypass (endo-ACAB) can be differentiated from the endoscopic coronary artery bypass grafting (endo-CABG) and the hybrid coronary revascularisation. In endo-ACAB, an off-pump bypass is created between the LIMA and LAD through multiple small holes (Fig. 9.2). In endo-CABG, an on-pump bypass is created between both the LIMA, RIMA and > 1 stenotic/occluded coronary arteries. Hybrid revascularisation combines minimally invasive coronary artery bypass surgery (of the LAD) and a percutaneous coronary intervention of a non-LAD lesion [30]. These novel treatment options have the advantage of reducing perioperative blood loss, postoperative pain, hospital admission duration and accelerating patient recovery and return to work [31].

Theoretically these minimally invasive care strategies could be recommended for patients with an eligible coronary anatomy, who are considered too high risk for open cardiopulmonary bypass surgery via midline sternotomy, including those with a high risk of deep sternal wound infection (diabetes mellitus, morbid obesity), severely impaired left ventricular systolic function, chronic kidney disease, significant carotid or neurological disease, severe aortic calcification, prior sternotomy and lack of venous conduits [32].

The patient presented here was morbidly obese and suffered from diabetes mellitus type 2 and chronic kidney disease. The coronary angiography showed a proximal complex LAD lesion and a 90 % stenosis of the RCA, a lesion pattern eligible for hybrid revascularisation. He was symptomatic postoperatively (dyspnoea on exertion NYHA II–III) and presented with sternal wound healing problems, atrial fibrillation and peripheral neuropathy. Research in the authors' own cardiac rehabilitation centre confirmed minimal invasive bypass procedures to result in reduced wound problems and reduced pain [33]. Future research should focus on the effect of these new treatment options on the other hazards associated with conventional bypass grafting.

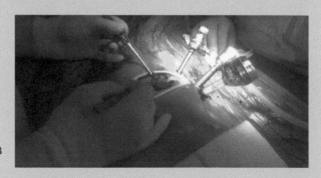

Fig. 9.2 Endo-ACAB procedure

Case (Part 5)
The patient restarts rehabilitation after electrical conversion of his atrial fibrillation to sinus rhythm. His program consists of three times weekly moderate continuous exercise training (5 min. warm-up, 30 min. at an intensity between the 1st and 2nd ventilatory thresholds and a 5 min. cool-down), educational sessions and psychological counselling. After six and twelve weeks of training, follow-up visits are planned in which repeat CPETs are performed. At both follow-up visits, the aerobic capacity improves steadily.

Question

What is specific about the cardiac rehabilitation program in cardiac surgery patients?

1. Preoperative preparation: smoking cessation at least six weeks prior to surgery, inspiratory muscle training for six weeks preoperatively in patients at high risk of respiratory complications.
2. Attention to wound healing: not infrequently, delayed healing of the sternal or saphenectomy wounds is present, which may cause difficulties in the first weeks of training. On the other hand, the avoidance of weight lifting for the first weeks after surgery causes a more pronounced atrophy of the muscles of the thorax and shoulder girdle. This is important for patients who have a job which demands significant strength. In this population, the training programme should incorporate strengthening exercises of the upper limbs starting from week 6 after surgery (when healing is complete) [34].
3. In some centres patients are invited for ambulatory rehabilitation only after a waiting period of 6–12 weeks, to allow for complete healing of the sternum. Unpublished data from our centre shows that an early start of an adapted rehabilitation programme (1–2 weeks after discharge) is safe and speeds up recovery without causing an increase in sternal problems. Also psychological recovery is helped by an early start of rehabilitation.
4. Vocational counselling is important after cardiac surgery, as many patients have doubts about their ability to return to work. The rehabilitation team should identify those patients who might have difficulties by specifically asking for it at the start of the rehabilitation programme. The training programme as well as the psychological counselling should be adapted to the specific demands of the job, and early contact with the company doctor is useful to increase the chances of a successful reintegration in the work setting. In cardiac surgery patients, a part-time return to work (with continued rehabilitation during this transition period) can be helpful

Case (Part 6)

After successful completion of the cardiac rehabilitation programme, the patient was advised to continue exercise training, to conform to guidelines introduced earlier during centre-based cardiac rehabilitation and also to sustain the prescribed healthy lifestyle behaviour. Despite the patient's good intentions, at the one-year follow-up visit, a return to prior unhealthy lifestyle and deterioration of aerobic capacity was noted (Fig. 9.3).

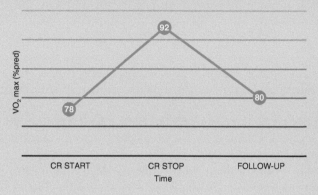

Fig. 9.3 Evolution of VO$_2$ max during patient follow-up. VO$_2$, oxygen consumption; CR start, start of cardiac rehabilitation program; CR stop, end of cardiac rehabilitation program; follow-up: VO$_2$ at one-year follow-up visit

Question

What can we do to enable cardiac patients to sustain health lifestyle behaviour and aerobic capacity?

Despite the proven effectiveness of classical cardiac rehabilitation programmes for coronary artery disease patients, long-term benefits are often poor. This is mainly due to lack of adherence to prescribed secondary prevention programme lifestyle behaviour and exercise training [35]. As demonstrated in the GOSPEL trial, a multifactorial continued reinforced intervention for coronary artery disease patients can improve long-term cardiovascular risk factor control, healthy lifestyle habits and pharmacological therapy compliance [36]. Also, novel care delivery strategies such as cardiac telerehabilitation have been put forward as a valid means to improve patient's adherence to secondary prevention guidelines [37]. In telerehabilitation, the patient is not restricted to the hospital or rehabilitation centre environment for cardiac rehabilitation but rehabilitates remotely by using one or several devices monitoring and communicating patient-specific information to the caregivers. These caregivers in turn have the possibility to provide patients with tailored feedback by email, SMS and/or messages included in a mobile smartphone-based application, based on received data. Prior research (Telerehab II and Telerehab III trials) concluded that an additional patient-specific, comprehensive telerehabilitation programme can lead to a bigger improvement in both physical fitness (VO2peak) and associated health-related quality of life, compared to centre-based cardiac rehabilitation alone at one-year follow-up [38–40]. The cardiac telereabilitation programme reduced cardiovascular readmission rates and proved to be cost-effective (incremental cost-effectiveness ratio [ICER] = -21,707 €/QALY) [41].

Conclusion

A specific cardiac rehabilitation early after cardiac surgery is very important to help the patient in his/her recovery. Attention to typical postoperative complications and the psychological response to the surgery as well as a training programme adapted to the physical possibilities of the patient are needed. In patients too high risk for open coronary artery bypass surgery via midline sternotomy, including those at risk of deep sternal wound infection, minimally invasive alternatives (endo-ACAB, endo-CABG, hybrid revascularisation) can be considered. Novel care delivery strategies such as cardiac telerehabilitation provide a valid means to improve cardiac patients' long-term adherence to secondary prevention programme recommendations.

References

1. Dronkers J, Veldman A, Hoberg E, der Waal C V. Prevention of pulmonary complications after upper abdominal surgery by preoperative intensive inspiratory muscle training: a randomizes controlled pilot study. Clin Rehabil. 2008;22:134–42.
2. Nomori H, Kobayashi R, Fuyuno G, Morinaga S, Yashima H. Preoperative respiratory muscle training. Assessment in thoracic surgery patients with special reference to postoperative pulmonary complications. Chest. 1994;105:1782–8.
3. Hulzebos EH, Helders PJM, Favié NJ, De Bie RA, de la Rivière A B, NLU VM. Preoperative intensive inspiratory muscle training to prevent postoperative pulmonary complications in high risk patients undergoing CABG surgery. JAMA. 2006;296:1851–7.
4. Hulzebos EH, Van Meeteren NLU, van den Buijs BJWM, de Bie RA, de la Rivière A B, PJM H. Feasibility of preoperative inspiratory muscle training in patients undergoing coronary artery bypass surgery with high risk of postoperative pulmonary complications: a randomised controlled pilot study. Clin Rehabil. 2006;20:949–59.
5. Fasol R, Schindler M, Schumacher B, Schlaudraff K, Hannes W, Seitelberger R, Schlosser V. The influence of obesity on perioperative morbidity: retrospective study of 502 aortocoronary bypass operations. Thorac Cardiovasc Surg. 1992;40:126–9.
6. Light RW. Pleural effusions after coronary artery bypass graft surgery. Curr Opin Pulm Med. 2002;8:308.
7. Shenkman Z, Shir Y, Weiss YG, Bleiberg B, Gross D. The effects of cardiac surgery on early and late pulmonary functions. Acta Anaesthesiol Scand. 1997;41:1193–9.
8. Ragnarsdóttir M, Kristjánsdóttir Á, Ingvarsdóttir I, Hannesson P, Torfason B, Cahalin LP. Short-term changes in pulmonary function and respiratory movements after cardiac surgery via median sternotomy. Scand Cardiovasc J. 2004;38:46–52.
9. Locke TJ, Griffiths TL, Mould H, Gibson GJ. Rib cage mechanics after median sternotomy. Thorax. 1990;45:465–8.
10. Wheatcroft M, Shrivastava V, Nyawo B, Rostron A, Dunning J. Does pleurotomy during internal mammary artery harvest increase post-operative pulmonary complications? Interactive CardioVasc Thorac Surg. 2005;4:143–6.

11. El-Ansari D, Waddington G, Adams R. Relationship between pain and upper limb movement in patients with chronic sternal instability following cardiac surgery. Physiother Theory Pract. 2007;23:273–80.

12. El-Ansari D, Adams R, Toms L, Elkins M. Sternal instability following coronary artery bypass grafting. Physiother Theory and Pract. 2000;16:27–33.

13. Matte P, Jacquet L, Van Dyck M, Goenen M. Effects of conventional physiotherapy, continuous positive airway pressure and non-invasive ventilatory support with bilevel positive airway pressure after coronary artery bypass grafting. Acta Anaesthesiol Scand. 2000;44(1):75–81.

14. Crowe JM, Bradley CA. The effectiveness of incentive spirometry with physical therapy for high-risk patients after coronary artery bypass surgery. Phys Ther. 1997;77:260–8.

15. Tripp H, Bolton R. Phrenic nerve injury following cardiac surgery: a review. J Card Surg. 1998;13:218–23.

16. O-Yurvati AH, Carnes MS, Clearfield MB, Stoll ST, McConathy WJ. Hemodynamic effects of osteopathic manipulative treatment immediately after coronary artery bypass graft surgery. J Am Osteopath Assoc. 2005;105(10):475–81.

17. D. Bharucha, R. Marinchak. Arrhythmias after cardiac sugery: atrial fibrillation and atrial flutter. UpToDate. Version 16.3. Oktober 2008.

18. Maisel R, Stevenson WG. Atrial fibrillation after cardiac surgery. Ann Intern Med. 2001;135:1061.

19. Doehner W, von Haehling S, Anker S. Protective overweight in cardiovascular disease: moving from 'paradox' to 'paradigm'. Eur Heart J. 2015;36:2729–32.

20. Angeras O, Albertsson P, Karason K, Ramunddal T, Matejka G, James S, Lagerqvist B, Rosengren OE. Evidence for obesity paradox in patients with acute coronary syndromes: a report from the Swedish Coronary Angiography and Angioplasty Registry. Eur Heart J. 2012;34:345–53.

21. Dawson DM et al. Perioperative Nerve Lesions. Arch Neurol. 1989;46:1355–60.

22. Sharma AD et al. Peripheral nerve injuries during cardiac surgery. risk factors, diagnosis, prognosis, and prevention. Anesth Analg. 2000;91:1358–69.

23. Lederman RJ et al. Peripheral nervous system complications of coronary artery bypass graft surgery. Ann Neurol. 1982;12(3):297–301.

24. Vasquez-Jimenez JF et al. Injury of the common peroneal nerve after cardiothoracic operations. The Ann Thorac Surg. 2002;73:119–22.

25. Kettering K. Minimally invasive direct coronary artery bypass grafting: a meta-analysis. J Cardiovasc Surg (Torino). 2008;49:793–800.

26. Head J, Kieser T, Falk V, Huysmans H, Kappetein A. Coronary artery bypass grafting: Part 1-the evolution over the first 50 years. Eur Heart J. 2013;34:2862–72.

27. Bonatti J, Lehr E, Schachner T, et al. Robotic total endoscopic double-vessel coronary artery bypass grafting-state of procedure development. J Thorac Cardiovasc Surg. 2012;144:1061–6.

28. Wiedemann D, Bonaros N, Schachner T, et al. Surgical problems and complex procedures: Issues for operative time in robotic totally endoscopic coronary artery bypass grafting. J Thorac Cardiovasc Surg. 2012;143:639–47.

29. Argenziano M, Katz M, Bonatti J, et al. Results of the prospective multicenter trial of robotically assisted totally endoscopic coronary artery bypass grafting. Ann Thorac Surg. 2006;81:1666–75.

30. Panoulas V, Colombo A, Margonato A, Maisano F. Hybrid coronary revascularization. Promising, but yet to take off. J Am Coll Cardiol. 2015;65:85–97.

31. Bonatti J, Zimrin D, Lehr E, et al. Hybrid coronary revascularization using robotic totally endoscopic surgery: perioperative outcomes and 5-year results. Ann Thorac Surg. 2012;94:1920–6.

32. Bonatti J, Lehr E, Vesely M, Friedrich G, Bonaros N, Zimrin D. Hybrid coronary revascularization: which patients? When? How? Curr Opin Cardiol. 2010;25:568–74.

33. Hansen D, Roijakkers R, Jackmaert L, Robic B, Hendrikx M, Yilmaz A, Frederix I, Rosseel M, Dendale P. Compromised cardiopulmonary exercise capacity in patients early after endoscopic

atraumatic CABG (endo-ACAB) surgery: implications for rehabilitation and treatment. 2016 Submitted.

34. Bjarnason-Wehrens B, Mayer-Berger W, Meister ER, Baum K, Hambrecht R, Gielen S. Recommendations for resistance exercise in cardiac rehabilitation. Recommendations of the German federation for cardiovascular prevention and rehabilitation. Eur J Cardiovasc Prev Rehabil. 2004;11:352–61.

35. Hansen D, Dendale P, Raskin A, Schoonis A, Berger J, Vlassak I, Meeusen R. Long-term effect of rehabilitation in coronary artery disease patients: randomized clinical trial of the impact of exercise volume. Clin Rehabil. 2010;24:319–27.

36. Giannuzzi P, Temporelli P, Marchioli R, Maggioni A, Balestroni G, Ceci V, Chieffo C, Gattone M, Griffo R, Schweiger C, Tavazzi L, Urbinati S, Valagussa F, Vanuzzo D. Global secondary prevention strategies to limit event recurrence after myocardial infarction results of the GOSPEL Study, a multicenter, randomized controlled trial from the Italian Cardiac Rehabilitation Network. Arch Intern Med. 2008;168:2194–204.

37. Frederix I, Vanhees L, Dendale P, et al. A review of telerehabilitation for cardiac patients. J Telemed Telecare. 2015;21:45–53.

38. Frederix I, Van Driessche N, Dendale P, et al. Increasing the medium-term benefits of hospital-based cardiac rehabilitation by physical activity telemonitoring in coronary artery disease patients. Eur J Prev Cardiol. 2015;22:150–8.

39. Frederix I, Van Craenenbroeck EM, Vrints C, et al. Telerehab III: a multi-center randomized, controlled trial investigating the long-term effectiveness of a comprehensive cardiac telerehabilitation program - Rationale and study design. BMC Cardiovasc Disord. 2015;15(1):29.

40. Frederix I, Hansen D, Van Craenenbroeck E, et al. Medium-term effectiveness of an internet-based, comprehensive and patient--specific telerehabilitation program with short message service support for cardiac patients: randomized controlled trial. J Med Internet Res. 2015;17(7):e185.

41. Frederix I, Hansen D, Van Craenenbroeck E, et al. Effect of comprehensive cardiac telerehabilitation on 1-year cardiovascular rehospitalisation rate, medical costs and quality of life: a cost-effectiveness analysis. Eur J Prev Cardiol. 2015; [Epub ahead of print]

Congestive Heart Failure: Stable Chronic Heart Failure Patients

10

Massimo F. Piepoli

10.1 Learning Objectives

The learning objectives of this case are as follows:

- Knowing neglected causes of heart failure
- Knowing the benefit of optimised medical treatment in heart failure
- Knowing the benefit of cardiac rehabilitation and secondary prevention in heart failure patients
- Knowing the indication of exercise prescription heart failure patient

Case History

December 2007.

A 64-year-old male patient arrived at the emergency department because of recent occurrence of shortness of breath, started in the last 2 months, but progressive, and most recently very severe disabling, since it was appearing for mild exercise. The last day the dyspnoea was presenting even at rest and during the night, such as paroxysmal nocturnal dyspnoea. This was associated with severe palpitation at rest.

M.F. Piepoli
Heart Failure Unit, Cardiology, Guglielmo da Saliceto Hospital, 29121 Piacenza, Italy
e-mail: m.piepoli@alice.it

© Springer International Publishing AG 2017
J. Niebauer (ed.), *Cardiac Rehabilitation Manual*,
DOI 10.1007/978-3-319-47738-1_10

When interrogated by the triage nurse, he denied any relevant event in his past and no cardiovascular events in his relatives (parents, brothers and sisters), but he admitted the presence of important risk factors: he was taking no exercise at all, he was slightly overweight (88 kg, 175 cm height, BMI 28.7) and during the last 4 years, he was on blood pressure medications (ramipril 5 mg od in the morning). On admission, his blood pressure was 100/70 mmHg, heart rate around 100 beats/min, no body temperature and O_2 saturation 96.5 %.

On physical examination the physician recorded that he was pale, slightly sweating, hyperventilating, with orthopnoea, an irregularly irregular pulse and peripheral ankle oedema. At the heart examination, the apex was slightly displaced on the left and a moderate, pansystolic murmur was heard on the apex, while on the lung examination, bilateral rales within the mid- and basal fields.

As first measure, the physician asked for an ECG (Fig. 10.1), a chest X-ray (Fig. 10.2) and routine blood test, which included full blood count, serum electrolyte concentration, kidney function markers, b-type natriuretic peptide (BNP) and cardiac enzymes (Fig. 10.3).

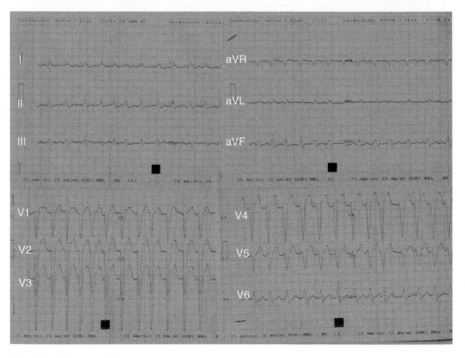

Fig. 10.1 Electrocardiogram

Fig. 10.2 Chest X-ray

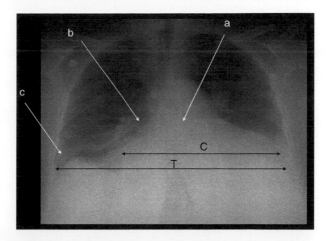

Fig. 10.3 Blood test

Blood test	Value	Reference value
Hb	13.1 gr/dl	13-17
Hct	41.1 %	40-52
BUN	65 mg/dl	10-50
Creatinine	1.56 mg/dl	0.6-1.4
Na	131.0 mEq/l	135-146
K	3.2 mEq/l	3.6-5.0
Cl	101 mEq/l	97-110
GOT/AST	38 U/l	10-31
GPT/ALT	40 U/l	10-31
LDH	189 U/l	120-240
CK/CPK	161 U/l	<149
CK MB	3.1 ng/ml	<2.8
Tn 1	0.3 ng/ml	<0.1
BNP	525 pg/ml	<100

10.2 Tests

10.2.1 12 Lead ECG (Fig. 10.1)

Report

Absence of regular atrial activity. Irregular and abnormally elevated ventricular rate, i.e. 147 /min: [normal value of heart rate: 50–100 /min]. Normal QRS axis: +60°. Abnormal QRS prolongation (110 ms), with repolarisation abnormalities compatible with incomplete left bundle branch block (LBBB) (Table 10.1).

Table 10.1 The criteria to diagnose a LBBB on the ECG

The heart rhythm must be supraventricular in origin

The QRS duration must be ≥ 120 ms

There should be a QS or RS complex in lead V1

There should be a monophasic R wave in leads I and V6

The T wave should be deflected opposite the terminal deflection of the QRS complex. This is known as appropriate T wave discordance with bundle branch block. A concordant T wave may suggest ischaemia or myocardial infarction

In our case: QRS duration was 110 ms, so the diagnosis of incomplete LBBB. T wave was concordant suggesting ischaemia.

In conclusion: Atrial fibrillation with elevated heart rate response. Ventricular repolarisation compatible with left ventricular overload / subendocardial ischaemia.

10.2.2 Chest X-Ray Anterior-Posterior View (Fig. 10.2)

Report

Enlarged heart: cardio/thoracic ratio >0.5 (reference value [r.v.] < 0.5); bilateral pulmonary congestion; bilateral pleural fluid accumulation

10.2.3 Blood Test (Fig. 10.3)

Report

Normal haemoglobin level, mild kidney dysfunction (creatinine and nitrogen elevation), electrolyte concentration reduction, elevated values of BNP, normal values of cardiac enzymes.

On the basis of these results, to confirm the diagnosis of heart failure, following the ESC Guidelines on Heart Failure, [1] it was decided to take an echocardiographic examination (Figs. 10.4 and 10.5).

10.2.4 Echocardiography-2D Parasternal View (Fig. 10.4)
10.2.5 Echocardiography-2D and Colour Doppler, Two-Chamber, Apical View (Fig. 10.5)
10.2.6 Echocardiography Parasternal View (Figs. 10.4 and 10.5)

Report

A poorly contracting, enlarged left ventricle is evident [end diastolic diameter 65 mm (r.v. < 45 mm), end systolic diameter 55 mm (r.v. < 35 mm), ejection fraction 28 % (r.v. > 55 %)] with enlarged left atrium (46 mm; r.v. < 40 mm). Instead, normal wall thickness of IVS (9 mm) and posterior wall (8 mm) (r.v. < 11 mm) are present.

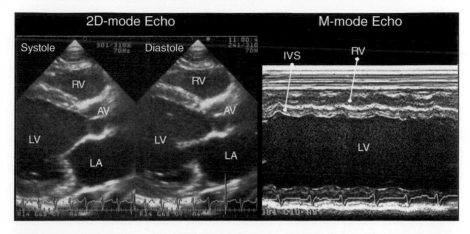

Fig. 10.4 On the left, bi-dimensional (2D)-mode long-axis views in systole and diastole; on the right, M-mode views at the level of the ventricles. *AV* aortic valve, *IVS* interventricular septum, *LA* left atrium, *LV* left ventricle, *RV* right ventricle

Fig. 10.5 Evidence of moderate mitral regurgitation: the presence of colour flow in left atrium during systolic *LV* contraction, occupying half of the left atrium area, is compatible with significant mitral disease

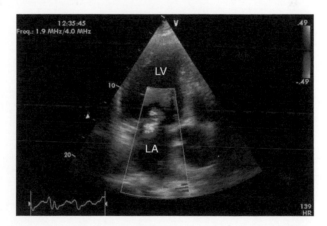

Concerning the mitral valve is evident a reduced surface of closure of the leaflets, that associated with enlarged valve annulus causes functional moderate mitral regurgitation.

After hospital admission, the patient was immediately started on furosemide infusion, low-dose beta-blocker, ACE inhibitor, oral anticoagulants and low molecular weight heparin. After 24 h a progressive clinical improvement was evident (reduction of dyspnoea, loss of 4 kg in weight) with disappearance of X-Ray sign of congestion and pleural fluid accumulation.

After clinical stabilisation, it was decided to attempt cardioversion earlier than the recommended 3 weeks of effective anticoagulant therapy, and therefore a transoesophageal echocardiography was performed which excluded the presence of thrombi and thus reduced the thromboembolic risk (Fig. 10.6).

Therefore the patient underwent successful electrical cardioversion (Fig. 10.7: post-cardioversion ECG).

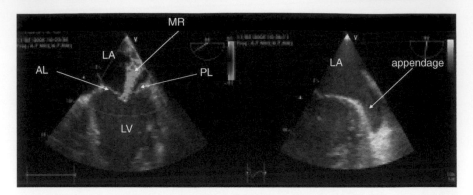

Fig. 10.6 Transoesophageal 2D echo and colour Doppler imaging. On the left, transverse plane, at mid-oesophagus level, four-chamber view with evidence of the left atrium (*LA*) and ventricle (*LV*) and mitral valve leaflets (anterior, *AL*, on the left; posterior, *PL*, on the right) with regurgitant jet in *LA*. On the right longitudinal long axis view at upper oesophagus level with the evidence of *LA* and left appendage, free of thromboembolic structures

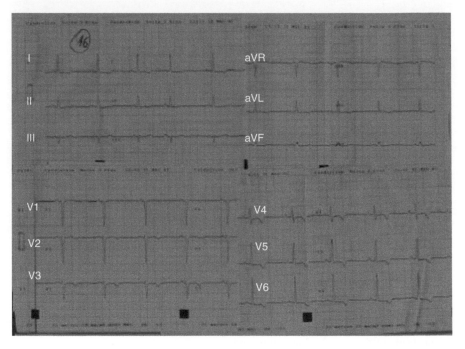

Fig. 10.7 Now p wave in front of QRS complex, with the same axis/polarity of the QRS, is present, indicating a regular organised atrial activity, i.e. sinus rhythm. T wave inversion is present in the anterior leads, suggesting a subendocardial ischaemia

10.2.7 Post-cardioversion 12-Lead ECG (Fig. 10.7)

Question 1
Which is the most likely cause of heart failure in this patient?

1. Ischaemic heart disease
2. Idiopathic DCMP
3. Valvular DCMP
4. Tachycardiomyopath

Answer

1. We cannot exclude the possibility of an ischaemic aetiology of the dilated cardiomyopathy, especially if we consider the signs of subendocardial ischaemia in the pre- and post-cardioversion ECG tracing (although these ECG changes are not uncommon after an AF episode).
2. Idiopathic dilated cardiomyopathy cannot be excluded, or in case of the absence of significant severe coronary artery disease, we may consider the past history of hypertension as a potential cause.
3. This seems an unlikely cause of the disease, according to the finding of the echocardiogram.
4. Sustained chronic tachyarrhythmias often cause a deterioration of cardiac function known as tachycardia-induced cardiomyopathy or tachycardiomyopathy. The exact incidence of tachycardia-induced cardiomyopathy in the general population is unknown, but in selected studies of patients with atrial fibrillation, approximately 25 % to 50 % of those with left ventricular dysfunction had some degree of tachycardia-induced cardiomyopathy. It is an important clinical entity due to the high incidence and potential reversibility of the disease process. In a patient with a negative history of ischaemic heart disease, this clinical entity should be considered Fig. 10.8 [2].

Before discharge, the patient underwent cardiac catheterisation (Figs. 10.9 and 10.10) including coronary angiogram and left ventriculography, which excluded the presence of significant coronary artery disease but confirmed a poorly functioning dilated left ventricle.

Two weeks after discharge, the patient underwent first an *echocardiographic control* (Fig. 10.11), with evidence of small improvement in left ventricular systolic function (35 %).

Question 2
Which exercise protocol would you recommend?

1. Cycle ergometer 10 watts/ /min
2. Cycle ergometer 30 watts/ /min
3. Treadmill Balke protocol
4. Treadmill Bruce protocol

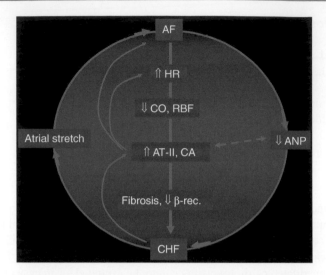

Fig. 10.8 Presents the pathophysiology linking atrial fibrillation and heart failure: heart failure may induce atrial remodelling including stretching of the fibres, which may trigger atrial fibrillation (*AF*). By increasing heart rate (*HR*) response, *AF* may determine reduction in cardiac output (*CO*), renal blood flow (*RBF*) with compensatory responses (including activation of the angiotensin (*AT-II*) and catecholamine (*CA*) systems). These changes induce myocardial fibrosis, beta-receptor downregulation and reduced vasodilating natriuretic peptide (*ANP*), all factors involved in the pathogenesis of heart failure (*Modified from Crijns et al, EHJ 1997*)

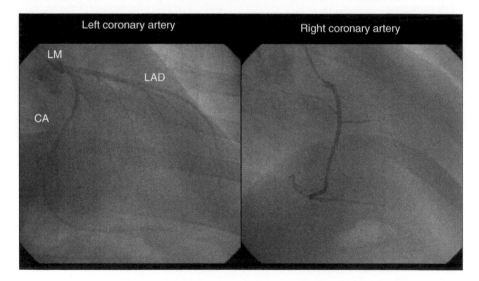

Fig. 10.9 Normal coronary angiogram. *LM* left main, *LAD* left anterior descending coronary artery, *CA* circumflex coronary artery, *RCA* right coronary artery

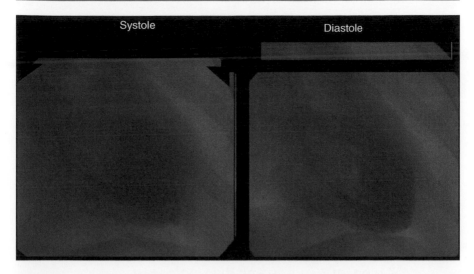

Fig. 10.10 Left ventricle angiogram in systole and diastole: Small difference in volumes between the systolic (*left picture*) and diastolic (*right picture*) phases is consistent with poor left ventricular systolic function

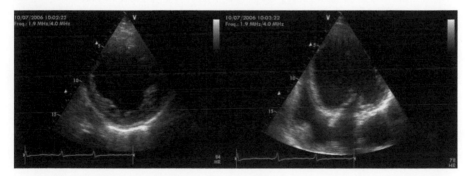

Fig. 10.11 Echocardiogram 2 weeks after cardioversion. Left: 2D echo, parasternal short axis view of the LV; on the right, 2D echo apical view of four chambers, showing a global spherical remodelling of the LV); subsequently, a cardiopulmonary exercise testing (CPET) was performed to evaluate the extent of exercise limitation and possible cardiac transplant list enrolment and/or to plan an exercise training programme

Answer

The choice was the cycle ergometer using 10w/min protocol, based on the presence of clinical syndrome on symptomatic heart failure of these patients which requires a simple, easy and safe test and which provides useful information to set up a rehabilitation protocol based on cycle ergometer (Figs. 10.12 and 10.13).

Question 3

Which of the following CPET parameters are most valuable in heart failure assessment?

EXERCISE PROTOCOLS

Cycle Ergometry
  Incremental or ramp
  Approximately 10 minutes
  Pedaling frequency of 60 rpm
  1-3 minutes resting data
  1-3 minutes unloaded pedaling
  Increase at 5-30 W/minute

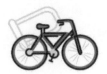

Treadmill
Speed constant and grade is increased (Balke Protocol)
  2 mph, 0% grade and than the grade is
  increased 2-3% every minute
Speed and grade are both increased (Bruce Protocol)
  1.7 mph, 10% grade and than increased
  by 0.8 mph and 2% grade every 3 minutes

Comparison of Cycle versus Treadmill

	Cycle	Treadmill
$\overset{\bullet}{V}O_2$ max	lower	higher
Leg muscle fatigue	often limits	less limiting
Work rate quantification	yes	estimation
Weight bearing in obese	less	more
Noise and artifacts	less	more
Safety issues	less	more

Figs. 10.12 and 10.13 Compares the characteristics of different exercise protocol and the differences between cycle versus treadmill exercise protocols

1. Peak oxygen consumption (peak VO$_2$)
2. Ventilatory response to exercise (Ve/VCO$_2$ slope)
3. Exercise duration
4. Heart rate response

Answer

The leading ventilatory parameters assessed on cardiopulmonary exercise testing are (1) Oxygen consumption at peak exercise (peak VO$_2$) and at anaerobic threshold (AT), (2) Ventilatory response to exercise (Ve/VCO$_2$ slope), because of their strong prognostic values, and they provide important information to set up a training programme.

Exercise duration and heart rate response are less valuable, since the first parameter is affected by the exercise protocol and the second by the pharmacological therapy (Figs. 10.14 and 10.15).

Question 4 How good is the correlation between peak VO$_2$ and left ventricular ejection fraction (LVEF) in heart failure?

1. Very good (R > 0.7)
2. Fairly good (R 0.7–0.6)
3. Poor (R 0.4–0.5)
4. Not at all

Answer

There are several pieces of evidences showing the absence of any correlation between haemodynamic dysfunction of the left ventricle (such as LVEF) and reduced exercise intolerance (Fig. 10.16).

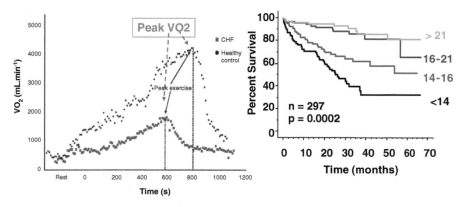

Fig. 10.14 Shows how to compute peak VO$_2$ and its important prognostic value in term of survival: a value above 18 ml/kg/min is considered a good prognostic indicator, while values below 11 ml/kg/ min are ominous sign and indication for enrolment in cardiac transplantation list [3] (Modified from Francis et al., Heart 2000)

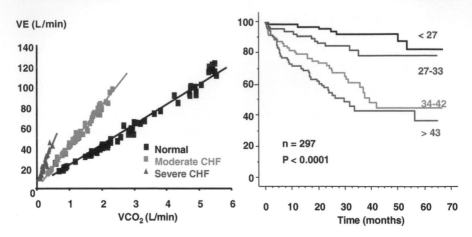

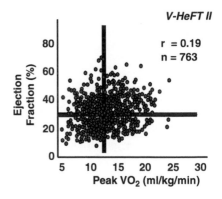

Fig. 10.15 Shows how to compute the Ve/VCO$_2$ slope and its important prognostic value: value above 34 are considered abnormal (Modified from Francis et al. Heart (2000))

Fig. 10.16 Lack of correlation between LVEF and exercise tolerance, measured as peak VO$_2$. The results from one of the largest heart failure trials, such as the V-HeFT II study, are presented

The following figures are presenting the result from the cardiopulmonary exercise testing (CPET) in our patient:

Three important phases of the texts have been highlighted, i.e. baseline, anaerobic threshold and peak exercise with relative findings.

The Fig. 10.18 is showing the results of the text in graphical forms.

CPET Report

- *Exercise protocol*: cycle 10 watts/min
- *Exercise duration:* 6 min: stop at 2 min 60 watts for shortness of breath (SOB)
- *Complication*: None (no arrhythmias, or disabling symptoms)
- *Peak exercise* was reached at 60 watts, with RQ > 1.1, VO$_2$ 13.3 ml/kg/min [54 % predicted VO$_2$max (r.v.: 24.4)], VO$_2$ 0.92 L/min [44 % predicted VO$_2$max (r.v.:2.1)], BP 120/80 mmHg, HR 122 bpm [78 % predicted HRmax (r.v.:156)]
- *Anaerobic threshold* was reached with VO$_2$ 11.6 ml/kg/min (47 % predicted VO$_2$max) or VO$_2$ 0.81 L/min (40 % predicted VO$_2$max)

CPET results

	Phase	Time	Work load	VO2 ml/kg/min	VO2 L/min	VCO2 L/min	RQ	VE L/min	HR Bpm
Baseline →	Baseline	1.9	0	2.9	0.208	0.190	0.91	12.7	55
	Exercise	2.9	10	5.1	0.357	0.301	0.84	16.9	71
	Exercise	3.9	20	7.1	0.497	0.455	0.92	21.9	92
	Exercise	4.9	30	9.5	0.655	0.641	0.98	30.6	101
AT →	Exercise	5.9	40	11.6	0.811	0.845	1.04	34.1	111
	Exercise	6.9	50	12.8	0.896	0.988	1.10	40.8	115
Peak →	Exercise	7.9	60	13.3	0.928	1.162	1.25	46.7	122
	Recover.	8.9	0	5.5	0.385	0.482	1.25	15.5	78

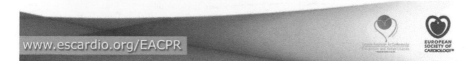

www.escardio.org/EACPR

Fig. 10.17 Minute by minute CPET results are shown in numerical forms, i.e. the phase, the times of the text, workload, O_2 consumption in relative value (VO_2 ml/kg min, adjusted for the body weight) and absolute value (L/min), CO_2 production (VCO_2 L/min), respiratory quotient (RQ, i.e. the ratio of VCO_2/VO_2), minute ventilation (L/min) and heart rate

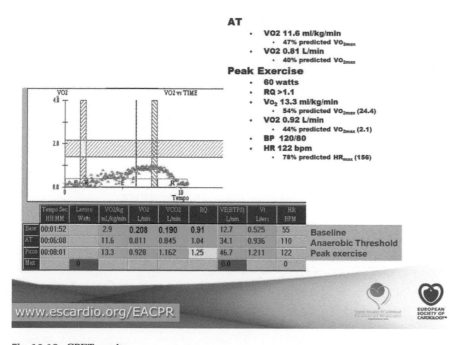

AT
- **VO2 11.6 ml/kg/min**
  - 47% predicted VO_{2max}
- **VO2 0.81 L/min**
  - 40% predicted VO_{2max}

Peak Exercise
- **60 watts**
- **RQ >1.1**
- **Vo_2 13.3 ml/kg/min**
  - 54% predicted VO_{2max} (24.4)
- **VO2 0.92 L/min**
  - 44% predicted VO_{2max} (2.1)
- **BP 120/80**
- **HR 122 bpm**
  - 78% predicted HR_{max} (156)

Fig. 10.18 CPET results

Fig. 10.19 CPET results:
Ve/VCO$_2$ slope

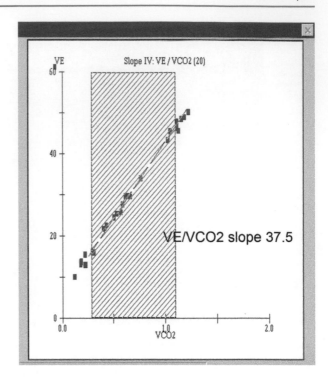

r.v. are reference values for age, sex, body mass index.

Thus our patient is presenting severe exercise limitations: Peak VO$_2$ 13.3 ml/kg/
min (Figs. 10.17 and 10.18) and abnormally elevated ventilatory response to exercise (normal value < 34) VE/VCO$_2$ 37.5 (Fig. 10.19).

Question 5
Which is the correct recommendation for medication for this patient?

1. Carvedilol, enalapril, spironolactone, furosemide, amiodarone, aspirin
2. All above but warfarin instead of aspirin
3. All above plus valsartan
4. All above but sotalol instead of carvedilol and amiodarone

Answer

2. There are some controversies, but also evidence-based facts:

- Beta-blockers, angiotensin-converting enzyme (ACE) inhibitors or angiotensin
  receptor blockers (ARB), aldosterone antagonists, diuretics constitute the cornerstone of heart failure therapy (ESC Guideline, Class of recommendation I) [1].
- Warfarin is preferred to aspirin in the setting of permanent, persistent, or paroxysmal atrial fibrillation, because reduced the risk of thromboembolic events
  (ESC Guideline, Class of recommendation I).

- Both ACEIs and ARBs appear to be equally effective in the prevention of AF, in patients with systolic left ventricular dysfunction or LV hypertrophy [4].
- Combination of beta-blockers, angiotensin-converting enzyme (ACE) inhibitors, angiotensin receptor blockers (ARB) and aldosterone antagonists is contraindicated because of side effect and mortality [1, 5].
- In the setting of atrial fibrillation and heart failure and low ejection fraction, amiodarone is the only effective anti-arrhythmic option (ESC Guideline, Class of recommendation 1).

The patient underwent an exercise training programme home based on bicycle, with periodic hospital-based control (Class I recommendation, Level of Evidence A: Fig. 10.20).

Question 6
Why is exercise training programme recommended in heart failure patients with reduced systolic function?

1. Because it reduces hospitalisation
2. Because it improves quality of life
3. Because it improves quantity of life
4. All above

Recommendations	Class[a]	Level[b]
It is recommended that regular aerobic exercise is encouraged in patients with HF to improve functional capacity and symptoms.	I	A
It is recommended that regular aerobic exercise is encouraged in stable patients with HFrEF to reduce the risk of HF hospitalization.	I	A

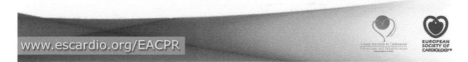

www.escardio.org/EACPR

Fig. 10.20 Recommendation for exercise training in heart failure (European Society of Cardiology Guidelines)

Answer

1. Structured exercise training programme improves exercise capacity, quality of life (reduces breathlessness and fatigue) and autonomic control and reduces hospitalisation (ESC Guideline Class of Recommendation I (Fig. 10.20) [1].

The HF-Action trial findings have risen some doubt, but its several limitation makes its findings at least inconclusive. In fact although it is the most comprehensive study to date, examining the effects of exercise upon patients with heart failure have addressed important points but left unsolved several issues: it confirms the safety of a home-based exercise training programme in CHF patients, but its lack of improvement in survival could be easily attributed to its several limitations, outlined by the authors themselves (study population too young and too healthy, lack of titration of the training programme, poor compliance and as a consequence, insufficient training effect).

Question 7

Which is the correct recommendation for physical activity to start with in this patient?

1. 15–20 min. of bicycle home based 3–5 days per week at moderate to high intensity (based on heart rate at 50–60 % peak VO_2)
2. At least on 1 day of the weekend physical activity of 1–2 h in outdoor cycling
3. At least every day 10–20 mins outdoor jogging
4. Each week at least 1 training in a swimming club

Answer

1. *Correct answer*: Six months of regular aerobic exercise training at moderate intensities (50–60 % of VO_{2peak}) and volumes (150 min per week) are associated with small but significant improvements (falls) in end-diastolic volume and end-systolic volume in patients with CHF, whereas these volumes increased in the inactive CHF volunteers, indicating that moderate-intensity exercise training is safe and may also promote reverse remodelling of the left ventricle in CHF. Intense exercise regimens (both aerobic and strength) are associated with sharp increases in platelet reactivity, whereas moderate-intensity training is associated with relatively counterbalanced stimuli to the thrombogenic and fibrinolytic systems. Therefore, patients with CHF, particularly those with (a history of) atrial fibrillation (like in our case), unstable atherosclerotic plaque or shortly after coronary artery stenting, should avoid high-intensity exercise. For many other reasons, high-intensity exercise should not normally be included in exercise programmes for patients with CHF.

The application of a tolerated workload from cycle ergometer training to outdoor cycling as well as jogging is not possible because of environmental factors influencing cardiovascular stress (e.g. head wind, slopes, temperature).

During swimming, head-up immersion and the hydrostatically induced volume shift result in an increased volume loading of the left ventricle, with increase of heart volume, and pulmonary capillary wedge pressure. Swimming slowly (20–25 m/min) results in measurements of heart rate, blood lactate and plasma catecholamines similar to those measured during cycle ergometry at workloads of 100–150 W. Because of these findings, chronic heart failure patients with diastolic and systolic dysfunctions should swim only after consultation with their physician.

Pragmatically, a sedentary lifestyle often contributes to the development of CHF, with many individuals harbouring long-term aversions to exercise. It is more likely that they will accept, and then enthusiastically adopt, healthful enduring exercise if that exercise is at relatively comfortable intensities [6].

10.3 Scheme of Home-Based Exercise Training Programme

Three to five weekly sessions on cyclette with the following protocol: 5–10 min unloading warming up, 15–20 min at heart rate corresponding to 50–60 % of heart rate at peak VO_2 and 5–10 min unloading cooling down.

At the start of the training programme, we performed a maximal symptom-limited CPET (to exclude any contraindication to training programme and to assess exercise capacity) and an echocardiogram.

Every 3–6 months of the training programme and/or after change in medication, i.e. ß-blocker or clinical condition, a repetition of maximal symptom-limited cardiopulmonary exercise testing was planned to check the patient compliance, to exclude contraindication and to adjust the workload of the cyclette.

Every 1–3 months, a hospital clinical control was planned to exclude any risk, which may contraindicate the prolongation of the home-based training programme.

The patient was enrolled in a bicycle home-based ET programme, with periodic hospital control, with the intensity of exercise of 30 watts, 15–30 min/day, at least 3 x/week, and the load was progressively increased to 50 watts after 3 months (Fig. 10.21).

After the 6-month training period, the patient was still in sinus rhythm, asymptomatic, NYHA class I and well compensated. Echocardiogram showed improvement in LVEF with only mild global hypokinesia (51 %), with normal left atrial size and no mitral regurgitation (Fig. 10.22). Cardiopulmonary exercise testing documented improvements in exercise tolerance (peak VO_2 15.4 ml/kg/min (+15 %) (Fig. 10.23) and ventilatory response to exercise: VE/VCO$_2$ 34.6 (r.v. < 34) (Fig. 10.24).

Phase	Time	Work load	VO2 ml/kg/min	VO2 L/min	VCO2 L/min	RQ	VE L/min	HR Bpm
Baseline	1.9	0	2.9	0.208	0.190	0.91	12.7	55
Exercise	2.9	10	5.1	0.357	0.301	0.84	16.9	71
Exercise	3.9	20	7.1	0.497	0.455	0.92	21.9	92
Exercise	4.9	30	9.5	0.655	0.641	0.98	30.6	101
Exercise	5.9	40	11.6	0.811	0.845	1.04	34.1	111
Exercise	6.9	50	12.8	0.896	0.988	1.10	40.8	115
Exercise	7.9	60	13.3	0.928	1.162	1.25	46.7	122
Recover.	8.9	0	5.5	0.385	0.482	1.25	15.5	78

ET → (Exercise, Time 3.9)

Peak → (Exercise, Time 7.9)

www.escardio.org/EACPR

Fig. 10.21 Shows how the CPET findings were used for planning the ET programme in our patients

Fig. 10.22 Echo-cardiographic examination after ET

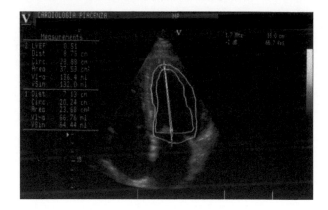

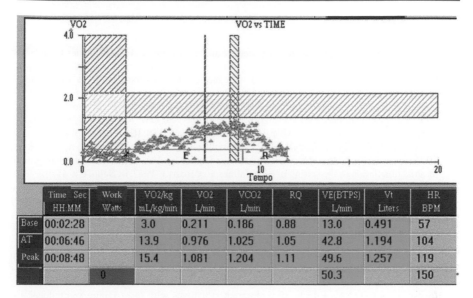

	Time Sec HH:MM	Work Watts	VO2/kg mL/kg/min	VO2 L/min	VCO2 L/min	RQ	VE(BTPS) L/min	Vt Liters	HR BPM
Base	00:02:28		3.0	0.211	0.186	0.88	13.0	0.491	57
AT	00:06:46		13.9	0.976	1.025	1.05	42.8	1.194	104
Peak	00:08:48		15.4	1.081	1.204	1.11	49.6	1.257	119
		0					50.3		150

Fig. 10.23 CPET results after ET

Fig. 10.24 Improvement in ventilatory response to exercise (Ve/VCO2 slope) after ET

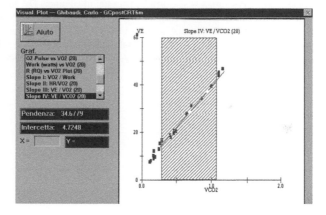

References

1. 2016 ESC Guidelines for the diagnosis and treatment of acute and chronic heart failure: The Task Force for the diagnosis and treatment of acute and chronic heart failure of the European Society of Cardiology (ESC)Developed with the special contribution of the Heart Failure Association (HFA) of the ESC. Ponikowski P, Voors AA, Anker SD, Bueno H, Cleland JG, Coats AJ, Falk V, González-Juanatey JR, Harjola VP, Jankowska EA, Jessup M, Linde C, Nihoyannopoulos P, Parissis JT, Pieske B, Riley JP, Rosano GM, Ruilope LM, Ruschitzka F, Rutten FH, van der Meer P. Eur Heart J. 1. May 20. pii: ehw128. [Epub ahead of print].
2. Walker NL, Cobbe SM, Birnie DH. Tachycardiomyopathy: a diagnosis not to be missed. Heart. 2004;90(2):e7; Crijns HJ, Van den Berg MP, Van Gelder IC, Van Veldhuisen DJ. Management of atrial fibrillation in the setting of heart failure. Eur Heart J. 1997;18 Suppl C:C45–9.
3. Corrà U, Piepoli MF, Adamopoulos S, Agostoni P, Coats AJ, Conraads V, Lambrinou E, Pieske B, Piotrowicz E, Schmid JP, Seferović PM, Anker SD, Filippatos G, PP P. Cardiopulmonary exercise testing in systolic heart failure in 2014: the evolving prognostic role: a position paper from the committee on exercise physiology and training of the heart failure association of the ESC. Eur J Heart Fail. 2014;16(9):929–41.
4. Healey JS, Baranchuk A, Crystal E, Morillo CA, Garfinkle M, Yusuf S, Connolly SJ. Prevention of atrial fibrillation with angiotensin-converting enzyme inhibitors and angiotensin receptor blockers: a meta-analysis. J Am Coll Cardiol. 2005;45(11):1832–9.
5. Investigators CHARM. Effects of candesartan in patients with heart failure and reduced LV systolic function taking angiotensin-converting enzyme inhibitor: the CHARM-Added trial. Lancet. 2003;362:767–71.
6. Piepoli MF, Conraads V, Corrà U, Dickstein K, Francis DP, Jaarsma T, McMurray J, Pieske B, Piotrowicz E, Schmid JP, Anker SD, Solal AC, Filippatos GS, Hoes AW, Gielen S, Giannuzzi P, Ponikowski PP. Exercise training in heart failure: from theory to practice. A consensus document of the Heart Failure Association and the European Association for Cardiovascular Prevention and Rehabilitation. Eur J Heart Fail. 2011;13(4):347–57.

Cardiac Rehabilitation in Patients with Implantable Cardioverter Defibrillator

11

L. Vanhees, V. Cornelissen, J. Berger, F. Vandereyt, and P. Dendale

In this particular report, we choose to present this rather exceptional case, who had a sedentary employment but with high levels of leisure time physical activity. This patient had a first stable period of many years after the first ICD implantation. However, when the ICD device was replaced because of battery failure, the patient experienced several electrical storms, for which he received psychological treatment because of fear of shock delivery in general and reticence towards exercise in particular.

Subsequent to the presentation of this case and the discussion regarding items which have to be considered when rehabilitating this patient, we will compare this case to expected results and possible complications during a cardiac rehabilitation programme, based on current scientific literature.

Case Report: Period 1

A 37-year-old male patient was sent to the cardiology department because of a 2-year lasting complaint of dizziness and intermittent loss of sight during severe exercise training. He did not perceive palpitations and received pharmacological treatment for possible vestibular problems.

Examination with resting ECG and symptom limited bicycle ergometry showed a possible former anteroseptal infarction (Fig. 11.1) and frequent premature ventricular beats (PVB).

L. Vanhees (✉) • V. Cornelissen
Department of Rehabilitation Sciences, Biomedical Sciences, KU Leuven, Leuven, Belgium
e-mail: luc.vanhees@kuleuven.be

J. Berger • F. Vandereyt • P. Dendale
Rehabilitation and Health Centre, Jesse Hospital, Hasselt, Belgium

© Springer International Publishing AG 2017
J. Niebauer (ed.), *Cardiac Rehabilitation Manual*,
DOI 10.1007/978-3-319-47738-1_11

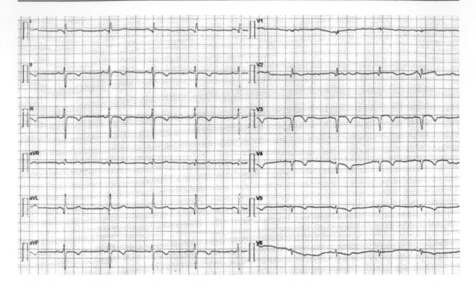

Fig. 11.1 Resting ECG showing possible former anteroseptal infarction

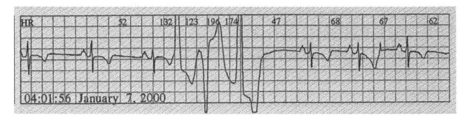

Fig. 11.2 Example of a documented triplet

To unmask an eventual Brugada syndrome, the patient received 100 mg Tambocor. Although there were no arguments for Brugada syndrome, the test revealed frequent PVB's with multifocal couplets and triplets (Fig. 11.2).

Electrophysiological examination reproduced the symptoms, where echography revealed no suspicion for arrhythmogenic right ventricular dysplasia (ARVD), nor were late potentials found. Treatment with amiodarone (200 mg; 2/day) was then started. After 6 weeks of pharmacological treatment, a control examination showed that the patient still experienced the same symptoms together with high nausea and photo sensibility indicating a low tolerability for the medication. Electrophysiological examination still induced symptoms and arrhythmias in spite of the use of amiodarone and indicated a right ventricular origin. Therefore, the option of ICD implantation (implantable cardioverter defibrillator) became plausible. Patient-specific characteristics can be found in Table 11.1.

Four months after the first cardiac examination, a single chamber ICD was implanted with one lead in the right ventricular apex. Four weeks after implantation, this patient was included in a cardiovascular rehabilitation programme where a

Table 11.1   Patient characteristics before ICD implantation

Age/gender	38/male
Socio-demographics	
Occupation	International truck driver
Social	Married, two children
Physical activity regular competitive soccer and tennis	
Clinical examination	
Height(cm)	177
Weight (kg)	71
BMI (kg/m²)	22.7
Blood pressure (systolic/diastolic)	120/80
Resting heart rate (beats/min)	55
Auscultation heart	Normal
Auscultation lungs	Normal
Medical history	Appendectomy (not recent)
Blood parameters	
Echography	Normal; ejection fraction: 65%
Resting ECG	Sinus rhythm; left anterior semi bloc, Q waves in V2, V3 and V4, flat repolarization anterolateral, negative T wave inferolateral
Electrophysiological examination	Inducible non-sustained ventricular tachycardia (200–220 beats/min) with right ventricular origin and reproducibility symptoms
MRI	Localized anterior wall hypokinesia
ECG monitoring	Very frequent PVBs and a few episodes of polymorphic ventricular tachycardia

baseline symptom-limited exercise test was undertaken. Results from this test are presented in Table 11.2.

Question   Which items do we have to take into account when testing and training a patient with an ICD device?

1. Device settings:

When testing or training an ICD patient, the level of exercise that could cause a defibrillation shock or anti-tachycardia pacing intervention should be avoided. The design of an exercise programme should always be preceded by a maximal or symptom-limited exercise test. Despite the fear of patients with an ICD and the risk of harmful and threatening symptoms, the exercise test has a key role in the evaluation of arrhythmias, the ICD device, peak heart rate and exercise tolerance and medical therapy (Fig. 11.3).

The testing protocol should consist of a standardized graded exercise tolerance test on a motor-driven treadmill or bicycle ergometer with assessment of ECG, blood pressure and oxygen uptake. The golden standard for the assessment of the

Table 11.2 Results from baseline symptom limited exercise test

Rest	
Heart rate (beats/min)	79
Systolic blood pressure (mmHg)	122
Diastolic blood pressure (mmHg)	87
Peak exercise	
VO$_2$ (mL/min)	2,058
VO$_2$ (mL/min/kg)	29
VO$_2$ predicted value (%)	72
Oxygen pulse (mL/beat)	13.2
Oxygen pulse predicted value (%)	79
Load (W)	165
Load predicted value (%)	75
Heart rate (beats/min)	156 (safety threshold 162–172)
Heart rate predicted value (%)	86
Systolic blood pressure (mmHg)	165
Diastolic blood pressure (mmHg)	75
RER	1.19
VE	63.4
Anaerobic threshold VO$_2$ (mL/min)	1,031
ECG	Several runs of nsVT starting from 120 W

RER respiratory exchange ratio, *VE* ventilation, *nsVT* non-sustained ventricular tachycardia

functional capacity is peak oxygen uptake [1]. A submaximal test (terminating the test at a given percentage of predicted maximum heart rate) is not recommended. Firstly because medications affect the age-predicted maximum of the heart rate, as a result of which it would only give an estimate of the actual exercise tolerance. Secondly it would not give the opportunity to evaluate the reactions of cardiac rhythm and the ICD on maximal exercise. The participant reaches a maximum cardiorespiratory response by continuing the exercise test till exhaustion or fatigue. In some studies, the point where the patient reached a heart rate threshold of cut-off point minus 10–30 beats was one of the endpoints of the test, in order to avoid discharge of the ICD. [2–5]. However, Lampman and colleague stated that when the cut-off point is situated below the age-predicted maximum (220 minus age), the ICD should temporarily be switched off during the exercise test [6]. This way, the patient could reach his or her true maximum without being at risk for inappropriate shocks. A similar strategy was used in the study from Belardinelli et al., where the minimal firing rate of the ICD device was set 20 beats above the peak heart rate achieved during maximal exercise testing [5]. However, it seems more logical to perform a maximal exercise test with the ICD activated, because that way you can gather information about the reaction of the cardiac rhythm and the ICD to exercise. Also the result of the exercise test can give confidence to the patient that exercise at a predetermined level is safe and can be performed in the controlled environment of a cardiac rehabilitation centre. A recent study evaluated the safety of symptom-limited exercise testing in 400 ICD patients [7]. They performed exercise testing until symptoms or until the

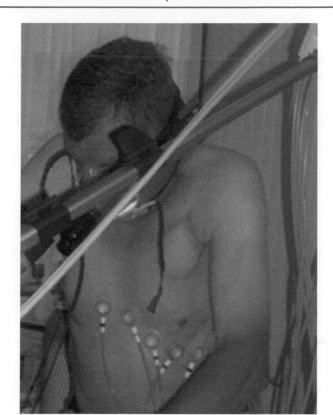

Fig. 11.3   Implantable cardioverter defi brillator (ICD) patient during exercise testing

Table 11.3   ICD device parameters

Device characteristics		Therapy
VF zone (beats/min)	250–500	6 DS (35 J)
VT zone (beats/min)	182–250	Three burst pacing; three ramp pacing; 5 DS (35 J)
Brady pacing (beats/min)	34	WI pacing

VF ventricular fibrillation, *VT* ventricular tachycardia, *DS* defibrillation shock

achievement of a heart rate 20 beats below the VT zone while remaining on pharmacological treatment. Most of the patients stopped exercise because of exhaustion (±70 %) or dyspnoea (±25 %). Signs of ischaemia were very rare, no ICD shock or antitachycardia pacing occurred and only in 16 out of the 400 patients exercise testing had to be stopped prematurely because of reaching the HR threshold without being exhausted. These results show that maximal or symptom-limited exercise testing in ICD patients with optimal pharmacological treatment is safe and feasible, but should only be performed in a professional and medical environment with continuous emphasis on safety measures. To ensure this safety precaution, information concerning the device settings should be available, and (Table 11.3) during testing and training, a (donut) magnet needs to be in the immediate vicinity of the patient to be able to interrupt eventual inappropriate interventions of the ICD.

In the beginning of a training programme, ECG monitoring during exercise is advisable to be able to document eventual exercise induced arrhythmias. The rehabilitation team should be well instructed about emergency measures in this particular patient population. They also have to know that they do not incur a risk by touching a patient while his ICD discharges, to avoid reactions of fear from the team members in case of an emergency.

2. Lead displacement:

Except from general safety recommendations when working with ICD patients, like thorough knowledge of the patient and the implanted device, the proximity of specialized ICD care and of course the active knowledge of the emergency procedure, some specific recommendations when training ICD patients are important. For the ICD lead to well grow in, a time interval of 4 weeks is mandatory before initiating any form of physical training and especially exercises which include movement of the left arm, as the ICD device is mostly implanted in the left pectoral muscle region. And although one would expect the ICD lead to have grown in, left arm hyperextension, arm ergometry and upper body strength exercises are to be postponed for at least 6 weeks after implantation. When exercises would include this left arm, low mobilization range and low intensity is mandatory. The patient needs correct information from the rehabilitation team to know which movements are acceptable.

3. Psychological and educational needs:

Apart from complications related to surgery, most post-operative stress is caused by the possibility of experiencing an electrical shock and the lack of treatment of the underlying cause for implantation. It is logical to think that the implantation of a lifesaving device would make the patient confident of the improved life expectancy and relieve the fear of sudden death. But living with the possibility of receiving a defibrillating shock at any time can be emotionally devastating. Compared to the general population, quality of life and psychosocial adjustment are poor in patients with an ICD [8–10]. According to Sears et al. [9], ICD-specific fears and symptoms of anxiety are the most common symptoms experienced by patients with ICD. Moreover, 13–38 % of these patients experience diagnosable levels of anxiety. ICD-specific fears include fear of shock, fear of device malfunction, fear of death and fear of embarrassment. The health-related quality of life is also negatively associated with fear of exercise [8]. When comparing two groups of ICD patients according to the experience of a defibrillating shock, Jacq et al. concluded that exposure to shocks may lead to an increased risk of anxiety and depressive symptoms [11].

Social and working life can also be negatively influenced as there is a limitation in physical activity, due to the fear that stress or emotions might alert the device. Others may worry about their body image or avoid exercise and sexual activity because of fears of arrhythmias and discharge of the ICD. In some countries, driving is even, at least temporarily, prohibited. Also partners of ICD patients report feelings of helplessness and uncertainty about what to do if, or when, the ICD discharges. They worry about the reliability of the ICD and about their own position if their partner should die. This may commonly result in overprotection of the ICD patient, and partners often restrict or restrain them from doing physical activities. The importance of involving, educating and equipping partners with the relevant information and skills so that they can empower and support the patient to reach informed decisions should not be underestimated [12, 13]. In the absence of such interventions, the potential for misconceptions, misguided beliefs and marital conflicts can increase, perpetuating further uncertainty, fear and loss of control as well as precipitating physical symptoms. Various studies report on the psychological benefits for patients with an ICD after psychological intervention or comprehensive cardiac rehabilitation. Kohn et al. [14] studied cognitive behavioural therapy in patients with an ICD in a randomized controlled trial. They concluded that cognitive behavioural therapy was associated with decreased levels of depression and anxiety, and increased adjustment, particularly among those patients who received a shock [14]. Fitchet et al. reported decreased anxiety scores after 12 weeks of comprehensive cardiac rehabilitation (CR), including psychosocial counselling, in a randomized controlled trial [4]. These data demonstrate the importance of planning and organizing psychosocial support for patients with an ICD in comprehensive cardiac rehabilitation. However, a recent review concluded that more randomized controlled studies are warranted to better highlight the impact of CR and exercise training on anxiety, depression and quality of life [15]. But although more and more patients are treated with an ICD device, the referral from hospitals to cardiac rehabilitation centres is still negatively influenced by the fear of inappropriate shock delivery during exercise. The beneficial effects of cardiac rehabilitation in terms of secondary prevention and on physiological and psychosocial functioning of cardiac patients in general are well established [16].

4. Vocational counselling:

In many countries, the law forbids patients with an ICD to drive trucks or transport people as a profession. This item needs to be addressed already in the pre-implantation period and from the beginning of the ambulatory rehabilitation programme. Reorientation or retraining for other professions can help the patient in finding a new job, which is a prerequisite for many to return to a "normal" life. Also counselling concerning sports participation is needed. Competition is to be avoided, but low level exercise such as doubles tennis, cycling, etc. can be performed [17].

Before even starting with the actual physical training component of the cardiac rehabilitation programme, our patient was hospitalized because of recurrent VT for which he received three defibrillating shocks. Although no life-threatening arrhythmias were induced by maximal exercise testing, our patient reached a peak heart rate of 77 % of the predicted value compared to 86 % in the exercise test few days before, perhaps indicating some avoidance towards heavy exercise. To prevent the further need for ICD interventions, as our patient is relatively physically active (tennis and soccer), a beta-blocking agent was provided (Emconcor 5 mg). Six weeks after starting the rehabilitation programme with a frequency of two times a week, our patient was retested, showing the following results (Table 11.4), indicating a small increase in maximal oxygen uptake capacity (VO2) but a 36 % improvement in workload. When reviewing the peak heart rate, some doubts about medication compliance could be mentioned. Because of a return to full-time employment, our patient prematurely dropped out of the rehabilitation programme.

Period 2 The patient was followed at the outpatient pacemaker clinic for years without having received discharges, but with infrequent anti-tachycardia pacing episodes. After 8 years, the ICD had to be replaced because of battery depletion. The characteristics from the second ICD device are shown in Table 11.5.

Six months afterwards, the patient experienced several consecutive shocks in 1 day due to a very rapid ventricular tachycardia, independent from physical activity. Treatment with amiodarone and beta-blockers did not control the

Table 11.4 Results from maximal exercise testing after 6 weeks of training

Rest	
Heart rate (beats/min)	65
Systolic blood pressure (mmHg)	110
Diastolic blood pressure (mmHg)	70
Peak exercise	
VO$_2$ (mL/min)	2,219
VO$_2$ (mL/min/kg)	31.7
VO$_2$ predicted value (%)	79
Oxygen pulse (mL/beat)	14.9
Oxygen pulse predicted value (%)	90
Load (W)	225
Load predicted value (%)	104
Heart rate (beats/min)	172 (safety threshold 162–172)
Heart rate predicted value (%)	94
Systolic blood pressure (mmHg)	170
Diastolic blood pressure (mmHg)	94
RER	1.28
VE	76.2
Anaerobic threshold	
VO$_2$ (mL/min)	1,041
ECG	Several runs of nsVT starting from 200 Watt

RER respiratory exchange ratio, *VE* ventilation, *nsVT* non-sustained ventricular tachycardia

Table 11.5 Second ICD device parameters

Device characteristics		Therapy
VF zone (beats/min)	240–500	6 DS (35J)
VT zone (beats/min)	194–240	Four burst pacing; four ramp pacing; WI pacing
Brady pacing (beats/min)	34	

VF ventricular fibrillation, *VT* ventricular tachycardia, *DS* defibrillation shock

Table 11.6 Results from maximal cycle ergometry during period with several electrical storms

Rest	
Heart rate (beats/min)	71
Systolic blood pressure (mmHg)	130
Diastolic blood pressure (mmHg)	77
Peak exercise	
Load (W)	160
Load predicted value (%)	75
Heart rate (beats/min)	124 (safety threshold 174–184)
Heart rate predicted value (%)	72
Systolic blood pressure (mmHg)	153
Diastolic blood pressure (mmHg)	82
ECG	Several episodes of nsVT; ST depression with horizontal or descendant ST slope in aVL (−1.1 mm)

nsVT non-sustained ventricular tachycardia

arrhythmia, and the patient experienced several series of discharges (up to 8 in 1 day). A new coronarography showed no stenosis, and echography still showed a zone of apical akinesia. He underwent a right ventricular ablation procedure and was sent again for ambulatory cardiac rehabilitation. Psychologically our patient was extremely anxious, especially in regard to exercise because of the experience with many electrical storms, independent from any form of physical activity. A bicycle ergometry test indicated a limited (motivation towards) maximal exercise capacity (Table 11.6).

Question How do we approach this patient in a second rehabilitation programme?

1. Exercise prescription:

The participation in low-intensity exercises in the safety of a well-supervised cardiac rehabilitation programme is very important to regain confidence in doing exercise in "real life". A slow increase of the exercise level with in the beginning

ECG monitoring will help the psychological recovery of the patient. At this moment however, it is unknown if participation in a rehabilitation programme also reduces the risk of severe arrhythmias, device discharge or death. Up to now, the scientific literature and experience in large rehabilitation centres do not show signs of increased risk of discharge, but definite information will have to await the results of the above-mentioned trial.

2. Heart rate monitoring during exercise:

Again, it is imperative that the rehabilitation team has perfect knowledge of the settings of the ICD in a particular patient and eventual changes in medication which might influence the heart rate response during exercise. On the other hand, the ambulatory rehabilitation is a very good setting to optimize the pacing settings in patients who are pacemaker dependent or have chronotropic incompetence. As most pacemakers have a built in sensor which respond to different physical stimuli (motion, acceleration, vibration, impedance), different exercises may provoke different pacing rates. A bicycle test is not the optimal way to test the sensor rate, whereas a treadmill test will reproduce better the response during daily life. Asking the patient which exercises he or she does at home is essential to optimize the activity sensor settings.

3. Psychological approach after an electrical storm:

The anxiety of the patient is explained in part by the fact that he has a device that is implanted to save his life, but that can hurt him badly in doing so. The electrical storms with several discharges, while conscious causes a sensation of helplessness, which needs to be addressed by the psychologist team. The implanted device literally makes it impossible to "run away" from the problem. Therefore, as many patients are getting a prophylactic ICD for non-ischaemic reasons, the "normal" educational material needs to be adapted specifically to the ICD patients.

4. Exercise avoidance:

Avoidance of exercise is a typical problem after frequent discharges. Therefore, supervised exercise and psychological counselling should address the questions which exercises are allowed and which have to be avoided or postponed.

Before the patient could start in his second cardiac rehabilitation programme, a new right ventricular ablation procedure was indicated because of the high incidence of life-threatening arrhythmias and associated electrical storms. Meanwhile this patient was offered to participate in the psychological sessions for ICD patients (Fig. 11.4), because of the tremendous exercise avoidance and fear for device discharges. After each session, our patient had to fill in the following questionnaire (Fig. 11.5) assessing his concerns. This relatively recent questionnaire gives an indication to which extent an ICD patient has certain concerns [18].

Figure 11.6 shows the results from this questionnaire in the course of the five sessions at which our patient participated, indicating a relatively high level of concerns. At this moment, this patient deals with severe psychological problems because of the fear of ICD discharges, limiting his general public functioning (Fig. 11.6).

After the ablation procedure, our patient will re-enter the cardiac rehabilitation programme and has the intention of finishing the full 3 months of rehabilitation.

Question Which results can we expect from a multidisciplinary cardiac rehabilitation programme?

Table 11.7 provides an overview of the studies that have examined the influence of exercise training in ICD patients [2–5, 19–22].

Week 1: Information and education about ICD
Introduction Cardiac Rehabilitation - benefits and efficacy
Introduction to and importance of exercise/activity
Experiental-Comparison Activity - demonstration of 'safe' amounts of exercise/work
How the ICD has changed peoples lives - elicitation of concerns/avoided activities/impact of ICD on patient and family.

Week 2: Review of last session - importance of exercise/life changes since ICD
Risk factors for CHD - what are yours and how can we help you?
Introduction to goal setting and pacing - setting individual goal plans
Introduction to relaxation and breathing - benefits and efficacy in reducing adrenaline and stabilising heart rate.

Week 3: Review of last session - importance of exercise/life changes since ICD/goal setting and pacing/relaxation and breathing.
Goal review - individual
Exercise goal review - group
How what we think can affect our heart rate - cognitive-behavioural model and negative effect of concerns and misconceptions

Week 4: Review of last session - exercise/life changes since ICD/goal setting and pacing/relaxation and breathing/CBT model
Goal review - individual
Exercise goal review - group
CBT Model - self-talk and how to change it - practical exercises in session.
Q + A session with family members - separate to participants - elicitation of concerns/avoided activities/impact of ICD on family.

Week 5: Review of last session - exercise/life changes since ICD/goal setting and pacing/relaxation and breathing/CBT model and self-talk/Q+A session.
Goal review - individual
Exercise goal review - group
Thoughts, feelings and behaviour - exploratory discussion, group solution finding to disclosed/reported difficulties.

Week 6: Review of last session - exercise/life changes since ICD/goal setting and pacing/relaxation and breathing/thoughts and feelings.
Goal review - individual
Exercise goal review - group
Programme review
Maintenance of change and coping with setbacks.

Fig. 11.4 Summary of session aims

The ICD Patient Concerns Questionnaire-ICD-C.

We want to know what things worry you about living with your ICD. It is important that you answer every question. Don't spent too long thinking about your answer. For each question please tick (✓) one box. Please don't leave any out.

I am worried about	Not at all	A little bit	Some what	Quite a lot	Very much so
1. My ICD firing					
2. My ICD not working when I need it to					
3. What I should do if my ICD fires					
4. Doing exercise in case it causes my ICD to fire					
5. Doing activities/hobbies that may cause my ICD to fire					
6. My heart condition getting worse if the ICD fires					
7. The amount of time I spend thinking about my heart condition and having an ICD					
8. The amount of time I spend thinking about my heart					
9. The ICD battery running out					
10. Working too hard/overdoings causing my ICD to fire					
11. Making love in case my ICD fires					
12. Having no warning my ICD will fire					
13. The symptoms/pain associcted with my ICD firing					
14. Being a burden on my partner/family					
15. Not being able to prevent my ICD from firing					
16. The future now that I have an ICD					
17. Problems occurring with ICD e.g. battery failure					
18. Getting too stressed in case my ICD fires					
19. Not being able to work/take part in activities and hobbies because I have an ICD					
20. Exercising too hard and causing my ICD to fire					

Fig. 11.5 ICD patient concerns questionnaire

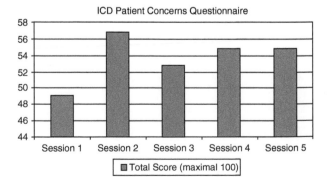

Fig. 11.6 Results from the ICD patient concerns questionnaire

Taking these results into account, some adapted recommendations for exercise training can be formulated, especially concerning upper extremity exercises. An ambulatory, supervised exercise training programme should contain three training sessions a week for at least 12 weeks with a duration of 60–90 mins and consist of a warming up, the main exercise part, and a cooling down. The warming up is a

Table 11.7 Components and results from several exercise programmes

Author	Study plan	No.	Training characteristics	Exercise tolerance	Complications
Vanhees (2001) [2]	Three months CCR	8	TF, 3 sessions/week TD, 90 min/session TI: [HRrest + 60–90 % (HRmax-HRrest)] with upper limit of HR= detection rate – 30 beats	Peak VO$_2$, +24 %	One asymptomatic VT with ICD intervention
Fitchet (2003) [4]	Twelve weeks CCR with aerobic exercise training	16	TF: not specified TD: not specified TI: HR of 60–75 % of age adjusted maximum with upper limit of HR=detection rate – 10 beats	Exercise time, +16 %	NO ICD discharges
Kamkc 2003 [19]	23±4 days with steady state and/or interval training	107	TF, 1–3 sessions/day TD, 15 min/session TI: not specified; upper limit of HR = detection rate – 20 beats	Excrcisc load, +100 %	No ICD interventions linked to physical training
Vanhees (2004) [3]	Three months CCR with aerobic exercise training	92	TF, 3 sessions/week TD, 90 min/session TI: Leuven (HRrest + 90–90 %[HRmax-HRrest]) with upper limit of HR= detection rate-20 beats TI: Leiden, 50–80 % max intensity	Peak VO$_2$, +17 %	Three ICD discharges after VT: patients dropped out of the study. One ICD discharge after VT. ONE VT without intervention One inappropriate shock
Belardinelli (2006) [5]	Eight weeks CCR	52	TF, 3 sessions/week TD, 60 mins/session TI, 60 % peak VO$_2$ Min firing rate set at +20 beats of HRmax achieved during exercise testing	Peak VO$_2$, +28 % Workload, +36 %	No adverse events

(continued)

Table 11.7 (continued)

Author	Study plan	No.	Training characteristics	Exercise tolerance	Complications
Dougherty (2008) [21]	Eight weeks CCR with aerobic exercise + home walking followed by 4 months home walking	10	TF, 3 supervised sessions/week TD: 60 mins/session TI: gradually increased to 60–80 % HRmax + 2 hours of home walking Following 8 weeks, 30 mins of walking on most days of the week	At 8 weeks: exercise time, +11 % No effect on peakVO$_2$	No adverse events
Dougherty (2015) [22]	8+16 weeks RCT (usual care vs aerobic exercise)	160 (76 usual care; 84 exercise group)	TF, 5 sessions/week TD, 60 min/session TI: gradually increased from 60–65 % HRres to 80–85 % HRres. upper limit of HR = detection rate – 20 beats During 16 weeks maintenance phase (150 mins/week at 80 % HRres)	Larger improvements in peakVO2 in aerobic group compared to usual care	No significant difference between both groups with regard to ICD shocks (tendency to more shocks in usual care group). Only one ICD therapy related to exercise

CCR comprehensive cardiac rehabilitation, *TF* training frequency, *TD* training duration, *TI* training intensity

period of calm physical activity of 5–10 mins, inducing the patient into cardiovascular adjustments and limiting the risk of arrhythmias or other cardiovascular complications. It can include low-intensity aerobic exercise and flexibility exercises. The cooling down is a mild exercise or relative rest of 5–10 mins, protecting the patient from possible complications in the early recovery period and to help the cardiovascular system to return slowly to a resting condition. The main part of the training session can contain aerobic exercises like walking, jogging, cycling, arm ergometry, rowing and predominantly isotonic callisthenics. The exercise intensity is individually determined for every patient, based on the participant's clinical status and the initial exercise tolerance assessed by the baseline exercise test. The interval for training heart rate (HR) is calculated, using the formula of Karvonen (HRtraining HRrest + 60–90 % × (HRpeak – HRrest)). Furthermore, ICD patients are restricted not to surpass the upper heart rate threshold, which was determined in the studies mentioned above as the lowest programmed detection rate minus 10, 20 beats. The cut-off rate is determined for each individual patient depending on the slowest ventricular tachycardia, and the exercise physiologist is responsible for knowing the cut-off rate for the device of each patient who participates in the rehabilitation programme. It is recommended to increase the exercise intensity progressively, based on feedback from the patient and on the results of further exercise tests. In our experience, we recommend an upper heart rate threshold during exercise training of the detection rate minus 20 beats/min. Patients with a history of ventricular arrhythmias provoked by ischaemia or heart failure exacerbations should also pay attention to the body position. It is recommended to perform exercise in an upright position rather than prolonged supine activities, because of lower left ventricular filling pressures in the upright position. Many patients receiving an ICD device are also typed as heart failure patients. Therefore, the addition of resistance training can be highly relevant for these patients with mostly a very poor physical condition. Conraads and colleagues already highlighted the importance of adding isodynamic exercises of specific muscle groups at moderate intensity [23]. By adding resistance training to the endurance training, amelioration of muscle strength and the application on daily encountered activities are possible. Again, arm exercises should be prescribed with special care and should especially be avoided the first 6 weeks after implantation.

The possibility of ECG monitoring should be available in the training room. During the first training sessions, the ECG monitoring assures confidence, freedom of movements and safety from shocks that may occur during exercise. It can give valuable information about heart rhythm, and it can make the patient confident in the safety of exercise. When there are no problems during the first sessions, other heart monitoring devices (e.g. Polar) give enough information to train safety. In the absence of a heart rate monitor, patients should palpate their peripheral pulse regularly during and after the exercises, in order to determine if the pulse is within the limits of the target heart rate. The rehabilitation environment should be light and airy and adequately equipped in order to encourage exercise. Although there is a specific need for close supervision and ECG monitoring during exercise activities, the same safety measures should be taken as in cardiac rehabilitation programmes for a general population of cardiac patients. Exercise training may provoke limited ventricular tachycardia in patients with an ICD during training and/or at the end of the post-training exercise programme. The diagnosis of ventricular tachyarrhythmia occurs when the heart rate exceeds the programmed cut-off rate, and consequently the therapy is delivered by the ICD. After a shock has been delivered, the ICD is interrogated within the next 24 h in order to locate the reason and to, if necessary, make adaptations to the ICD programmed characteristics. As soon as the patient is again clinically stable and feels confident to restart exercise training, the rehabilitation programme should be continued.

There is great emphasis on the individualization of risk factor management, a multidisciplinary approach to ensure provision of optimal care and the need for life-long exercise participation. Cardiologists, physicians, exercise physiologists, dieticians, psychologists and other professionals should collaborate to manage risk reduction through follow-up techniques, including office or clinic visits, attendance of cardiac rehabilitation sessions and mail or telephone contact to show interest in the patient, to keep the patient motivated for participation in the programme and to further reduce psychological stress.

References

1. Vanhees L et al. How to assess physical activity? How to assess physical fitness? Eur J Cardiovasc Prev Rehabil. 2005;12(2):102–14.
2. Vanhees L et al. Exercise performance and training in patients with implantable cardioverter-defibrillators and coronary heart disease. Am J Cardiol. 2001;87(6):712–5.
3. Vanhees L et al. Effect of exercise training in patients with an implantable cardioverter defibrillator. Eur Heart J. 2004;25(13):1120–6.
4. Fitchet A et al. Comprehensive cardiac rehabilitation programme for implantable cardioverter-defibrillator patients: a randomised controlled trial. Heart. 2003;89(2):155–60.
5. Belardinelli R et al. Moderate exercise training improves functional capacity, quality of life, and endothelium-dependent vasodilation in chronic heart failure patients with implantable cardioverter defibrillators and cardiac resynchronization therapy. Eur J Cardiovasc Prev Rehabil. 2006;13(5):818–25.
6. Lampman RM, Knight BP. Prescribing exercise training for patients with defibrillators. Am J Phys Med Rehabil. 2000;79(3):292–7.
7. Voss F et al. Safety of symptom-limited exercise testing in a big cohort of a modern ICD population. Clin Res Cardiol. 2016;105(1):53–8.
8. Sears Jr SF et al. Examining the psychosocial impact of implantable cardioverter defibrillators: a literature review. Clin Cardiol. 1999;22(7):481–9.
9. Sears Jr SF, Conti JB. Quality of life and psychological functioning of icd patients. Heart. 2002;87(5):488–93.
10. Pedersen SS, van den Broek KC, Sears Jr SF. Psychological intervention following implantation of an implantable defibrillator: a review and future recommendations. Pacing Clin Electrophysiol. 2007;30(12):1546–54.
11. Jacq F et al. A comparison of anxiety, depression and quality of life between device shock and nonshock groups in implantable cardioverter defibrillator recipients. Gen Hosp Psychiatry. 2009;31(3):266–73.
12. Dougherty CM, Thompson EA. Intimate partner physical and mental health after sudden cardiac arrest and receipt of an implantable cardioverter defibrillator. Res Nurs Health. 2009;32(4):432–42.
13. Albarran JW, Tagney J, James J. Partners of ICD patients--an exploratory study of their experiences. Eur J Cardiovasc Nurs. 2004;3(3):201–10.
14. Kohn CS, et al. The effect of psychological intervention on patients' long-term adjustment to the ICD: a prospective study. Pacing Clin Electrophysiol. 2000. 23(4 Pt 1): 450–6.
15. Isaksen K et al. Exercise training and cardiac rehabilitation in patients with implantable cardioverter defibrillators: a review of current literature focusing on safety, effects of exercise training, and the psychological impact of programme participation. Eur J Prev Cardiol. 2012;19(4):804–12.
16. Ades PA. Cardiac rehabilitation and secondary prevention of coronary heart disease. N Engl J Med. 2001;345(12):892–902.
17. Lampert R, Cannom D, Olshansky B. Safety of sports participation in patients with implantable cardioverter defibrillators: a survey of heart rhythm society members. J Cardiovasc Electrophysiol. 2006;17(1):11–5.
18. Frizelle DJ et al. Development of a measure of the concerns held by people with implanted cardioverter defibrillators: the ICDC. Br J Health Psychol. 2006;11(Pt 2):293–301.
19. Kamke W et al. Cardiac rehabilitation in patients with implantable defibrillators. Feasibility and complications. Z Kardiol. 2003;92(10):869–75.
20. Davids JS et al. Benefits of cardiac rehabilitation in patients with implantable cardioverter-defibrillators: a patient survey. Arch Phys Med Rehabil. 2005;86(10):1924–8.

21. Dougherty CM, Glenny R, Kudenchuk PJ. Aerobic exercise improves fitness and heart rate variability after an implantable cardioverter defibrillator. J Cardiopulm Rehabil Prev. 2008;28(5):307–11.
22. Dougherty CM et al. Prospective randomized trial of moderately strenuous aerobic exercise after an implantable cardioverter defibrillator. Circulation. 2015;131(21):1835–42.
23. Conraads VM et al. Combined endurance/resistance training reduces NT-proBNP levels in patients with chronic heart failure. Eur Heart J. 2004;25(20):1797–805.

The Rehabilitation in Cardiac Resynchronization Therapy

12

Dumitru Zdrenghea, Dana Pop, and Gabriel Guşetu

12.1 Introduction

Heart failure (HF), especially systolic heart failure, represents an increasingly important public health issue [1]. Due to a more effective management of many cardiac diseases, we encounter fewer complications and observe an increase in survival, heart failure now being diagnosed in older patients, therefore in patients that have multiple comorbidities such as renal, respiratory, or hematologic disease.

The decrease in left ventricular ejection fraction and cardiac output results in a decrease in physical performance and favors a sedentary lifestyle, reducing the exercise capacity even more.

Moreover, poor exercise capacity seems to be the consequence not only of abnormal cardiac hemodynamics but also of skeletal myopathy. This is due to sympathetic overstimulation, chronic activation of inflammatory pathways with inadequate muscle blood flow, malnutrition, and deconditioning and relies on structural changes such as decrease in mitochondria volume, in the amount of oxidative enzymes, and also in a shift in myofibril content from slow-twitch myosin heavy chain (type 1 and 2a) to fast-twitch myosin type 2b fibers [2], more glycolytic than the first ones. Muscular atrophy and evidence of abnormal myocyte apoptosis are often recorded [3, 4].

The patients' decreased exercise capacity needs to be improved by any means. Optimal pharmacological treatment has been proven to enhance the patients' QoL and life expectancy, but it has its limitations [5]. Cardiac transplant, although a valuable treatment in end stage heart failure, is restricted due to co-morbidities, limited

D. Zdrenghea (✉) • D. Pop • G. Guşetu, MD, PhD
University of Medicine and Pharmacy "Iuliu Haţieganu" Rehabilitation Hospital,
Cluj-Napoca, Romania
e-mail: dzdrenghea@yahoo.com

© Springer International Publishing AG 2017
J. Niebauer (ed.), *Cardiac Rehabilitation Manual*,
DOI 10.1007/978-3-319-47738-1_12

supply of donor hearts and complex postoperative care [6, 7]. Physical training, specially designed for patients with heart failure, has proven to be a cost-effective method to increase their exercise tolerance and quality of life (QoL) [8], even if the benefit is not as spectacular as in ischemic heart disease. Thus, six of the trials included in the ExTraMATCH meta-analysis yielded a 20 % increase of peak oxygen consumption (VO$_2$ peak) following physical training programs [9]. The program duration and training intensity should be adapted to the baseline clinical and hemodynamic parameters [10].

Furthermore, cardiac resynchronization therapy (CRT) applied in moderately to severely symptomatic patients with decreased LVEF (below 35 %) and significant mechanical dyssynchrony due to left bundle branch block has demonstrated, over the last two decades, additional benefits in terms of prognosis, quality of life, cardiac hemodynamics, and exercise capacity [11]. Thus, 1–3 months following CRT device implantation, large clinical trials, such as COMPANION and MUSTIC-SR [12], have extensively shown improvement in NYHA class and QoL scores, reduced hospitalizations, improvement in 6 MW distance, and in VO$_2$ peak and ventilatory threshold as markers of exercise performance. CRT accumulates these benefits without increasing myocardial oxygen consumption; by restoring left ventricle mechanical synchrony, it improves left ventricular ejection fraction and cardiac output and reduces mitral regurgitation.

Taking into account that CRT recipients are basically HF patients with a pacemaker, prescribing exercise according to the recommendations designed for people with HF should result in additional benefits in terms of aerobic performance. Indeed, a sub-study of COMPANION reported a 40 % increase in VO$_2$ peak in the group that combined CRT and 4 months of exercise training as compared to CRT alone that only led to a 16 % improvement [11].

Physical training, however, encounters some "technical" issues in CRT patients, which need to be taken into account in order to achieve the maximum benefit.

Case Report

A 56-year-old man (DOB 27 Aug 1959) with a 5-month history of idiopathic dilated cardiomyopathy (DCM) *was admitted in our department*. He was a non-smoker and had no alcohol consumption in the past. He had a son who died of heart failure at age 32, 2 months after the patients' diagnosis was established. Even though suggestive for a family form of DCM, genetic testing was not carried out. At the time of diagnosis (5 months earlier), a coronary angiography was performed and significant coronary artery disease was ruled out. Recommendations about lifestyle changes were made and medical treatment was initiated (carvedilol, perindopril, furosemide, spironolactone).

After 5 months of good adherence to non-pharmacological treatment and medication, the patient complained of poor exercise tolerance (dyspnea) during daily activities – NYHA III class; hence, he was addressed to the Cardiology Department of the Clinical Rehabilitation Hospital.

On physical examination no peripheral or respiratory signs of congestion were found: weight = 76 kg, height = 168 cm, and BP = 100/80 mmHg; standard 12-lead ECG showed sinus rhythm, 60 bpm; PR interval = 200 ms; and left bundle branch block – LBBB (QRS duration = 170 ms – Fig. 12.1). The cardiac ultrasound revealed an LVEF = 24 %, moderate functional mitral regurgitation, left ventricular mechanical delay (septal-to-posterior wall motion delay, SPWMD = 150 ms), interventricular mechanical delay (IVMD = 50 ms), and a global longitudinal strain (GLS) = −14.2 %, lower than normal.

During cardiopulmonary exercise testing (CPET) on cycle, 10 W/min *ramp* protocol, the patient achieved a peak VO_2 of 11 ml/kg/min (3, 1 METS), ventilatory threshold being lower than normal – 32 % of the predicted VO_2max.

We considered that the patient was eligible for CRT-D (cardiac resynchronization therapy with defibrillator). After the implantation of CRT-D device, we noted the narrowing of the QRS complex (150 ms – Fig. 12.2) and initial upward deflection in V1 and downward in V6 – criteria of a successful CRT. There were also improved: the LVEF (30 %), GLS (−17.2 %), and the ultrasound parameters of interventricular and intraventricular dyssynchrony (IVMD = 30 ms, SPWMD = 100 ms).

The patient was reevaluated 4 weeks later. Reassessment via cardiac ultrasound showed unmodified parameters, and the CPET demonstrated an increase in the peak VO_2 up to 12 ml/kg/min, representing a 9 % increase in oxygen uptake after CRT.

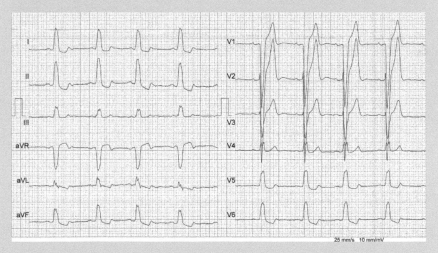

Fig. 12.1 MI, 56 years, male. Standard 12-lead rest ECG at admission. Sinus rhythm, HR = 60 bpm; PR= 200 ms; LBBB, QRS duration = 170 ms

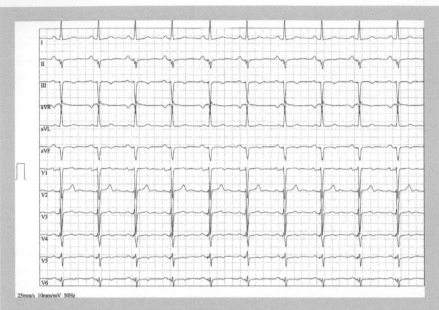

Fig. 12.2 MI, 56 years, male. Standard 12-lead rest ECG after the implantation of CRT-D device. The QRS complex shortened (150 ms) and records an initial positive (*upward*) deflection in V1 and negative (*downward*) deflection in V6, due to early activation of the posterolateral wall of the LV(criteria of successful CRT)

Question 1

Could CRT explain the increase in exercise capacity? Is CPET always required to assess the exercise capacity after CRT or is clinical evaluation accurate enough? Could an increase in peak VO$_2$ of 1 ml/kg/min be considered acceptable after CRT or is it inadequate?

Answer

Improvement of exercise capacity after CRT has been largely demonstrated [11, 13]. In heart failure patients with LBBB, the delayed activation of the left ventricular lateral wall induces a mechanical inter- and intraventricular dyssynchrony that additionally impairs the already decreased LVEF. Hemodynamic studies have shown, 1–3 months after CRT, improvement of the LVEF [14, 15], stroke volume, and SBP and reduction of the capillary pulmonary wedge pressure, mitral regurgitation [16], LV systolic and diastolic diameters [12, 17], and BNP concentrations [18]. Once these goals have been achieved, the neurohormonal blockade optimization [19] by drugs like beta-blockers, ACE inhibitors, or mineralocorticoid receptor antagonists becomes feasible.

In addition to cardiac hemodynamic improvement [20], CRT results in clinical benefits: increase of exercise capacity usually by one NYHA class, less hospitalizations [21], and better QoL scores [13]. All these benefits are usually recorded in the first 1–3 months after implantation [22].

Alongside enhanced cardiac hemodynamic, some peripheral mechanisms are also responsible for the increase in the patients' exercise capacity; the acute increase in systolic blood pressure has a sympathoinhibitory effect, exerted through stimulation of the carotid baroreceptors and probably of the cardiopulmonary baroreceptors and muscular ergoreceptors [11]. The sympathetic nerve overstimulation, resulting in arteriolar constriction and decreased capillary blood flow, is the cornerstone of skeletal myopathy in heart failure, inducing reactive oxygen species release (favored by local hypoperfusion), inflammatory cytokine synthesis [4], with further protein loss, and abnormal apoptosis. Both direct assessment of MSNA (muscle nerve sympathetic activity) [23] *or plasma epinephrine levels* [24] and studies of HRV (heart rate variability) [25, 26] as marker of autonomic imbalance proved the decrease of sympathetic overstimulation after CRT. The latter was noted 3 months following the implantation and was associated with increase in 6 MWT distance or peak VO_2 during CPET [11].

The vascular endothelial function, impaired in HF patients, seems to be another pathway positively influenced by CRT in terms of exercise capacity improvement. Thus, RH-PAT (reactive hyperemia peripheral arterial tonometry) index increases with 20 % after CRT is added to optimal pharmacologic therapy [27, 28].

After CRT, the CPET is not imperative; however, the accurate assessment of exercise capacity gain [29] and prognosis as well as the best rehabilitation program outlines rely on the CPET parameters; therefore, it is recommended whenever possible.

In our patient, the exercise capacity was moderately increased (a VO_2 max improvement of only 1 ml/kg/min) at the lower border of the reported ranges (1.1–2.3 ml/kg/min), directly related to the baseline LVEF and duration of the disease [14, 30].

Question 2

What are the possible determinants of less than expected improvement in exercise capacity after CRT?

- Technical issues related to the implantation of the CRT device
- Sedentary lifestyle at the onset of the disease
- Comorbidities: obesity, chronic respiratory disease, anemia, etc.

Answer

In clinical trials, about 30 % of patients have no benefit from CRT (CRT nonresponders) [31]. Certain documents concerning the best approach to CRT nonresponders have shown that reevaluation of the CRT device (including pacing lead position and programmed parameters) should be considered along with optimization of the pharmacologic therapy as the main steps in this "troubleshooting algorithm" in order to achieve and maintain the clinical outcome [32].

The suboptimal technical results of CRT are primarily related to LV pacing lead placement limitations, caused by particular anatomy of the coronary sinus branches, scar proximity, or phrenic nerve stimulation, but also to suboptimal atrioventricular (AV) and right ventricle-to-left ventricle (RV-LV) delay [33].

In our patient, the poor improvement in exercise capacity was not determined by technical issues, all the parameters tested soon after implantation and at 4 weeks post-procedural evaluation being within normal range.

On the other hand, some clinical issues such as preexisting sedentary lifestyle and physical deconditioning could lead to a weaker and delayed response to CRT, but our patient has an active lifestyle.

Furthermore, the CRT non-responders should be evaluated for other well-known conditions such as chronic kidney disease, worsening of mitral regurgitation, new-onset atrial fibrillation, or myocardial ischemia (in the setting of coronary artery disease). All of them were ruled out in our case.

The third category includes conditions unrelated to abnormal cardiac performance, but certainly very common among HF patients [32]. These conditions are able to decrease the benefits of CRT.

Obesity increases oxygen consumption at rest; thus, the maximal effort capacity is reduced but our patient has normal weight. Chronic respiratory diseases, especially COPD [34, 35], contribute to the decrease in peak VO_2 by impairing the respiratory phase of oxygen transportation. Our patient performed spirometry, which showed normal values, and the ventilatory parameters were also within normal range during CPET; thus, a respiratory cause was improbable.

Anemia is another well-known cause for reduced effort capacity in heart failure patients. It could be the result of erythropoietin deficit, in this case erythropoietin treatment representing a feasible option for improving clinical status. More often anemia is due to iron deficit, which occurs long before the onset of anemia. This is why screening for iron deficiency by serum ferritin determination and parenteral iron replacement is largely recommended in HF patients [36].

In our patient, a moderate anemia was recorded (Hb = 10.3 g/dl, ferritin 30 ng/ml) as well as an iron deficiency of 489 mg. We therefore administered iv Ferinject (500 mg/10 ml), and after 4 weeks, the normalization of hemoglobin was achieved (Hb = 13.1 g/dl). An additional dose of 500 mg was administered to restore the iron reserve. This was followed by an improvement in clinical status. The patient noticed a better effort capacity and quality of life. Therefore we considered the patient can be included now in a physical training program.

Question 3

What is the rationale of cardiac rehabilitation in CRT recipients considering that the resynchronization therapy by itself improves the exercise capacity?

Answer

The physical training in resynchronized HF patients is recommended because it further enhances exercise tolerance [37]. The COMPANION trial has reported an improvement of 24 % in exercise capacity [11], regardless of baseline characteristics of patients or disease severity.

These benefits result mainly from improvement of peripheral mechanisms involved during exercise, including skeletal muscle abnormalities (peripheral sympathetic nerve activity, inflammatory cytokines, endothelial dysfunction) [37, 38], the last being recorded after at least 3 months of cardiac rehabilitation [38]. Therefore, for the same myocardial oxygen consumption and cardiac output, endurance training provides additional benefits in terms of exercise capacity measured by parameters such as peak oxygen consumption (peak VO_2). Reverse left ventricular remodeling and increasing of cardiac output were also reported [12].

So, our patient was enrolled in a cardiac rehabilitation program designed for heart failure patients. The physical training was initiated in the Outpatient Department of the Clinical Rehabilitation Hospital.

A 6-month program consisting of three sessions/week was initiated. According to current guideline recommendations, each session was planned to consist of 5 mins warm-up and cool-down period and progressive 15–30 mins training on cycle, with progressive increase in exercise workload from 50 % peak VO_2 (HR = 80 bpm) to 70 % peak VO_2 (HR = 90–95 bpm). To calculate training HR, the heart rate reserve (HRR) was used because peak HR during CPET was low (treatment with carvedilol). During the rest of the days of the week, walking 2–3 km/hour, for 15–30 mins, was recommended.

Medical advice regarding lifestyle changes (dietary energy content, salt intake, smoking, and alcohol forbidden) was provided.

During cycle ergometer training, even if the heart rate increased appropriately, he tolerated the exercise poorly and complained of dyspnea, especially once the HR exceeded 80 bpm.

Question 4

How can the unexpectedly decreased exercise tolerance be explained?

Answer

The debate comprises several issues:

- The severe impairment of the left ventricle systolic performance. The negative correlation between the LVEF and the resting heart rate has been demonstrated; furthermore, the lower the LVEF [39], the lower the maximal exercise heart rate and the heart rate reserve.
- In our patient, however, the LVEF significantly improved (from 24 to 30 %) and the resting heart rate was normal. Moreover, during exercise, the heart rate increased normally, even if the patient complained of dyspnea.
- The skeletal myopathy in heart failure [4]. The decreased oxidative capacity of skeletal muscle is an important limiting factor of exercise capacity especially in elderly or in patients with longer disease duration. It is not the case of our middle-aged patient with a 6-month history of heart failure and without any suggestive symptoms of myopathy (muscular weakness/pain).
- The loss of biventricular pacing during exercise. The greatest benefits of CRT observed during the follow-up of large cohorts were associated with a biventricular pacing exceeding 98 % of all ventricular beats [40]. When the biventricular pacing is lost (due to atrial fibrillation or, in sinus rhythm, because of an AV conduction faster than the programmed AV interval), the LBBB, ventricular

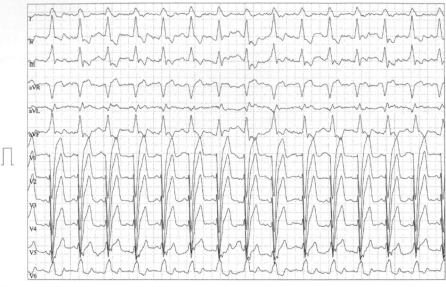

Fig. 12.3 MI, 56 years, male. On the ECG recorded during training sessions, at HR above 80/min, the LBBB reappears because PR shortens to 150 ms, less than the programmed AV delay (160 ms)

dyssynchrony, and the hemodynamic disturbances will reappear and the benefit of CRT is lost. This can occur during exercise (including physical training) above a certain heart rate because of increased sympathetic stimulation.

The ECG monitoring of the patient during training has shown shortening of the intrinsic PR interval to 150 ms, when the heart rate exceeded 80 bpm. Whereas the programmed AV delay was 160 ms, the biventricular pacing was lost, and on the surface (standard 12-lead) ECG, the initial LBBB reappeared (Fig. 12.3). Therefore the AV delay was refined by choosing a rate-responsive AV delay corresponding to 130 ms for a heart rate range of 80–120 bpm.

As seen in Fig. 12.4, after reprogramming the AV interval, the biventricular pacing was preserved during physical training, up to a heart rate of 108 bpm. Given the improvement of the symptoms (dyspnea), he was able to complete his 6-month training program.

At the end of the training program, CPET showed a 25 % improvement in peak VO_2 (from 12 to 15 ml/kg/min – Fig. 12.5) and also the maintaining of biventricular pacing all along exercise testing.

Conclusion

CRT is an effective additional tool in the management of systolic heart failure patients, in the setting of LBBB and LVEF <35 %. By improving cardiac hemodynamics but also the skeletal myopathy and peripheral mechanisms which intervene during exercise, physical training enhances the benefits of CRT. Whenever physical training fails to increase the exercise capacity, the

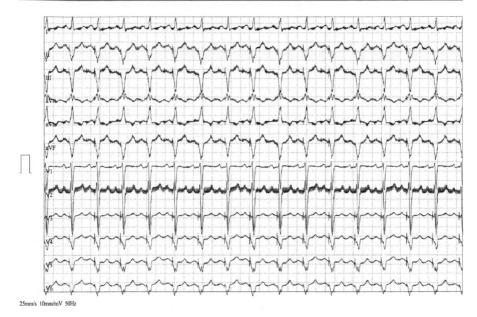

25mm/s 10mm/mV 50Hz

Fig. 12.4 MI, 56 years, male. The AV delay was programmed at 130 ms. During the entire training session, the biventricular pacing is preserved, up to a HR of 108 bpm

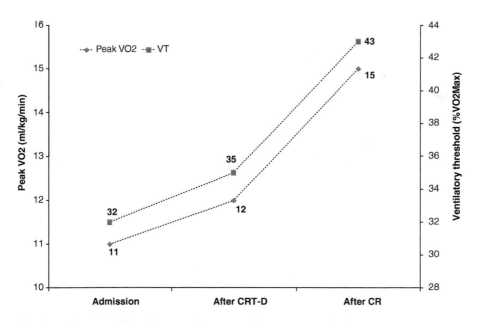

Fig. 12.5 The peak VO_2 and VT at admission and improvement after CRT-D implantation and after the training program

underlying causes, as anemia or loss of biventricular pacing during exercise, have to be reviewed.

That's why always before or during the exercise training is recommended to check by CPET, exercise testing, or by ECG monitoring of the training sessions, if during the entire session the biventricular pacing is preserved.

References

1. Cook C, Cole G, Asaria P, Jabbour R, Francis DP. The annual global economic burden of heart failure. Int J Cardiol. 2014;171(3):368–76.
2. Piepoli MF, Crisafulli A. Pathophysiology of human heart failure: importance of skeletal muscle myopathy and reflexes. Exp Physiol. 2014;99(4):609–15.
3. Ivakine EA, Cohn RD. Maintaining skeletal muscle mass: lessons learned from hibernation. Exp Physiol. 2014;99(4):632–7.
4. Middlekauff HR. How does cardiac resynchronization therapy improve exercise capacity in chronic heart failure? J Card Fail. 2005;11(7):534–41.
5. Gandhi PU, Szymonifka J, Motiwala SR, Belcher AM, Januzzi Jr JL, Gaggin HK. Characterization and prediction of adverse events from intensive chronic heart failure management and effect on quality of life: results from the pro-B-type natriuretic peptide outpatient-tailored chronic heart failure therapy (PROTECT) study. J Card Fail. 2015;21(1):9–15.
6. Ashraf O, Sharif H. Cardiac failure, transplantation and donation: current perspectives. J Cardiovasc Surg (Torino). 2015;56(4):661–9.
7. Toyoda Y, Guy TS, Kashem A. Present status and future perspectives of heart transplantation. Circ J. 2013;77(5):1097–110.
8. Taylor RS, Piepoli MF, Smart N, Coats AJ, Ellis S, Dalal H, et al. Exercise training for chronic heart failure (ExTraMATCH II): protocol for an individual participant data meta-analysis. Int J Cardiol. 2014;174(3):683–7.
9. Piepoli MF, Davos C, Francis DP, Coats AJ. Exercise training meta-analysis of trials in patients with chronic heart failure (ExTraMATCH). BMJ. 2004;328(7433):16.
10. Vromen T, Kraal JJ, Kuiper J, Spee RF, Peek N, Kemps HM. The influence of training characteristics on the effect of aerobic exercise training in patients with chronic heart failure: a meta-regression analysis. Int J Cardiol. 2016;208:120–7.
11. De Marco T, Wolfel E, Feldman AM, Lowes B, Higginbotham MB, Ghali JK, et al. Impact of cardiac resynchronization therapy on exercise performance, functional capacity, and quality of life in systolic heart failure with QRS prolongation: COMPANION trial sub-study. J Card Fail. 2008;14(1):9–18.
12. Duncan A, Wait D, Gibson D, Daubert JC. Left ventricular remodelling and haemodynamic effects of multisite biventricular pacing in patients with left ventricular systolic dysfunction and activation disturbances in sinus rhythm: sub-study of the MUSTIC (Multisite Stimulation in Cardiomyopathies) trial. Eur Heart J. 2003;24(5):430–41.
13. Turley AJ, Raja SG, Salhiyyah K, Nagarajan K. Does cardiac resynchronisation therapy improve survival and quality of life in patients with end-stage heart failure? Interact Cardiovasc Thorac Surg. 2008;7(6):1141–6.
14. Seifert M, Schlegl M, Hoersch W, Fleck E, Doelger A, Stockburger M, et al. Functional capacity and changes in the neurohormonal and cytokine status after long-term CRT in heart failure patients. Int J Cardiol. 2007;121(1):68–73.
15. Schuchert A, Muto C, Maounis T, Ella RO, Polauck A, Padeletti L. Relationship between pre-implant ejection fraction and outcome after cardiac resynchronization therapy in symptomatic patients. Acta Cardiol. 2014;69(4):424–32.

16. Chan KL, Tang AS, Achilli A, Sassara M, Bocchiardo M, Gaita F, et al. Functional and echocardiographic improvement following multisite biventricular pacing for congestive heart failure. Can J Cardiol. 2003;19(4):387–90.
17. Donal E, Leclercq C, Linde C, Daubert JC. Effects of cardiac resynchronization therapy on disease progression in chronic heart failure. Eur Heart J. 2006;27(9):1018–25.
18. Piepoli MF, Villani GQ, Corra U, Aschieri D, Rusticali G. Time course of effects of cardiac resynchronization therapy in chronic heart failure: benefits in patients with preserved exercise capacity. Pacing Clin Electrophysiol. 2008;31(6):701–8.
19. Kachboura S, Ben Halima A, Ibn Elhadj Z, Marrakchi S, Chrigui R, Kammoun I, et al. Cardiac resynchronization therapy allows the optimization of medical treatment in heart failure patients. Ann Cardiol Angeiol. 2014;63(1):17–22.
20. Schlosshan D, Barker D, Pepper C, Williams G, Morley C, Tan LB. CRT improves the exercise capacity and functional reserve of the failing heart through enhancing the cardiac flow- and pressure-generating capacity. Eur J Heart Fail. 2006;8(5):515–21.
21. Linde C, Gold MR, Abraham WT, St John Sutton M, Ghio S, Cerkvenik J, et al. Long-term impact of cardiac resynchronization therapy in mild heart failure: 5-year results from the REsynchronization reVErses Remodeling in Systolic left vEntricular dysfunction (REVERSE) study. Eur Heart J. 2013;34(33):2592–9.
22. Pires LA, Abraham WT, Young JB, Johnson KM. Clinical predictors and timing of New York Heart Association class improvement with cardiac resynchronization therapy in patients with advanced chronic heart failure: results from the Multicenter InSync Randomized Clinical Evaluation (MIRACLE) and Multicenter InSync ICD Randomized Clinical Evaluation (MIRACLE-ICD) trials. Am Heart J. 2006;151(4):837–43.
23. Kuniyoshi RR, Martinelli M, Negrao CE, Siqueira SF, Rondon MU, Trombetta IC, et al. Effects of cardiac resynchronization therapy on muscle sympathetic nerve activity. Pacing Clin Electrophysiol. 2014;37(1):11–8.
24. Grassi G, Vincenti A, Brambilla R, Trevano FQ, Dell'Oro R, Ciro A, et al. Sustained sympathoinhibitory effects of cardiac resynchronization therapy in severe heart failure. Hypertension. 2004;44(5):727–31.
25. Adamson PB, Kleckner KJ, VanHout WL, Srinivasan S, Abraham WT. Cardiac resynchronization therapy improves heart rate variability in patients with symptomatic heart failure. Circulation. 2003;108(3):266–9.
26. Fantoni C, Raffa S, Regoli F, Giraldi F, La Rovere MT, Prentice J, et al. Cardiac resynchronization therapy improves heart rate profile and heart rate variability of patients with moderate to severe heart failure. J Am Coll Cardiol. 2005;46(10):1875–82.
27. Enomoto K, Yamabe H, Toyama K, Matsuzawa Y, Yamamuro M, Uemura T, et al. Improvement effect on endothelial function in patients with congestive heart failure treated with cardiac resynchronization therapy. J Cardiol. 2011;58(1):69–73.
28. Tesselaar E, Schiffer A, Widdershoven J, Broers H, Hendriks E, Luijten K, et al. Effect of cardiac resynchronization therapy on endothelium-dependent vasodilatation in the cutaneous microvasculature. Pacing Clin Electrophysiol. 2012;35(4):377–84.
29. Mehra MR, Greenberg BH. Cardiac resynchronization therapy: caveat medicus! J Am Coll Cardiol. 2004;43(7):1145–8.
30. Chwyczko T, Sterlinski M, Maciag A, Firek B, Labecka A, Jankowska A, et al. Impact of cardiac resynchronisation therapy on adaptation of circulatory and respiratory systems to exercise assessed by cardiopulmonary exercise test in patients with chronic heart failure. Kardiol Pol. 2008;66(4):406–12.
31. Zhang Q, Zhou Y, Yu CM. Incidence, definition, diagnosis, and management of the cardiac resynchronization therapy nonresponder. Curr Opin Cardiol. 2015;30(1):40–9.
32. Aranda Jr JM, Woo GW, Schofield RS, Handberg EM, Hill JA, Curtis AB, et al. Management of heart failure after cardiac resynchronization therapy: integrating advanced heart failure treatment with optimal device function. J Am Coll Cardiol. 2005;46(12):2193–8.
33. Bax JJ, Abraham T, Barold SS, Breithardt OA, Fung JW, Garrigue S, et al. Cardiac resynchronization therapy: Part 1--issues before device implantation. J Am Coll Cardiol. 2005;46(12):2153–67.

34. Guder G, Brenner S, Stork S, Hoes A, Rutten FH. Chronic obstructive pulmonary disease in heart failure: accurate diagnosis and treatment. Eur J Heart Fail. 2014;16(12):1273–82.
35. Yoshihisa A, Takiguchi M, Shimizu T, Nakamura Y, Yamauchi H, Iwaya S, et al. Cardiovascular function and prognosis of patients with heart failure coexistent with chronic obstructive pulmonary disease. J Cardiol. 2014;64(4):256–64.
36. Avni T, Leibovici L, Gafter-Gvili A. Iron supplementation for the treatment of chronic heart failure and iron deficiency: systematic review and meta-analysis. Eur J Heart Fail. 2012;14(4):423–9.
37. Patwala AY, Woods PR, Sharp L, Goldspink DF, Tan LB, Wright DJ. Maximizing patient benefit from cardiac resynchronization therapy with the addition of structured exercise training: a randomized controlled study. J Am Coll Cardiol. 2009;53(25):2332–9.
38. Conraads VM, Vanderheyden M, Paelinck B, Verstreken S, Blankoff I, Miljoen H, et al. The effect of endurance training on exercise capacity following cardiac resynchronization therapy in chronic heart failure patients: a pilot trial. Eur J Cardiovasc Prev Rehabil. 2007;14(1): 99–106.
39. Haennel RG. Exercise rehabilitation for chronic heart failure patients with cardiac device implants. Cardiopulm Phys Ther J. 2012;23(3):23–8.
40. Hayes DL, Boehmer JP, Day JD, Gilliam 3rd FR, Heidenreich PA, Seth M, et al. Cardiac resynchronization therapy and the relationship of percent biventricular pacing to symptoms and survival. Heart Rhythm. 2011;8(9):1469–75.

Exercise Training in Congenital Heart Diseases

13

Birna Bjarnason-Wehrens, Sigrid Dordel,
Sabine Schickendantz, Narayanswami Sreeram,
and Konrad Brockmeier

13.1 Introduction

Congenital malformations of the heart and vessels occur in 5–9 per 1000 live births [1–4]. The data from the European Surveillance of Congenital Anomalies central database (EUROCAT) show the average prevalence in Europe to be 7.2 per 1000 live births varying between countries [3]. The spectrum of congenital malformations of the heart and vessels is diverse. Defects can roughly be categorised into left-to-right shunt lesions, cyanotic lesions, obstructive lesions and complex lesions associated with common mixing and single ventricle physiology [1] (Fig. 13.1). Table 13.1 shows the most frequent congenital heart diseases comprising approximately 80 % of all malformations [1, 2].

About 10–15 % of the congenital malformations of the heart and vessels do not require correction. Between 70 and 80 % of all congenital heart defects can be corrected or palliated in the long term, and an increasing number of therapeutic procedures can be performed by interventional catheterisation techniques, avoiding the need for open-heart surgery [1]. Definitive therapeutic procedures are increasingly carried out in early infancy, to avoid long-term complications resulting from the haemodynamic burden or from chronic cyanosis [5–7]. In 2002, a total of 27,772 operations for the treatment of congenital malformations of the heart and vessels were performed in Europe. Germany leads the European statistic. In 2014, 5779 cardiac operations for congenital heart defects were performed in Germany, 4775 of those using the heart-lung machine. Significantly, almost half of all

B. Bjarnason-Wehrens (✉) • S. Dordel
Institute for Cardiology and Sports Medicine, German Sportuniversity Colgene,
Am Sportpark Müngersdorf 6, Cologne 50933 Germany
e-mail: bjarnason@dshs-koeln.de

S. Schickendantz • N. Sreeram • K. Brockmeier
Department of Peadiatric Cardiology, University of Cologne,
Kerpener Str. 62, Salzburg 50937 Germany

© Springer International Publishing AG 2017
J. Niebauer (ed.), *Cardiac Rehabilitation Manual*,
DOI 10.1007/978-3-319-47738-1_13

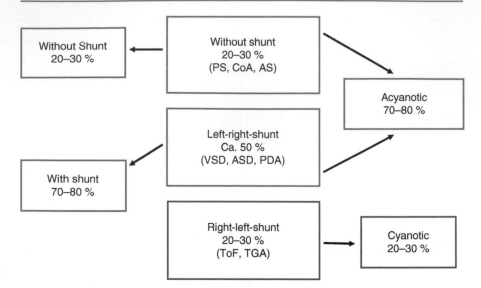

Fig. 13.1 Classification of congenital heart defects according to defects with or without shunt and with or without cyanosis (Definition of abbreviations, see Table 13.1) [20]

Table 13.1 The most frequently diagnosed congenital heart diseases [1, 2]

Acyanotic defects	
Obstructions in valves or vessels	*Primary left-to-right shunt*
Pulmonary stenosis (PS) 6–13 %	Ventricular septal defects (VSD) (isolated) 14–16 %
Coarctation of the aorta (CoA) 8–11 %	Atrial septal defects (ASD) 4–10 %
Aortic stenosis (AS) 6–9 %	Persistent ductus arteriosus (PDA) 10–15 %
Cyanotic lesions	
Right-to-left shunt	*Complex lesions*
Tetralogy of Fallot (ToF) 9–14 %	Single ventricle physiology, e.g. hypoplastic left heart syndrome (HLHS) 4–8 %
Transposition of the great arteries (TGA) 10–11 %	

operations were performed on neonates and infants. In addition, there were 5100 catheter interventions [8]. Progress in treatment of congenital heart disease has led to a dramatic reduction of mortality [6–10]. Population-based data from the USA demonstrate 39 % reduction in mortality from heart defects (all ages) in the period from 1979 to 1997 [4]. Mortality rates demonstrate further decline up to 2007 [4, 8] that since then have been stable on the low level. Age at death is increasing, suggesting that more affected persons are living to adolescence and adulthood [8, 9]. Results of the UK central cardiac audit database, valid for the year 2001, show the 1-year survival rate for children undergoing operation before 1 year of age at 90 % and for therapeutic catheterisation at 98.1 % [10]. In Norway in 2011, the 1-year survival for children undergoing operation was 96.5 % and the 5-year 95.0 % [6]. In Germany mortality from congenital cardiac malformations (operated or unoperated) has decreased by approximately 60 % between 1990 and 2014. This decrease was seen in all age groups. The greatest decline was seen in the group of neonates (70 %) [8]. In Finland the 60-year survival in CHD patients was found to be 70 % versus 86 % for the general population [7]. Thus the population of adult patients with congenital heart diseases (ACHD) is continuously growing. Due to the remarkable improvement in survival, this also applies to the group of patients with more complex disease. The precise number of ACHD patients in Europe is unknown [11].

With improved survival, the focus of follow-up care has to shift from assessment of procedure-related mortality towards assessment of long-term quality of life. A review from Marino et al. [12] revealed high prevalence of developmental disorders/deficits in children with CHD. This applies to attention performance, psychosocial strengths as well as deficits in gross and fine motor development. Preventive diagnosis and treatment have to be initiated early, aiming to find deficits and alleviate them through the use of specific therapeutic/rehabilitative measures [13–15]. Motor development and physical activity are one of the fields on which diagnosis and treatment must focus, in particular to what extent physical activity should be recommended in order to improve the quality of life [13–18].

This chapter will focus on the impact of physical activity and exercise training in children, adolescents and adults with congenital heart disease.

13.2 The Impact of Physical Activity and Exercise Training in Children and Adolescents with Congenital Heart Diseases

Children have a basic need for motor activity. This elementary need to move is biologically based and guaranteed by the dominance of central nervous excitation processes. Movement serves as a catalyst in the child's development, especially in younger children. A high level of movement ensures the advancement of the child's physical development, especially the locomotor system, which through movement gains the impulses needed for its normal development [19, 20]. In contrast, physical inactivity in childhood is abnormal – regardless of whether it is due to physical, emotional, psychosocial or cognitive factors [20]. Establishing contacts self-confidently, thoughtfulness, cooperation, benchmarking, competence, abiding by rules and participating in group activities are important behaviours which preschool children mainly learn by taking part in active games with peers. As early as preschool age, good motor abilities, skilfulness and strength improve a child's social reputation with his/her group of peers, thereby improving self-confidence and supporting the development of emotional stability and positive self-image; this is even more pronounced at early school age [19]. Thus the children's perceptual and motor experience not only determines their physical and motor development but also decisively influences their emotional, psychosocial and cognitive development. Deficiency in this field might affect the children's entire personal development in a negative way [19–21].

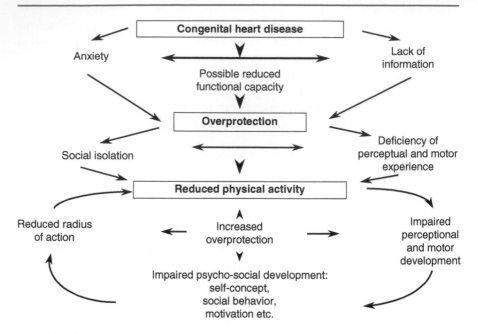

Fig. 13.2 Conditional network of possible causes and effects of physical inactivity in children with congenital heart diseases (CHD) [20]

Often, cardiac disease means a restriction of the affected child's perceptual and motor experience. Complex and severe heart defects may, at least temporarily, cause reduced symptom-limited exercise tolerance and therefore require a certain amount of rest. Times of inpatient examinations or corrective operations are always periods of more or less strict immobilisation. Depending on their duration and the child's age and mental stability, cardiac disease can lead to developmental stagnation or regression. Great uncertainty exists especially with regard to the danger to which one might expose children by allowing them to engage in physical activity. This is often – unnecessarily – also the case with children whose physical capacities are grossly normal [20, 21]. Figure 13.2 shows the conditional network of possible causes and effects of physical inactivity in children with heart diseases.

Relatively few studies [19, 21–25] have focused on the motor development in children with congenital malformed heart (Fig. 13.3). All studies but one [25] performed have demonstrated that deficits in motor development can be expected in a relatively large group of affected children and adolescents. In a large study [21] the motor development in 194 subjects with congenital malformations of the heart was compared with that of a representative control group of healthy peers. The classification of the motor development demonstrated 58.7 % of the children with heart disease to have moderate to severe deficits in gross motor skills and 31.9 % to have severe deficits (Fig. 13.4). In the group of children with CHD, no differences were found for gender, but older children and adolescents (aged 11–15 years) had more

The body-coordination-test for children (KTK)
Schilling F. Körperkoordinationstest für Kinder. KTK Manual. Weinheim: 1974

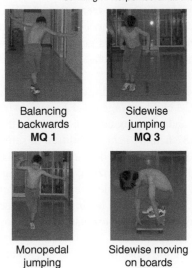

MQ	Classification
131-145	high motor deverlopment
116-130	good motordeverlopment
86-115	normal motor deverlopment
71-85	moderate motor disturbances
56-70	sever motor disturbances
< 56	below classification level

Balancing
backwards
MQ 1

Sidewise
jumping
MQ 3

Monopedal
jumping
MQ 2

Sidewise moving
on boards
MQ 4

Fig. 13.3 The body coordination test for children. Classification of motor development depending on the motor quotient adjusted for age and gender (Schilling F. Körperkoordinationstest für Kinder. KTK Manual. Weinheim: 1974) [21]

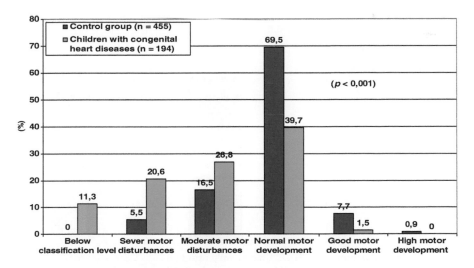

Fig. 13.4 Classification of the motor development in children with congenital heart disease compared to a representative group of healthy pears [21]

severe deficits compared to younger children (5–10 years of age; $p < 0.01$). The mean age- and gender-adjusted motor quotient was significantly lower in the group of children with CHD compared to the control group. This was seen in the children with significant residual sequelae as well as in those with no or mild residual sequelae (Fig. 13.5). This is especially noticeable since there is no reason for any restriction of physical activity in the children with mild uncorrected lesions or without residual sequelae after previous surgery.

Another large study investigated the motor competence in children with complex congenital heart disease [18]. The results of 120 children (aged 7–12 years) who had undergone a surgical repair with multiple and complex correction within the first year of life were compared with that of 387 healthy school children at same age. Children with CHD scored significantly worse for manual dexterity, ball skills, grip strength, quadriceps muscle strength and static and dynamic balance (Fig. 13.6). Compared with the healthy peers, children with complex congenital heart disease had 5.8-fold (95 % confidence interval, 3.8–8.8) risk of having some degree of impaired motor competence. The risk for having severe motor disturbances was 11-fold (95 % confidence interval, 5.4–22.5) [18].

The results of studies investigating the exercise tolerance of children and young adults with various forms of congenital heart diseases demonstrate that depending on the severity of the defect, the success of corrective procedures and the presence and degree of residual sequelae, physical performance may be limited [26–38]. However, the findings show that even children with mild uncorrected lesions or

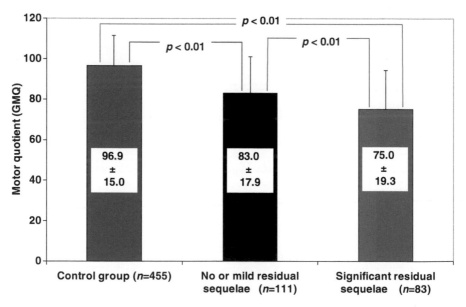

Fig. 13.5 The mean motor quotient in children with no or mild residual sequelae compared to those having significant residual sequelae and to a representative group of healthy peers

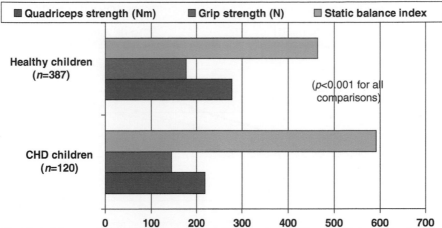

Fig. 13.6 Mean results in quadriceps and handgrip strength as well as static balance (low balance index indicates good abilities to perform the balance task) in children with complex congenital heart disease compared with healthy peers (According to Holm et al. [18])

without residual sequelae after previous surgery may reveal a substantial reduction in their physical performance [27, 28, 37].

Fredriksen et al. [27] compared the peak oxygen uptake (VO_{2peak}) of 169 children and adolescents (91 boys, 78 girls, aged 8–16 years) with congenital heart disease with that of a representative control group of 196 healthy pears. The results demonstrated that patients with CHD exhibited lower VO_{2peak} values in all age groups, with declining values for boys after the age of 12–13 years (Fig. 13.7). While patients with tetralogy of Fallot had lower VO_{2peak} values, they made approximately the same progress with age as healthy peers. A marked decline in VO_{2peak} was seen in patients with transposition of the great arteries after the age of 12–13 years. These results have been confirmed in more recently published studies showing reduced exercise capacity in children, adolescents and young adults (aged 6–25 years) with various CHD diagnosis. They revealed VO_{2peak} to be markedly reduced by 60–82 % of that predicted [33, 35, 36, 38].

Some studies have evaluated the physical activity patterns in children and adolescents with CHD and [38–43] and in the majority of the cases found it to be reduced compared to healthy pears.

A study investigating the activity patterns of 54 children and adolescents (aged 7–14 years) after neonatal arterial switch operation using 24 h continuous heart rate monitoring revealed that these patients do not meet the guideline for physical activity. Compared to the results of 124 age-matched healthy children, the CHD group was significantly less active. This was true for moderate and vigorous activities. The results revealed only 19 and 27 % of the CHD patients engaged in more than 30 min a day of moderate activity and 20 min a day in vigorous activity, respectively [42]. McCrindle et al. [43] demonstrated that in children and adolescents after Fontan procedure, the measured time spent in moderate and vigorous activity was markedly

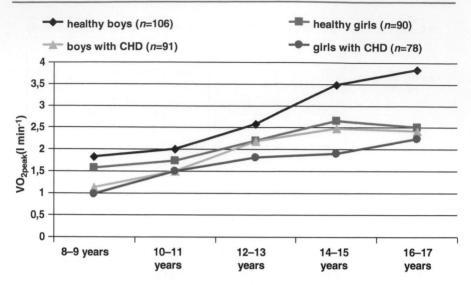

Fig. 13.7 Mean results of VO$_{2peak}$ (1 min^{-1}) for healthy boys and girls compared to boys and girls with congenital heart disease (According to Fredriksen et al. [27])

below normal at all age. This was seen particularly in female patients and was not significantly related to self-reported activity levels or to VO$_{2peak}$ levels [43].

O'Bryne et al. [38] evaluated the habitual exercise habits in 88 subjects (12.6 ± 3.3 years) with conotruncal abnormalities. They revealed median amount of weekly exercise to be 4 h (interquartile range 0–2, 2–4, 4–9.7, and 9.7–24 h/week). The VO$_{2peak}$ was 76 ± 21 % of that predicted. They found hours of weekly habitual exercise to be correlated with exercise performance. Arvidsson et al. [40] evaluated the physical activity level and physical performance in 32 children aged 9–11 years and 25 adolescents aged 14–16 years with CHD. They found a significant correlation between physical activity level and VO$_{2peak}$ in 9–11-year-old girls and 14–16-year-old boys and girls but not in the group of 9–11-year-old boys with CHD.

Obesity is also a common comorbidity in children with congenital heart diseases [44]. Findings from Stefan et al. [45] demonstrated exercise-intolerant and activity-restricted children experienced larger increases in the absolute body mass index (BMI) and the BMI percentile than children with neither exercise intolerance nor activity restrictions. In 110 children with congenital heart disease (mean age 8.4 years), activity restriction was the strongest predictor of the risk of being overweight and obese at follow-up [45].

These results emphasise the importance of encouraging children and adolescents with congenital heart disease to engage more in physical activity and exercise training in order to avoid sedentary behaviour in adulthood and prevent atherosclerotic cardiovascular disease.

The impact of a congenital cardiac malformation on the development of the affected child depends on the type and severity of the malformation, as well as the timing and success of therapeutic measures. For some complex malformations with single ventricle physiology, only palliative solutions are available. Lesions such as tetralogy of Fallot [46], atrioventricular septal defect [47] and transposition of the great arteries [46] can be successfully corrected in infancy with good long-term outcome. After successful correction in infancy, most of the children born with cyanotic congenital malformations are able to participate in all normal age-appropriate physical activities with their healthy peers [13–15, 48–54]. While in children with significant postoperative clinical findings some restrictions regarding physical activity might be recommended, the group of children with no or mild residual sequelae do not require any restrictions and should be taking part in normal physical activity. Although it is well recognised that neurological impairment might be caused by pre-/postoperative persistent low cardiac output, acidosis and/or hypoxia or from ischaemia related to surgery and be associated with later neurological deficits [55–59], this alone does not explain the deficits in motor development observed in children with congenital heart diseases. The main studies cited did exclude all children with recognised syndromes, disabilities or comorbidities, which might have affected their motor development. It is more likely that a significant proportion of the deficits in motor development observed are primarily due to lack of efficient bodily perception and movement experience due to restrictions in physical activity. Overprotective behaviour in the children's parents and teachers could be an important reason for the observed deficits. Mothers of children with congenital heart disease report higher levels of vigilance with their children than mothers of healthy children same aged [60]. Anxiety and overprotecting parents' attitude might reduce the child's exposure to peers, not least regarding physical activity, which might influence the child's social competence, motor development and cause retardation [61]. Parents of children with congenital heart disease are more likely to report elevated levels of parenting stress compared to the normal population [62–64]. This high level of stress is unrelated to the severity of the child's disease but tends to be higher in parents with older children when it becomes more difficult for them to set limits and maintain control [65]. Mothers are most concerned not only about the medical prognosis of their child but also regarding the child's quality of life including aspects like functional and physical limitations [65].

13.3 Recommendations for Physical Activity

Numerous groups of experts have provided recommendations concerning exercise for children with CHD [13–15, 50–53, 66]. These recommendations can contribute to avoiding unnecessary exclusion of children and adolescents with heart disease from physical activity and sport. Moreover, they can minimise children's, parents' and teachers' insecurity in regard to the affected child's physical abilities. In keeping with these recommendations, all youth with CHD who fulfil the necessary requirements should have the opportunity to participate in physical activity and, if needed, take part in specially adapted programmes of physical education. For the assessment of aptitude and classification, the primary heart defect is less important

Table 13.2 Classification according to current cardiac situation and postoperative clinical findings [20, 66]

Group 0	*Patients with haemodynamically significant cardiac defects before cardiac surgery/ interventions (including ablation)*
Group 1	*Patients after heart surgical/catheter interventional operations*
1.1	No residual sequelae (complete correction)
1.2	With mild residual sequelae
1.3	With significant residual sequelae
1.4	Patients with complex heart defects after palliative interventions
1.4a	Such as the Fontan operation or the Mustard operation for TGA, where separation of systemic and pulmonary circulation has been achieved
1.4b	Patients in whom the two circulatory systems have not been separated (e.g. aortopulmonary shunt operation)
Group 2	*Patients with heart defects not requiring operation*
2.1	Shunt lesions with insignificant left-to-right-shunt such as small atrial or ventricular septal defect
2.2	Insignificant valvular defects/anomalies such as congenital bicuspid aortic valve
2.3	Clinically insignificant arrhythmias/changes in ECG
2.4	Clinically insignificant myocardial changes
Group 3	*Patients with inoperable heart defects*
Group 4	*Patients with chronic cardiomyopathy*
4.1	Clinically significant
4.2	Clinically insignificant
Group 5	*Patients with problematic long-term/permanent therapy*
5.1	Pacemaker
5.2	Anticoagulants
5.3	Antiarrhythmics
5.4	Anticongestives
Group 6	*Patients after heart transplantation*

Table 13.3 Recommendation for exercise training according to the classification of the severity of the current clinical situation [66]

Group	Severity	Category	Recommendation for exercise
0	Cardiac defects requiring surgery	0	No ports
A	No residual sequelae (complete correction)	1.1	Unlimited
B	Mild residual sequelae	1.2; 2.1; 2.2; 2.3; 2.4; 4.2	Unlimited
C	Clinically significant residual sequelae	1.3; 5.1; 5.2; 5.3	No competitive sports
D	Severe clinically significant residual sequelae	1.4a;1.4b; 3; 4.1; 5.4; [6]	Limited sports
E	Vitally threatening findings		No sports

than the current clinical status and potentially deleterious residual defects (Tables 13.2 and 13.3).

For many of the affected children, no restriction of physical activity and sport is recommended [13–15, 49–50, 53, 66]. This group includes all children and adolescents whose heart defects were definitively corrected in infancy or early childhood (persistent ductus arteriosus, small atrial septal defect, ventricular septal defect), who do not have symptom-limited reduction of exercise capacity (*Group 1.1*). Even in patients with mild residual defects (*Group 1.2*) (such as moderate aortic valve disease), normal load can be permitted in physical education and physical activities in leisure time. This also applies to children and adolescents whose cardiac defects do not require surgery (*Group 2*, for instance, small septal defects or insignificant valvular stenosis) [20, 66]. Patient *groups 1.1*, *1.2 and 2* do need temporary participation in remedial programmes and/or adapted physical education if a restriction of physical fitness and/or psychomotor deficits exists. In this context, the indication for participation in special exercise-based rehabilitation groups may also result from psychosocial reasons [54].

Despite the reduction in mortality and improved haemodynamic outcomes of surgery and interventional catheterisation, a considerable number of affected children and adolescents have haemodynamically significant residual defects, which may impair their expectancy and quality of life. For them, participation in special exercise-based rehabilitation groups is most recommended. For patients with significant findings, complex heart defects subsequent to palliative interventions, inoperable heart defects, chronic cardiomyopathy, complex arrhythmia or after heart transplantation, participation in physical activity cannot generally be advocated. Here, a decision for each individual patient has to be made in consultation with the attending paediatric cardiologist. Patients with complex heart defects after palliative operations (*Group 1.4*) represent a special group. In a great number of them (*Group 1.4a*), a separation of the systemic and pulmonary circulations can be performed, and thus no cyanosis persists. However, some patients remain cyanotic (*Group 1.4b*). For these groups, and for children receiving anticoagulant therapy or with implanted devices (pacemakers, ICDs) or at a risk of sudden death, special and sometimes individual recommendations have to be made [13–15, 49–50, 53, 66]. Possible contraindications for participation in physical activities are summarised in Table 13.4.

Prior to starting a physical training programme, a thorough cardiological examination has to be performed in order to classify diagnosis and severity of the disease (Table 13.5). The objective of this examination is to determine the

Table 13.4 Contraindications for participation in physical activities [20, 66]

Contraindications for participation in physical activity may result from the following:
Acute myocarditis
Children/adolescents with heart defects which acutely require surgery
Significant coarctation and/or heart failure NYHA class III/IV (preoperative)
Severe pulmonary hypertension
Severe cyanosis
Complex arrhythmia
Severe cardiomyopathy, obstructive hypertrophic cardiomyopathy

Table 13.5 Required preliminary examinations to determine the possibility of participation in physical activity and exercise training [13–15, 20, 66]

Initial examination:
Precise knowledge of patient's clinical history
General physical examination
ECG at rest
Echocardiography
Ergometry[a](spiroergometry, if needed), especially in case of cyanotic lesions with transcutaneous
O_2 measurement, 6 min running test or 6 min walking test if needed with ECG monitoring (as an alternative for younger children)
Long-term ECG
Facultative: stress echocardiography[a]
Control checkups (at least yearly)
Clinical history
General clinical examination
ECG at rest
Echocardiography
Endurance testing[a]

[a]Starting at age 5–6

patient's individual symptom-limited exercise tolerance and the risk of exercise-related sudden cardiac death associated with the individual's specific disease [13–15].

In addition to the required preliminary examinations (Table 13.5), physical activity participation should be assessed at the initial examination as well as at every control checkup. For children up to 10–12 years of age, regular assessment of motor development and different motor skills is recommended [14, 15].

13.4　Physical Activity in Children and Adolescents with CHD

Improvement of physical activity in children with CHD should start as early as possible. In this way, deficits in perceptual and motor experience and their negative consequences can be minimised. Children need to be provided with the opportunity to act out their basic need for physical activity and should only be stopped if there is a specific danger of sudden death. They should participate in physical activity (indoors and outdoors) with their peers in an unrestricted fashion, as far as possible. This applies to play and guided activity in kindergarten, school and/or sports clubs [14–15, 20, 50, 66].

Recommendation for physical activity and exercise training has to include information about the type, contents, intensity, duration and frequency of exercise. The appropriate type of exercise is of main importance. Predominantly static exercise can result in high stress on the systemic and pulmonary circulations, which can have extreme effects on the haemodynamic function in congenital heart disease.

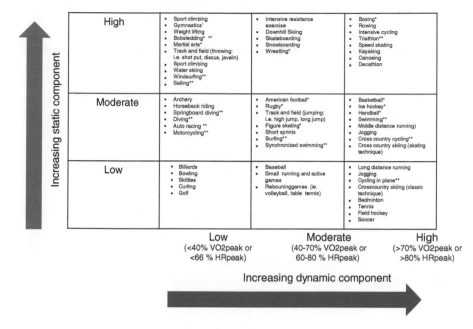

Fig. 13.8 Classification of selected organised sports and exercise based on peak static and dynamic components during participation (increasing static component; increasing dynamic component). * = Risk of bodily collision, ** increased risk if syncope occurs (Modified according to [15, 67])

Predominantly dynamic type of exercise, however, reduces the afterload and can therefore be expected to have a protective effect [15, 66]. Selected forms of exercise and games in childhood with a high dynamic/low static component are running, skipping, jumping, cycling, swimming, inline skating, skateboarding, running games, ball games and so-called small active games. Types of exercise with a high static/low dynamic component are, for example, climbing, swinging, leaning on both arms, pulling, pushing, martial arts such as judo and gymnastics, e. g. on the high bar or the parallel bars (leaning on both arms, hanging) [15, 66]. Figure 13.8 shows classification of selected organised sports and exercise based on peak static and dynamic components during participation.

Recommendation on exercise intensity should be established and controlled based on the results of an exercise stress test done on a bicycle/treadmill ergometer including ECG and blood pressure monitoring. In physical activities and exercises with high dynamic components, i.e. aerobic endurance activities, heart rate, breathing and rate of individually perceived exertion can be used to assess appropriate intensity (Chap. 4).

Participation in specific supervised programmes for the promotion of motor abilities can help to limit motor deficits and prepare and support the integration of children into their peer group [19]. The special aims of such programmes are to develop individual perception of potential limitations and establish the boundaries of their exertional tolerance. In connection with acquiring age-appropriate knowledge about the disease-specific situation and the resulting symptom-limited capacity, this leads to a realistic self-estimation. In combination with this positive self-concept, emotional and psychosocial stability as well as a proper social integration, a realistic self-evaluation represents the most efficient protection from overload in daily life, physical activity and sport [19]. This is of special importance in adolescents with CHD since the specific behaviour patterns in youth often cause them to consciously disregard their body signals in order to avoid the 'embarrassment' a necessary physical break would bring about. By doing this, they expose themselves to potential danger. Prevention of this danger can – besides appeals to the adolescent's rationality – only be achieved through an early stabilisation of personality and the improvement of self-responsibility and self-confidence.

Results of empirical studies show that the physical performance and motor skills of children and adolescents with CHD can be enhanced through regular engagement in autonomous or supervised physical activity [19, 25, 31, 35, 68–71]. These results also demonstrate that such participation not only improves physical performance (Fig. 13.9) and motor abilities but also positively influences the child's emotional, psychosocial and cognitive development. The participation of 16 patients (aged 8–17 years) with complex congenital heart disease (11 Fontan patients and 5 with other CHD) in a 12-week exercise-based cardiac rehabilitation programme (1 h twice a week) revealed a significant improvement of exercise capacity. VO_{2peak} rose from 26.4 ± to 30.7 ± mL/kg per min and ventilatory anaerobic threshold from 26.4 ± to 30.7 ± mL/kg per min. No changes were seen in the control group. No rehabilitation-related complications or

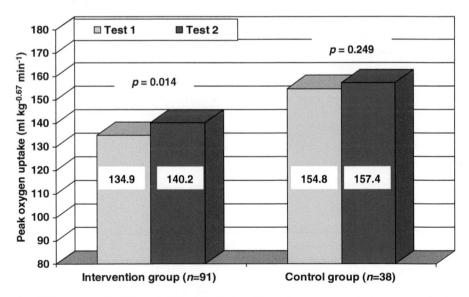

Fig. 13.9 Changes in VO_{2peak} (mL/kg$^{-0.67}$ min^{-1}) achieved by an exercise-based intervention in children with various congenital heart diseases compared to a control group (According to Fredriksen et al. [70]). Study group of children and adolescents (aged 10–16 years) with various congenital heart diseases. Intervention: participation in a 2-week inpatient exercise-based rehabilitation programme or 5-month outpatient programme twice a week

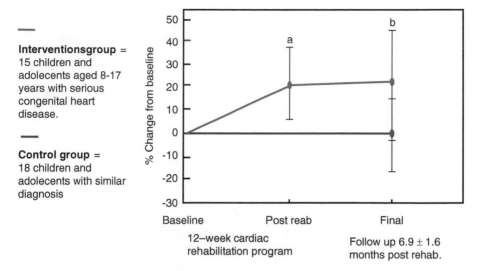

Interventionsgroup =
15 children and adolecents aged 8-17 years with serious congenital heart disease.

Control group =
18 children and adolecents with similar diagnosis

Fig. 13.10 Changes in VO$_{2peak}$ (compared to baseline) over time for intervention group and control group (a = $p < 0.05$ vs. baseline, b = $p < 0.05$ vs. control group) (According to Rhodes et al. [68])

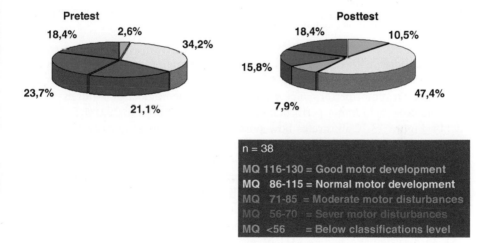

Fig. 13.11 Changes in classification of the motor development in children with congenital heart disease as a result of an 8-month specific psychomotor training programme (*MQ* motor quotient) (According to Dordel et al. [19]). Study group of 38 children and adolescents aged 7–14 with diverse CHD. Intervention: 8 months (75 min once a week) specific psychomotor training programme

adverse effects were observed [69]. Both groups were reinvestigated 6.9 ± 1.6 months after competition of the programme, and the results demonstrate sustained improvements in not only exercise function but also self-esteem and emotional status in the rehabilitation group [68] (Fig. 13.10).

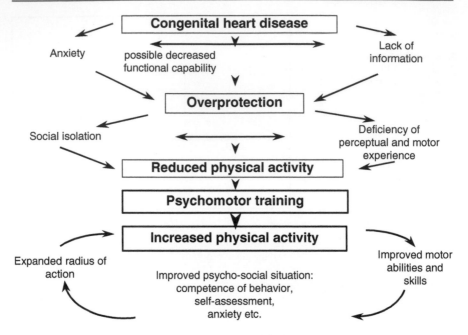

Fig. 13.12 Compensation of negative consequences of CHD by means of goal-oriented improvement of motor development (according to Bjarnason-Wehrens et al. [20])

In 31 children with various types of CHD who participated in 8-month specific psychomotor training programme (75 min once a week), significant improvements in their motor performance were achieved. The number of children classified with deficits in motor performance decreased from 54.8 to 29.0 % [17] (Fig. 13.11). Figure 13.12 illustrates how possibly negative consequences of the disease can be compensated through the improvement of motor abilities and skills by special motor training programmes. In 61 children with single ventricle physiology after Fontan (aged 6–11 years) who participated in 24 months of home-based rehabilitation programme, motor gross skill improved significantly by 49 %. The level of moderate-to-vigorous physical activity increased significantly and was measured 36 ± 31 min/week above the baseline result at 24-month evaluation [25]. In a systematic review [31] of effects of physical exercise training programmes in CHD children and young adults, the results of 31 articles (621 subjects) were analysed. Eighteen studies reported on occurrence of adverse events, but none of them reported negative findings related to the exercise programme. Twenty-four studies (177 subjects) reported results on VO_{2peak} with mean increase of 2.6 ml/kg/min. Significant improvement in 6 min walking distance was reported in two studies. Muscle strength was assessed in five studies, showing significant improvement in strength mediated by the programme in three studies [31]. Tikkanen et al. [35] published a systematic review evaluating the results of cardiac rehabilitation in congenital heart disease in patients under 18 years of age. Sixteen studies met the inclusion criteria. These studies were of heterogeneous methodology and variable quality. Aerobic exercise training and resistance training were the core components of the exercise-based rehabilitation programmes. They found great differences in the exercise contents as well as exercise intensity, frequency and duration. While most of the older studies only included aerobic exercises, the more currently published studies included combined aerobic and resistance exercise programme. None of the studies reported adverse events. The optimal structure of an exercise-based paediatric cardiac rehabilitation programme remains unclear [35].

13.5 Phase II Rehabilitation: Heart Groups for Children and Adolescents with CHD

In Germany special medically prescribed, supervised outpatient therapy services (children's heart groups) have been launched to promote psychomotor skills in children and adolescents with CHD [19, 54]. Children in need of this therapy are given the opportunity to be physically active in a medically supervised, 'protected area'. Here, potentially existing psychomotor deficits can be identified and treated. Simultaneously, conditions for a thorough integration into physical activity of peers (as, for instance, physical education at school) are established. Most children need only short-term participation (90–120 sessions or units). For children who, as a result of the severity of their disease, urgently require medical supervision during physical activity, longer-term participation (possibly for years) is desirable and practical in order to provide means for them to be physically active at all. To provide adequate individual attention, group sizes should be small (up to 10 children), and children should all approximately be of the same age. Table 13.6 summarises the main objectives of the specific psychomotor training programme provided in these groups [54]. The content of special motor training programmes primarily aims at improvement of perceptual and motor development in order to compensate for existing deficits. Positive experience of one's own body, its functions and capabilities constitutes the basis for developing a positive self-image, which in turn helps the children to cope with their disease and the possible restrictions connected with it. Based on differentiated body perception, children develop awareness for strain and learn to have the confidence to take breaks during group activities as often as needed. Moreover, all age-appropriate forms of activity should be made available for the children. At preschool and elementary school age, these are diverse coordinative tasks involving gross and fine motor skills (Figs. 13.13 and 13.14). Specific resistance and endurance training is neither necessary nor efficient up to the age of 8–10. Improved strength and cardiovascular performance at this age result from improved motor coordination.

Table 13.6 General and special objectives to be achieved by the participation in special medically prescribed, supervised psychomotor training programmes (children's heart groups) [19, 54]

General objectives are:

To eliminate or minimise impairments, disabilities and handicaps linked to the disease and to prevent possible secondary effect

To promote self-management and self-responsibility in terms of self-help

To promote equal participation in social life and to prevent prevention or counteract possible discrimination. It is particularly important to ensure and/or re-establish the affected person's integration into school, education, job, family and society

To enhance overall quality of life

To reduce disease-related morbidity

Special objectives are:

To improve physical performance

To improve perceptional and movement experience

To improve body coordination, endurance, strength, speed and flexibility

To improve motor skills

To improve sport-specific skills

To offer insight into the diversity of physical activity and sports available for peer groups

To give advices for movement-orientated leisure activities

To provide motivation for autonomous lifelong physical activity

To identify and compensate possible existing deficits in motor development

To improve social skills and social integration

To improve self-esteem and self-image and coping with the disease

To develop a realistic self-evaluation

To help coping with the disease

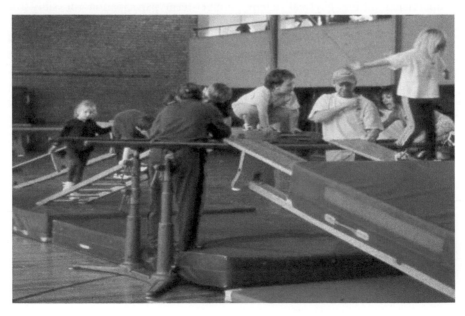

Fig. 13.13 Psychomotor training at preschool age in the children heart group

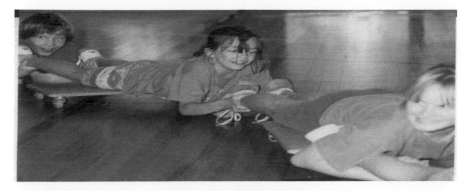

Fig. 13.14   Psychomotor training in the children heart group

Fig. 13.15   Modified games in the children heart group

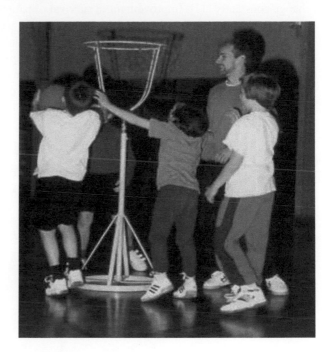

Even at early school age, but especially in adolescence, sport-specific skills are acquired and increasingly improved through diverse and varied physical activities depending on interests and available resources. An important goal is to offer insight into the diversity of physical activity and sports available to all youth (Fig. 13.15). This is meant to help them obtain specific skills and knowledge and thereby enable and motivate them to participate with their peers in physical activities and choose an adequate lifetime sport. Special attention has to be given to the danger of abdominal strain. Even at preschool age, children with specific risk factors should learn to avoid breath holding during exercise (see Chap. 4). Participation in a children heart groups can also help to minimise parents' concern and anxiety about their child being physically active and can thereby reduce overprotection [19, 54].

13.5.1 Exercise Training in Adult Patients with Congenital Heart Diseases (ACHD)

13.5.1.1 Epidemiology

Approximately 85 % of the patients born with congenital malformations of the heart and vessels survive into adult life [70]. Precise data on the size and composition of the population of adult patients with CHD are not available but can be assumed to change constantly [11]. Improvement in survival of patients with CHD has led to a continuously growing number of ACHD patients, in particular those with more complex disease [11]. In the Euro Heart Survey on adult congenital heart disease [73], the data of 4110 patients with eight diagnosis groups (ASD II, VSD, ToF, CoA, TGA, Marfan syndrome, Fontan circulation, cyanotic defects) were collected with follow-up of 5.1 years. The results demonstrate a predominately young population (median 27, range 23–37 years) with substantial morbidity (in particular

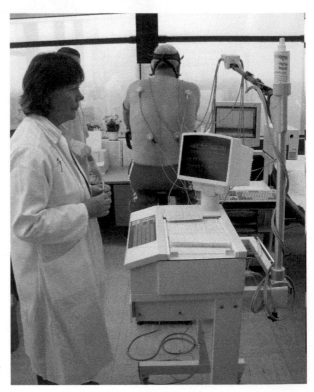

Fig. 13.16 Cardiopulmonary exercise testing

arrhythmias, endocarditis or a stroke/TIA) but low 5-year mortality. The majority of the patients had no or only mild functional limitation, and more than 60 % of them were classified in NYHA class I. Major differences was seen between the diagnosis groups with the worst outcomes in patients with cyanotic defects and patients with Fontan circulation. However, a noticeable number of patients in the group of 'milder' defects also suffered from cardiac symptoms [73]. These findings emphasise the importance of specialised care for adult born with congenital malformation of the heart and the vessel.

Relatively few data are available on exercise capacity and exercise tolerance in adult patients with congenital heart diseases (Fig. 13.16). These date demonstrate a reduced aerobic capacity in all groups investigated [74–83]. Most of these data focus on patients with complex congenital heart disease. Severely diminished exercise capacity has been demonstrated in adult [74–76, 78] as well as in adolescent patients after Fontan operation [78] showing VO_{2peak} which ranges from 14.8 to 26.3.8 mL/kg per min, corresponding to 32 % up to 65 % of predicted value. An early surgical procedure was associated with higher VO_{2peak} values. A retrospective analysis of the results of cardiopulmonary exercise test performed in adult patients with congenitally corrected transposition of the great arteries also revealed a severely reduced exercise capacity (VO_{2peak} 11 to 22 mL/kg per min; 30–50 % of predicted value). The results demonstrate normal mean resting heart rate but reduced heart rate response to exercise (79 % of predicted value) [79]. Similar results were found in 168 adult patients who had undergone surgical repair of tetralogy of Fallot with VO_{2peak} at 51 % and peak heart rate at 79 %, compared to predicted values. Exercise capacity decreased with increasing age and was also associated with the age at surgical repair [80]. Fredriksen et al. [77] compared the exercise capacity of

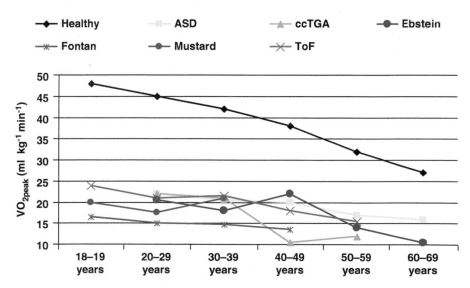

Fig. 13.17 Mean VO_{2peak} (mL/kg/min) value in adults with different congenital heart diseases and in different age groups compared to healthy subjects (According to Fredriksen et al. [78])

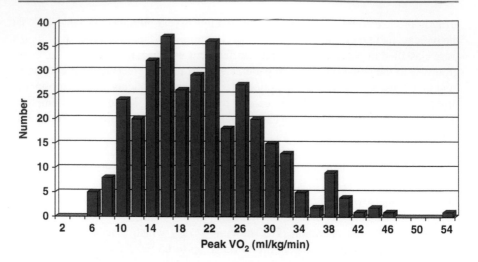

Fig. 13.18 Distribution of peak VO2 in asymptomatic adult patients with congenital heart diseases (According to Diller et al. [81])

475 adult patients (aged 16–71 years) with a wide spectrum of congenital heart diseases (ASD, ccTGA, ToF, Epseins anomaly, modified Fontan procedure, Mustard procedure). The results demonstrate considerably reduced exercise capacity (25–50 %) in all groups but with great variance between diagnosis groups (VO$_{2peak}$ range 6 to 45 mL/kg per min) showing the lowest values within in the Fontan group (Fig. 13.17). All patients achieved significantly lower maximal heart rate than predicted, and in all patients except those with ASD, forced vital capacity was lower than the predicted values [77]. Diller et al. [81] performed cardiopulmonary exercise testing in 335 adult patients (mean age 33 ±13 years) with wide spectrum of congenital heart diseases (ToF, Fontan procedure, Mustard procedure, complex anatomy, valvular disease, ASD, Eisenmenger, ccTGA, pulmonary atresia, aortic coarctation, Epseins anomaly, VSD). They found exercise capacity to be diminished in all patients, even in those who were allegedly asymptomatic (VO$_{2peak}$ 26.1 ± 8.2 mL/kg per min) (Fig. 13.18). The mean VO$_{2peak}$ was 21.7 ± 8.5 mL/kg per min compared to 45.1 ± 8.5 mL/kg per min in the healthy control group ($p < 0.001$). The results demonstrate great variance between diagnosis groups, with the highest values (28.7 ± 10.4 mL/kg per min) in patients after repair of aortic coarctation and the lowest (11.5 ± 3.6 mL/kg per min) in the Eisenmenger syndrome patients. Great variance was also seen within the diagnosis groups. Follow-up date (304 days; range 17–580 days) revealed peak VO$_2$ < 15.5 mL/kg/min to be associated with higher risk of hospitalisation or death (hazard ratio, 2.9; 95 % CI 2.2–7.4 $p < 0.0001$) and death alone (hazard ratio, 5.6; 95 % CI 1.4–31.2 $p < 0.02$) [79] (Fig. 13.19).

Kempny et al. [82] analysed the results of available studies ($n = 2286$, 23 papers) together with own results ($n = 2129$) in 4415 patients with wide spectrum of diagnosis and severity of CHD. They found exercise capacity measured using cardiopulmonary exercise test to be reduced in 80 % compared to references of healthy

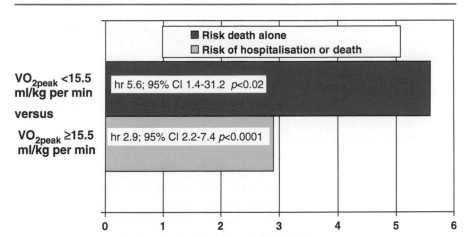

Fig. 13.19 Prognostic value of exercise intolerance in adult patients with congenital heart disease. Risk of death alone or risk of hospitalisation or death in patients with exercise intolerance (VO_{2peak} < 15 mL/kg/min vs. $VO_{2peak} \geq$ 15 mL/kg/min) according to Diller et al. [81]). Study group of 335 adult patients with wide spectrum of CHD. Follow-up of 304 days (range 17–580 days)

subjects, defined as 90 % of predicted peak VO_2. They revealed significant differences between subgroups: the highest values were found in the arterial switch TGA group (36.7 ± 9.1 mL/kg/min, 89 % of predicted values). The lowest values were found in the Eisenmenger syndrome patients (12.5 ± 3.9 mL/kg/min; 42.7% of predicted value) and those with complex heart disease (15.7 ± 5.6; 46 % of predicted value). Similar to Diller et al. [81], they found exercise capacity to be markedly reduced even in patients with simple lesion. Significant differences were also observed in VE/VCO$_2$ slope with the highest values in patients with low exercise capacity [82]. Both peak VO_2 and VE/VCO$_2$ slopes have been shown to correlate with NYHA class and quality of life and to be independent predictors of morbidity and mortality in patients with congenital heart diseases [81–84].

In patients with chronic heart failure, chronotropic incompetence (CI) has been demonstrated to be a predictor of cardiac death and all-cause mortality [85]. Norozi et al. [86] investigated the presence and risk of CI in 345 patients (aged 14–50 years) with diverse congenital heart disease. Chronotropic incompetence was defined as the failure to achieve ≥80 % of the predicted maximal heart rate response given by 220 – age (years) at peak exercise. The results revealed 34 % of the patients to have chronotropic incompetence. Patients with CI had higher NYHA class (1.7 ± 0.06 vs. 1.4 ± 0.03, $p < 0.001$), significant elevated N-BNP levels as well as reduced VO_{2peak} and VO_{2AT}. Resting heart rate and maximal heart rate achieved during exercise test were also significantly reduced. These results were reconfirmed after excluding patients, who received negative chronotropic medication [86]. Diller et al. [81] evaluated the heart rate response to exercise in 727 adult patients with varying diagnosis (mean age 33 ± 13 years). They diagnosed chronotropic incompetence in 62 % of the patients with the highest prevalence in patients after Fontan palliation (85 %), with Eisenmenger physiology (90 %) and with complex anatomy (81 %). The lowest prevalence was seen in patients with repaired ventricular septal defect. Patients with CI were more likely to have higher NYHA class and lower peak VO_2 (20.4 ±8.2 vs. 28.0 ± 9.9 mL/kg/min). During a median follow-up of 851 days after cardiopulmonary exercise testing, 38 patients died. The results demonstrate lower values of heart rate reserve, peak heart rate, heart rate recovery and peak VO_2 to be significantly associated with increased mortality.

Abnormal heart rate response to exercise was shown to be a powerful prognostic marker in adult patients with congenital heart disease, independent of arrhythmic medication and exercise capacity. Lower heart rate reserve was associated with greater risk of death in patients with complex anatomy, Fontan circulation and tetralogy of Fallot [87]. Thus, special attention has to be paid to chronotropic incompetence in adolescents and adult patients with congenital heart disease. This also applies to heart rate variability, which has been demonstrated to be reduced in this group of patients [87–89].

The overall 20-year risk of developing an atrial arrhythmia from age 20 years is 7 % and from age 55 years is 38 %. Several of these are complex atrial arrhythmias, which are not amenable to pharmacological control except with the use of multiple (and potentially negatively inotropic) medications. The results of catheter ablation are also variable. Often new surgical modifications (the atrial Maze operation, Fontan conversion) need to be considered. As this subgroup also has a high risk of sudden (potentially arrhythmic) cardiac death, exercise recommendations need to be weighed very carefully [90].

Beside the severity of the disease and the presence of clinically significant residual lesions, chronotropic incompetence and impaired lung function may contribute to the reduced aerobic capacity seen in adult patients with congenital heart diseases. Furthermore, few studies have reported skeletal muscle abnormalities in adults with Fontan circulation [91–94], suggesting that muscle wasting as known in heart failure patients might be common in this population. Cordina et al. [91] evaluated the skeletal muscle mass and muscle metabolic in 16 patients (30 ± 2 years) with Fontan circulation using dual x-ray absorptiometry (DXA) for lean mass quantification and calf muscle magnetic resonance spectroscopy. The results demonstrate reduced muscle mass and intrinsic muscle metabolic abnormalities in adults with Fontan circulation, showing a quarter of the group to have muscle wasting within sarcopenia range [91]. Muscle wasting was associated with reduced exercise capacity. Kröönström et al. [95] evaluated the muscle function in 315 adult patients with CHD (34 ± 13 years) using isotonic and isometric muscle function test. The results revealed CHD subjects to have lower isotonic muscle function in the upper and lower body compared to references of healthy subjects. Furthermore, higher NYHA classes II–IV were demonstrated to be a significant predictor for reduced isotonic muscle function.

However, exercise limitations might also be caused by factors like physical deconditioning due to low habitual physical activity level and lack of exercise experience in childhood, misperception about exercise restrictions as well as lack of interest and/or anxiety [72], while symptoms only account for approximately 30 % of all barriers to exercise [72].

13.5.1.2   Physical Activity in Adult Patients with Congenital Heart Disease

Sedentary lifestyle is assumed to be prevalent in adults with CHD. Current guidelines recommend 30 min of daily activity at individualised intensity for adults with CHD [96]. The habitual physical activity in this group is not well studied and the published results controversial. Dua et al. [97] assessed the physical activity of 61 adults with congenital heart diseases over 1 week using accelerometer. The range of physical activity was seen between normal and severely limited, declining with increasing severity of the disease. However, only 23 % of the asymptomatic patients (NYHA class I) engaged in more than 30 min a day of moderate activity. The results revealed that most of the patients were willing to participate in physical activity and exercise but were unsure about the safety and the benefits of such activities. Müller et al. [98] evaluated the physical activity levels using triaxial accelerometer in 330 adult CHD patients. They found 76 % of the patients to meet the recommendations of daily physical activity. In most of the patients, exercise capacity was reduced (73.7 ± 19.5 % of predicted). Sandberg et al. [99] assessed the habitual physical activity in 80 patients (40 simple lesions; 40 complex lesions) and compared to that of 42 age- and sex-matched controls using an Actiheart monitor which is a combined uniaxial accelerometer and heart rate monitor. The results demonstrate no significant differences in time spent with moderate-to-vigorous activity and sedentary time between the groups. Only 54 % of the patients with simple lesions, 45 % of those with complex lesions and 56 % of the controls did reach the current recommendation for physical activity. Tikkanen et al. [100] assessed physical activity and exercise capacity in 145 patients (33.5 ± 10.2 years) including follow-up over 13.2 months. At baseline 42 % reported low, 32.4 % occasional and 25.5 % frequent physical activity. Exercise capacity was significantly higher in the frequently active group (27.4 ± 4.0 vs. 21.4 ± 6.1 vs. 19.0 ± 5.0, respectively). At follow-up frequent physical activity was associated with retention or even improvement in exercise capacity. The results support the assumption that exercise capacity in adult CHD patients is not only limited by disease-related factors and regular physical activity has the potential to improve the often seen diminished exercise capacity in this group [101]. All together these results emphasise the importance of individualised activity recommendation for adult patient with CHD.

The results of a British study [102] demonstrate that in adult patients with CHD, the safety, efficiency as well as potential health benefits of physical activity and exercise training are usually not addressed by the physicians. Out of 99 adult CHD patients questioned, 71 % reported that this topic had never spontaneously been raised by none of their physicians. Only 19 % reported that they had been encouraged to be more physically active, and 11 % stated that they had been told to have no exercise limitation due to the cardiac disease. More commonly, patients were given advises which kinds of exercise were prohibited. On the other hand, only 37 % of the patients reported that they had addressed this topic by themselves while consulting their physician. Almost half of them assumed that all physical activity and exercise were safe for them, including patients with more severe CHD [102].

Gratz et al. [103] compared the self-reported health-related quality of life and the results of cardiopulmonary exercise test in 564 patients (14–73 years) with various CHD. In all diagnosis groups, even the simplest exercise capacity was significantly lower than in the control group of healthy subjects. Despite these limitations in exercise capacity, the patients reported excellent quality of life in most aspects. Reductions were only reported regarding physical aspects, with significant lower scores for physical functioning, while psychosocial aspects were not divergent to healthy population. Most of the patients severely overestimated their physical abilities, whereas almost none of them did underestimate their physical abilities. This was seen in all diagnosis groups. The reason for this misconception of physical abilities might be that the patients themselves as well as their families actively dissimulate limitations in subjective exercise capacity to improve their self-esteem. Lack in thorough knowledge about the disease, its treatment, prevention and contraindication especially regarding physical exertion might also contribute to this misconception and might result in precarious overexertion by the patients themselves [103].

Especially in young people with congenital heart disease, the ability to exercise is a fundamental measure of quality of life, perceived capacity for social acceptance, employment, sexual relations and procreation [72]. Recommendation regarding recreational physical activity, exercise training and sports (including competitive sports) should be a core component of the patients' education. Physical activity in youth is a major predictor of maintained fitness throughout life [96, 104]. Thus education regarding physical activity should begin as early as possible in school age and be intensified in early adolescent stage to avoid lack of exercise experience, poor coordination and physical deconditioning already at younger age and the transference of sedentary lifestyle into adulthood. If these adolescents need to be restricted in their physical activity, information about this should be given at early adolescent stage (10–12 years), allowing both the child and the parents to adapt to the new rules [50].

13.5.1.3 Exercise-Based Cardiac Rehabilitation in Adults with Congenital Heart Disease

Available data demonstrate that adults with congenital heart diseases do have subnormal up to severely limited exercise tolerance. It has also been demonstrated that low exercise tolerance in this group of patients is associated with higher risk of morbidity as well as mortality. Numerous studies have demonstrated the benefit of exercise training, especially endurance training in healthy individuals as well as for individuals with cardiovascular disease. This also applies to patients with chronic health failure where exercise training has been demonstrated to reduce symptoms and improve exercise tolerance and quality of life [105]. Therefore the obvious question is if exercise training could have similar effects in individuals with congenital malformations of the heart and the vessels. In several smaller studies, exercise-based cardiac rehabilitation programmes in children and adolescents with CHD have been shown to be safe and to improve exercise efficiency [31, 35, 68–70]. This has also been seen in patients with complex congenital heart disease

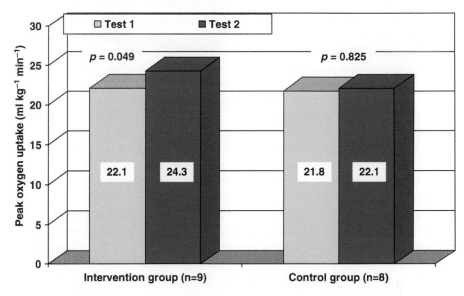

Fig. 13.20 Changes in VO$_{2peak}$ (mL/kg/min) achieved by exercise-based intervention in adult patients with tetralogy of Fallot compared to a control group (according to Therrien et al. (106)). Study group of adult patients with tetralogy of Fallot (mean age 35.0 ± 9.5 intervention vs. 43.4 ± 7.3 control group; $p = 0.07$). Intervention: participation in 12-week exercise-based rehabilitation programme three times a week including 20 min individualised aerobic training (60–85 % VO$_{2peak}$) on cycle ergometer and 20 min treadmill walking

resulting in sustained improvement in exercise tolerance without rehabilitation-related complications or adverse effects [31, 35, 68, 69]. However, the efficacy and safety of structured exercise-based rehabilitation programmes in adults with congenital heart defects are more or less unknown [72].

In a pilot study performed on adult patients with repaired tetralogy of Fallot, 16 individuals were randomised to an exercise ($n = 8$; mean age 35.0 ± 9.5 years) or a control group ($n = 9$; mean age $43.3 \pm 7.$ years). The exercise group participated in a 12-week exercise programme including one 50 min session once a week. The exercise programme included a 40 min endurance training (20 min cycle ergometry and 20 min treadmill walking) with relative intensity level of 60–85 % of peak VO$_2$. In addition patients were motivated to perform twice a week a home-based programme including brisk walking with relative intensity of 60–85 % of their maximal heart rate. The results demonstrate significant improvements in VO$_{2peak}$ (22.1 mL/kg/ min to 24.3 mL/kg/min; $p = 0.049$) in the exercise group, whereas it remained unchanged in the control group (21.8 mL/kg/min to 22.1 mL/kg/min; $p = 0.825$) (Fig. 13.20). No rehabilitation-related complications or adverse effects were reported [106].

Winter et al. [107] performed a randomised controlled clinical trial evaluating the efficacy of a 10-week exercise training versus control in adults with a systemic right ventricle. Analysis was performed for a sample of 46 patients (32+11 years;

intervention $n = 24$; control $n = 22$). The exercise training was home based and included three sessions of step aerobics per week.

Patients were advised to perform warm-up for 5 min at 60 % of maximal heart rate followed by 32 min interval training with five 4 min intervals with 75 % (up to 90 %) HRpeak alternated with four 3 min intervals at 60 % of HRpeak, followed by 5 min cool-down at 60 % of HRpeak. As a result of the intervention, VO_{2peak} improved by 7 % with significant difference compared to controls (3.4 mL/kg/min, 95 % CI: 0.2–6.7; $p < 0.04$), and significant improvement was also seen in OUES (170, 95 % CI: 105–236; $p < 0.001$). The control group showed no significant changes in cardiopulmonary exercise test results during follow-up.

NT-proBNP levels and quality of life remained unchanged during follow-up in both groups [104]. No adverse events occurred during training. The authors conclude that patients with a systemic RV should be encouraged to become physically active. Westhoff-Bleck et al. [108] randomised 48 patients (29.3 ± 3.4 years) after Mustard procedure to a 24-week home-based exercise intervention ($n = 24$) or control group ($n = 24$). The intervention group was advised to perform continuous aerobic exercise training on a cycle ergometer with low intensity (heart rate corresponding to 50 % VO_{2peak}) starting with 10 min exercise three times per week. During the 24-week intervention exercise, frequency and duration were increased gradually up to five sessions per week and 30 min exercise time. To improve adherence to training, patients received weekly phone calls. Exercise training was well tolerated, and no cardiac decompensation or arrhythmias while exercising was observed. The results demonstrate significant improvement in VO_{2peak} (3.8 ml/kg/min, 95 % CI: 1.8 to 5.7; $p = 0.001$), maximum exercise time, maximum workload as well as VO_2 and workload at aerobic threshold in the exercise group. An insignificant decrease in VE/VCO_2 slope was observed in the intervention group, whereas control revealed an insignificant incline. NT-proBNP levels remained unchanged during follow-up in both groups. Systemic ventricular function and volumes determined by cardiac magnetic resonance imaging remained unchanged in both groups. The intervention group showed significant improvement in NYHA classification ($p = 0.046$). The authors conclude that low intensity aerobic exercise training improves exercise capacity and can be performed safely in this group of patients. Dua et al. [109] evaluated the efficacy of a 10-week home-based exercise intervention in 50 adults with wide spectrum of CHD. The exercise intervention comprised an individualised progressive walking programme on 5 days a week. All patients were contacted twice a week by telephone call to assess progress and adverse effects and improve adherence to the programme. The participation leads to significant increase in treadmill test duration, physical activity and improvement in quality of life. No adverse effects were reported [109].

These promising results encourage implementing exercise rehabilitation programmes for stable adult patients in order to improve exercise tolerance as well as to oppose sedentary lifestyle common in these patients. Further studies are necessary to ascertain utility, efficacy and safety of structured exercise-based rehabilitation programme in adult CHD patients but also in order to find out if the participation in such programmes is associated with reduced symptoms, improved exercise tolerance and quality and length of life.

Adult patients with congenital malformations of the heart and the vessels are at risk to adapt a sedentary lifestyle and develop overweight and obesity. Reduced exercise capacity has been found in all diagnosis groups also in asymptomatic patients. In the majority of the patients, no exercise restriction is necessary [96, 110]. Physicians taking care of adult patients with CHD should address the topic physical activity and exercise training regularly. Mentoring the patient regarding his/her exercise tolerance and physical activities should be a part of every consultation. Based on the results of thorough medical examination, including cardiopulmonary exercise test (see Table 13.5), individual exercise prescriptions should be provided and updated regularly [96, 110]. An individual exercise prescription should emphasise the beneficial effects of physical activity and exercise training on exercise tolerance, physical limitations, risk modification, psychosocial factors and health concerns such as obesity [96, 110]. All patients who are not severely limited by symptoms at rest should be encouraged to have an active lifestyle [52, 96]. Exercise prescription should include information about target heart rate as well as other tools, which help the patient find out if the relative intensity of the activity performed is adequate for him/her. The 'breathing rule', an activity which can be carried out as long as breathing still permits comfortable speech, may also be helpful [110]. Recommendations for competitive athletes in adults with congenital heart diseases have been published [50, 52]. Currently only few data are available concerning recreational exercise in adult CHD patients. This also applies to results from exercise-based cardiac rehabilitation in this group of patients [72, 96]. All patients who do not need any restriction regarding physical activity and exercise training should be encouraged to take up regular exercise training, especially endurance training, and be provided with individual exercise prescription (see Chap. 4). The participation in structured medically supervised exercise training may be helpful to catch up limitations in exercise capacity and educate the patient in order to provide him/her with the knowledge and self-esteem necessary to take up physically active lifestyle and regular exercise training on his/her own. Patients with significant residual sequelae, complex heart defects after palliative intervention such as the Fontan operation or the Mustard operation for TGA might also benefit from medically supervised individually prescribed low-to-moderate intensity aerobic endurance training (see Tables 13.2 and 13.3).

References

1. Allen DH, Gutgesell HP, Clark EB, et al., editors. Moss and adams'heart disease in infants, children, and adolescents. Including the fetus and young adults. 6 ed. Philadelphia: Lippincott Williams & Wilkins; 2001.
2. American Heart Association; American Stroke Association. Heart Disease and Stroke Statistics. 2008 Update. American Heart Association; American Stroke Association; 2008. [web page] http://www.americanheart.org.
3. Dolk H, Loane M, Garne E, European Surveillance of Congenital Anomalies (EUROCAT) Working Group. Congenital heart defects in Europe prevalence and perinatal mortality, 2000 to 2005. Circulation. 2011;123:841–9.

4. American Heart Association; American Stroke Association. Statistical Fact Sheet. 2013 Update. Congenital cardiovascular defects. American Heart Association; American Stroke Association; 2013. [web page] http://www.americanheart.org.
5. Look JE, Keane JF, Perry SB, editors. Diagnostic and interventional catheterization in congenital heart disease (developments in cardiovascular medicine). 2 ed. Norwell: kluwer Academic Publisher; 2004.
6. Raissadati A, Nieminen H, Jokinen E, Sairanen H. Progress in late results among pediatric cardiac surgery patients: a population-based 6-decade study with 98 % follow-up. Circulation. 2015;131:347–53.
7. Erikssen G, Liestøl K, Seem E, Birkeland S, Saatvedt KJ, Hoel TN, Døhlen G, Skulstad H, Svennevig JL, Thaulow E, Lindberg HL. Achievements in congenital heart defect surgery: a prospective, 40-year study of 7038 patients. Circulation. 2015;131:337–46.
8. Deutsche Herzstiftung (Edt.) 27. Deutscher Herzbericht 2015. Sektorenübergreifende Versorgungsanalyse zur Kardiologie und Herzchirurgie in Deutschland, Frankfurt am Main: Eigenverlag; 2015 ISBN 978-3-9811926-6-7
9. Boneva RS, Botto LD, Moore CA, Yang Q, Correa A, Erickson JD. Mortality associated with congenital heart defects in the United States: trends and racial disparities, 1979-1997. Circulation. 2001;103:2376–81.
10. Sarubbi B, Pacileo G, Pisacane C, Ducceschi V, Iacono C, Russo MG, Iacono A, Calabro R. Exercise capacity in young patients after total repair of tetralogy of fallot. Pediatr Cardiol. 2000;21:211–5.
11. Baumgartner H, Bonhoeffer P, De Groot NMS, et al. ESC Guidelines for the management of grown-up congenital heart disease. The Task Force on the Management of Grown-up Congenital Heart Disease of the European Society of Cardiology (ESC) Endorsed by the Association for European Paediatric Cardiology (AEPC). Eur Heart J. 2010;31:2915–57.
12. Marino BS, Lipkin PH, Newburger JW, Peacock G, Gerdes M, Gaynor JW, Mussatto KA, Uzark K, Goldberg CS, Johnson WH, Li J, Smith SE, Bellinger DC, Mahl WT. Neurodevelopmental outcomes in children with congenital heart disease: evaluation and management. A scientific statement from the American Heart Association. Circulation. 2012;126:1143–72.
13. Longmuir PE, Brothers JA, de Ferranti SD, Hayman LL, Van Hare GF, Matherne GP, Davis CK, Joy EA, McCrindle BW, American Heart Association Atherosclerosis, Hypertension and Obesity in Youth Committee of the Council on Cardiovascular Disease in the Young. Promotion of physical activity for children and adults with congenital heart disease: a scientific statement from the American Heart Association. Circulation. 2013;127:2147–59.
14. Takken T, Giardini A, Reybrouck T, Gewillig M, Hövels-Gürich HH, Longmuir PE, McCrindle BW, Paridon SM, Hager A. Recommendations for physical activity, recreation sport, and exercise training in paediatric patients with congenital heart disease: a report from the exercise, basic & translational research section of the European Association of Cardiovascular Prevention and Rehabilitation, the European Congenital Heart and Lung Exercise Group, and the Association for European Paediatric Cardiology. Eur J Prev Cardiol. 2012;19:1034–1.
15. Hager A, Bjarnason-Wehrens B, Oberhoffer R, Hövels-Gürich H, Lawrenz W Dubowy KO, Paul T. Sport bei angeborenen Herzerkrankungen. In: Deutsche Gesellschaft für Kinder- und Jugendmedizin, editors. Leitlinen Kinder und Jugendmedizin. , München: Elsvier, Urban & Fischer Verlag; 2015, M40 S.1–18.
16. Bjarnason-Wehrens B, Dordel S, Schickendantz S, Krumm C, Bott D, Sreeram N, Brockmeier K. Motor development in children with congenital cardiac diseases compared to their healthy peers. Cardiol Young. 2007;17:487–98.
17. Bjarnason-Wehrens B, Schmitz S, Dordel S. Motor development in children with congenital cardiac diseases. Eur Cardiol. 2008;4:92–6.
18. Holm I, Fredriksen PM, Fosdahl MA, Olstad M, Vollestad N. Impaired motor competence in school-aged children with complex congenital heart disease. Arch Pediatr Adolesc Med. 2007;161:945–50.

19. Dordel S, Bjarnason-Wehrens B, Lawrenz W, Leurs S, Rost R, Schickendantz S, Sticker E. Efficiency of psychomotor training of children with (partly-) corrected congenital heart disease. Z Sportm. 1999;50:41–6.
20. Bjarnason-Wehrens B, Dordel S, Sreeram N, Brockmeier K. Cardiac Rehabilitation in Congenital Heart Disease. In: Perk J, Mathes P, Gohlke H, Monpére C, Hellemans I, McGee H, Sellier P, Saner H, editors. Cardiovascular prevention and rehabilitation. London: Springer; 2007. p. 361–75.
21. Bjarnason-Wehrens B, Dordel S, Schickendantz S, Krumm C, Bott D, Sreeram N, Brockmeier K. Motor development in children with congenital cardiac diseases compared to their healthy peers. Cardiol Young. 2007;17:487–98.
22. Unverdorben M, Singer H, Trägler M, Schmidt M, Otto J, Singer R, Vallbracht C. Impaired coordination in children with congenital heart disease – only hardly to be explained by medical causes. Herz/Kreisl. 1997;29:181–4.
23. Stieh J, Kramer HH, Harding P, Fischer G. Gross and fine motor development is impaired in children with cyanotic congenital heart disease. Neuropediatrics. 1999;30:77–82.
24. Majnemer A, Limperopoulos C, Shevell MI, Rosenblatt B, Rohlicek C, Tchervenkov V. Long-term neuromotor outcome at school entry of infants with congenital heart defects requiring open-heart surgery. J Pediatr. 2006;148:72–7.
25. Longmuir PE, Russell JL, Corey M, Faulkner G, McCrindle BW. Factors associated with the physical activity level of children who have the Fontan procedure. Pediatrics. 2011;161:411–7.
26. Iserin L, Chua TP, Chambers J, Coats AJ, Somerville J. Dyspnoea and exercise intolerance during cardiopulmonary exercise testing in patients with univentricular heart. The effects of chronic hypoxaemia and Fontan procedure. Eur Heart J. 1997;18:1350–6.
27. Fredriksen PM, Ingjer F, Nystad W, Thaulow E. A comparison of VO2(peak) between patients with congenital heart disease and healthy subjects, all aged 8-17 years. Eur J Appl Physiol Occup Physiol. 1999;80:409–16.
28. Sarubbi B, Pacileo G, Pisacane C, Ducceschi V, Iacono C, Russo MG, Iacono A, Calabro R. Exercise capacity in young patients after total repair of tetralogy of fallot. Pediatr Cardiol. 2000;21:211–5.
29. Wessel HU, Paul MH. Exercise studies in tetralogy of Fallot: a review. Pediatr Cardiol. 1999;20:39–47.
30. Paul MH, Wessel HU. Exercise studies in patients with transposition of the great arteries after atrial repair operations (Mustard/Senning): a review. Pediatr Cardiol. 1999;20:49–55.
31. Duppen N, Takken T, Hopman MT, ten Harkel AD, Dulfer K, Utens EM, Helbing WA. Systematic review of the effects of physical exercise training programmes in children and young adults with congenital heart disease. Int J Cardiol. 2013;168:1779–87.
32. Duppen N, Etnel JR, Spaans L, Takken T, van den Berg-Emons RJ, Boersma E, Schokking M, Dulfer K, Utens EM, Helbing W, Hopman MT. Does exercise training improve cardiopulmonary fitness and daily physical activity in children and young adults with corrected tetralogy of Fallot or Fontan circulation? A randomized controlled trial. Am Heart J. 2015;170:606–14.
33. Dulfer K, Helbing WA, Duppen N, Utens EM. Associations between exercise capacity, physical activity, and psychosocial functioning in children with congenital heart disease: a systematic review. Eur J Prev Cardiol. 2014;21:1200–15.
34. Motonaga KS, Punn R, Axelrod DM, Ceresnak SR, Hanisch D, Kazmucha JA, Dubin AM. Diminished exercise capacity and chronotropic incompetence in pediatric patients with congenital complete heart block and chronic right ventricular pacing. Heart Rhythm. 2015;12:560–5.
35. Tikkanen AU, Oyaga AR, Riaño OA, Álvaro EM, Rhodes J. Paediatric cardiac rehabilitation in congenital heart disease: a systematic review. Cardiol Young. 2012;22:241–50.
36. Opotowsky AR, Landzberg MJ, Earing MG, Wu FM, Triedman JK, Casey A, Ericson DA, Systrom D, Paridon SM, Rhodes J. Abnormal spirometry after the Fontan procedure is common and associated with impaired aerobic capacity. Am J Physiol Heart Circ Physiol. 2014;307:H110–7.

37. Chen CW. Su WJ, Wang JK, Yang HL, Chiang YT, Moons P. Physical self-concept and its link to cardiopulmonary exercise tolerance among adolescents with mild congenital heart disease. Eur J Cardiovasc Nurs. 2015;14:206–13.
38. O'Byrne ML, Mercer-Rosa L, Ingall E, McBride MG, Paridon S, Goldmuntz E. Habitual exercise correlates with exercise performance in patients with conotruncal abnormalities. Pediatr Cardiol. 2013;34:853–60.
39. Lunt D, Briffa T, Briffa NK, Ramsay J. Physical activity levels of adolescents with congenital heart disease. Aust J Physiother. 2003;49:43–50.
40. Arvidsson D, Slinde F, Hulthén L, Sunnegårdh J. Physical activity, sports participation and aerobic fitness in children who have undergone surgery for congenital heart defects. Acta Paediatr. 2009;98:1475–82.
41. Fredriksen PM, Ingjer E, Thaulow E. Physical activity in children and adolescents with congenital heart disease. Aspects of measurements with an activity monitor. Cardiol Young. 2000;10:98–106.
42. Massin MM, Hovels-Gurich HH, Gerard P, Seghaye MC. Physical activity patterns of children after neonatal arterial switch operation. Ann Thorac Surg. 2006;81:665–70.
43. McCrindle BW, Williams RV, Mital S, Clark BJ, Russell JL, Klein G, Eisenmann JC. Physical activity levels in children and adolescents are reduced after the Fontan procedure, independent of exercise capacity, and are associated with lower perceived general health. Arch Dis Child. 2007;92:509–14.
44. Norgaard MA, Lauridsen P, Helvind M, Pettersson G. Twenty-to-thirty-seven-year follow-up after repair for Tetralogy of Fallot. Eur J Cardiothorac Surg. 1999;16:125–30.
45. Stefan MA, Hopman WM, Smythe JF. Effect of activity restriction owing to heart disease on obesity. Arch Pediatr Adolesc Med. 2005;159:477–81.
46. Norgaard MA, Lauridsen P, Helvind M, Pettersson G. Twenty-to-thirty-seven-year follow-up after repair for tetralogy of fallot. Eur J Cardiothorac Surg. 1999;16:125–30.
47. Schaffer R, Berdat P, Stolle B, Pfammatter JP, Stocker F, Carrel T. Surgery of the complete atrioventricular canal: relationship between age at operation, mitral regurgitation, size of the ventricular septum defect, additional malformations and early postoperative outcome. Cardiology. 1999;91:231–5.
48. Hutter PA, Kreb DL, Mantel SF, Hitchcock JF, Meijboom EJ, Bennink GB. Twenty-five years' experience with the arterial switch operation. J Thorac Cardiovasc Surg. 2002;124:790–7.
49. Reybrouck T, Mertens L. Physical performance and physical activity in grown-up congenital heart disease. Eur J Cardiovasc Prev Rehabil. 2005;12:498–502.
50. Hirth A, Reybrouck T, Bjarnason-Wehrens B, Lawrenz W, Hoffmann A. Recommendations for participation in competitive and leisure sports in patients with congenital heart disease. A consensus document. Eur J Cardiovasc Prev Rehabil. 2006;13:293–9.
51. Mitchell JH, Maron BJ, Epstein SE. 16th bethesda conference: cardiovascular abnormalities in the athlete: recommendations regarding eligibility for competition. October 3-5, 1984. J Am Coll Cardiol. 1985;6:1186–232.
52. Graham Jr TP, Driscoll DJ, Gersony WM, Newburger JW, Rocchini A, Towbin JA. Task Force 2: congenital heart disease. J Am Coll Cardiol. 2005;45:1326–33.
53. Picchio FM, Giardini A, Bonvicini M, Gargiulo G. Can a child who has been operated on for congenital heart disease participate in sport and in which kind of sport? J Cardiovasc Med (Hagerstown). 2006;7:234–8.
54. Bjarnason-Wehrens B, Sticker E, Lawrenz W. Held K. Die Kinderherzgruppe (KHG) – Positionspapier der DGPR. Z Kardiol. 2005;94:860–6.
55. Bellinger DC, Wypij D, duDuplessis AJ, Rappaport LA, Jonas RA, Wernovsky G, Newburger JW. Neurodevelopmental status at eight years in children with dextro-transposition of the great arteries: the Boston Circulatory Arrest Trial. J Thorac Cardiovasc Surg. 2003;126:1385–96.
56. Newburger JW, Wypij D, Bellinger DC, du Plessis AJ, Kuban KC, Rappaport LA, Almirall D, Wessel DL, Jonas RA, Wernovsky G. Length of stay after infant heart surgery is related to cognitive outcome at age 8 years. J Pediatr. 2003;143:67–73.
57. Wernovsky G, Newburger J. Neurologic and developmental morbidity in children with complex congenital heart disease. J Pediatr. 2003;142:6–8.

58. Majnemer A, Limperopoulos C, Shevell M, Rosenblatt B, Rohlicek C, Tchervenkov C. Long-term neuromotor outcome at school entry of infants with congenital heart defects requiring open-heart surgery. J Pediatr. 2006;148:72–7.
59. Dunbar-Masterson C, Wypij D, Bellinger DC, Rappaport LA, Baker AL, Jonas RA, Newburger JW. General health status of children with D-transposition of the great arteries after the arterial switch operation. Circulation. 2001;104(12 Suppl 1):I138–42.
60. Carey LK, Nicholson BC, Fox RA. Maternal factors related to parenting young children with congenital heart disease. J Pediatr Nurs. 2002;17:174–83.
61. Kong SG, Tay JS, Yip WC, Chay SO. Emotional and social effects of congenital heart disease in Singapore. Aust Paediatr J. 1986;22:101–6.
62. Uzark K, Jones K. Parenting stress and children with heart disease. J Pediatr Health Care. 2003;17:163–8.
63. Morelius E, Lundh U, Nelson N. Parental stress in relation to the severity of congenital heart disease in the offspring. Pediatr Nurs. 2002;28:28–32.
64. DeMaso DR, Campis LK, Wypij D, Bertram S, Lipshitz M, Freed M. The impact of maternal perceptions and medical severity on the adjustment of children with congenital heart disease. J Pediatr Psychol. 1991;16:137–49.
65. Van Horn M, DeMaso DR, Gonzalez-Heydrich J, Erickson JD. Illness-related concerns of mothers of children with congenital heart disease. J Am Acad Child Adolesc Psychiatry. 2001;40:847–54.
66. Schickendantz S, Sticker EJ, Dordel S, Bjarnason-Wehrens B. Sport and physical activity in children with congenital heart disease. Dtsch Arztebl. 2007;104(9):A563–9.
67. Mitchell JH, Haskell W, Snell P, Van Camp SP. Task force 8: classification of sports. J Am Coll Cardiol. 2005;45:1364–7.
68. Rhodes J, Curran TJ, Camil L, Rabideau N, Fulton DR, Gauthier NS, Gauvreau K, Jenkins KJ. Sustained effects of cardiac rehabilitation in children with serious congenital heart disease. Pediatrics. 2006;118:e586–93.
69. Rhodes J, Curran TJ, Camil L, Rabideau N, Fulton DR, Gauthier NS, Gauvreau K, Jenkins KJ. Impact of cardiac rehabilitation on the exercise function of children with serious congenital heart disease. Pediatrics. 2005;116:1339–45.
70. Fredriksen PM, Kahrs N, Blaasvaer S, Sigurdsen E, Gundersen O, Roeksund O, Norgaand G, Vik JT, Soerbye O, Ingjer E, et al. Effect of physical training in children and adolescents with congenital heart disease. Cardiol Young. 2000;10:107–14.
71. Moons P, Barrea C, De Wolf D, Gewillig M, Massin M, Mertens L, Ovaert C, Suys B, Sluysmans T. Changes in perceived health of children with congenital heart disease after attending a special sports camp. Pediatr Cardiol. 2006;27:67–72.
72. Warnes CA, Williams RG, Bashore TM, Child JS, Connolly HM, Dearani JA, del Nido P, Fasules JW, Graham Jr TP, Hijazi ZM, et al. ACC/AHA 2008 Guidelines for the management of adults with congenital heart disease: a report of the American College of Cardiology/American Heart Association Task Force on Practice Guidelines (writing committee to develop guidelines on the management of adults with congenital heart disease). Circulation. 2008;118:e714–833.
73. Engelfriet P, Boersma E, Oechslin E, Tijssen J, Gatzoulis MA, Thilen U, Kaemmerer H, Moons P, Meijboom F, Popelova J, et al. The spectrum of adult congenital heart disease in Europe: morbidity and mortality in a 5 year follow-up period. The Euro heart Survey on adult congenital heart disease. Eur Heart J. 2005;26:2325–33.
74. Harrison DA, Liu P, Walters JE, Goodman JM, Siu SC, Webb GD, Williams WG, McLaughlin PR. Cardiopulmonary function in adult patients late after Fontan repair. J Am Coll Cardiol. 1995;26:1016–21.
75. Fredriksen PM, Therrien J, Veldtman G, Warsi MA, Liu P, Siu S, Williams W, Granton J, Webb G. Lung function and aerobic capacity in adult patients following modified Fontan procedure. Heart. 2001;85:295–9.
76. Iserin L, Chua TP, Chambers J, Coats AJ, Somerville J. Dyspnoea and exercise intolerance during cardiopulmonary exercise testing in patients with univentricular heart. The effects of chronic hypoxaemia and Fontan procedure. Eur Heart J. 1997;18:1350–6.

77. Fredriksen PM, Veldtman G, Hechter S, Therrien J, Chen A, Warsi MA, Freeman M, Liu P, Siu S, Thaulow E, et al. Aerobic capacity in adults with various congenital heart diseases. Am J Cardiol. 2001;87:310–4.

78. Paridon SM, Mitchell PD, Colan SD, Williams RV, Blaufox A, Li JS, Margossian R, Mital S, Russell J, Rhodes J. A cross-sectional study of exercise performance during the first 2 decades of life after the Fontan operation. J Am Coll Cardiol. 2008;52:99–107.

79. Fredriksen PM, Chen A, Veldtman G, Hechter S, Therrien J, Webb G. Exercise capacity in adult patients with congenitally corrected transposition of the great arteries. Heart. 2001;85:191–5.

80. Fredriksen PM, Therrien J, Veldtman G, Ali Warsi M, Liu P, Thaulow E, Webb G. Aerobic capacity in adults with tetralogy of Fallot. Cardiol Young. 2002;12:554–9.

81. Diller GP, Dimopoulos K, Okonko D, Li W, Babu-Narayan SV, Broberg CS, Johansson B, Bouzas B, Mullen MJ, Poole-Wilson PA, et al. Exercise intolerance in adult congenital heart disease: comparative severity, correlates, and prognostic implication. Circulation. 2005;112:828–35.

82. Kempny A, Dimopoulos K, Uebing A, Moceri P, Swan L, Gatzoulis MA, et al. Reference values for exercise limitations among adults with congenital heart disease. Relation to activities of daily life–single centre experience and review of published data. A comprehensive review of CPETstudies in more than 4400 ACHD patients. Eur Heart J. 2012;33:1386–96.

83. Tutarel O, Gabriel H, Diller GP. Exercise: friend or foe in adult congenital heart disease? Curr Cardiol Rep. 2013;15:416.

84. Dimopoulos K, Okonko DO, Diller GP, Broberg CS, Salukhe TV, Babu-Narayan SV, Li W, Uebing A, Bayne S, Wensel R, Piepoli MF, Poole-Wilson PA, Francis DP, Gatzoulis MA. Abnormal ventilatory response to exercise in adults with congenital heart disease relates to cyanosis and predicts survival. Circulation. 2006;113:2796–802.

85. Azarbal B, Hayes SW, Lewin HC, Hachamovitch R, Cohen I, Berman DS. The incremental prognostic value of percentage of heart rate reserve achieved over myocardial perfusion single-photon emission computed tomography in the prediction of cardiac death and all-cause mortality: superiority over 85 % of maximal age-predicted heart rate. J Am Coll Cardiol. 2004;44:423–30.

86. Norozi K, Wessel A, Alpers V, et al. Chronotropic incompetence in adolescents and adults with congenital heart disease after cardiac surgery. J Card Fail. 2007;13:263–8.

87. Butera G, Bonnet D, Sidi D, et al. Patients operated for tetralogy of Fallot and with non-sustained ventricular tachycardia have reduced heart rate variability. Herz. 2004;29:304–9.

88. Massin MM, Derkenne B, von Bernuth G. Correlations between indices of heart rate variability in healthy children and children with congenital heart disease. Cardiology. 1999;91:109–13.

89. McLeod KA, Hillis WS, Houston AB, et al. Reduced heart rate variability following repair of tetralogy of Fallot. Heart. 1999;81:656–60.

90. Bouchardy J, Therrien J, Pilote L, Ionescu-Ittu R, Martucci G, Bottega N, Marelli AJ. Atrial arrhythmias in adults with congenital heart disease. Circulation. 2009;120:1679–86.

91. Cordina R, O'Meagher S, Gould H, Rae C, Kemp G, Pasco JA, Celermajer DS, Singh N. Skeletal muscle abnormalities and exercise capacity in adults with a Fontan circulation. Heart. 2013;99:1530–4.

92. Brassard P, Poirier P, Martin J, et al. Impact of exercise training on muscle function and ergoreflex in Fontan patients: a pilot study. Int J Cardiol. 2006;107:85–94.

93. Greutmann M, Le TL, Tobler D, et al. Generalised muscle weakness in young adults with congenital heart disease. Heart (Br Cardiac Soc). 2011;97:1164–8.

94. Inai K, Saita Y, Takeda S, et al. Skeletal muscle hemodynamics and endothelial function in patients after Fontan operation. Am J Cardiol. 2004;93:792–7.

95. Kröönström LA, Johansson L, Zetterström AK, Dellborg M, Eriksson P, Cider Å. Muscle function in adults with congenital heart disease. Int J Cardiol. 2014;170:358–63.

96. Budts W, Börjesson M, Chessa M, van Buuren F, Trindade PT, Corrado D, Heidbuchel H, Webb G, Holm J, Papadakis M. Physical activity in adolescents and adults with congenital heart defects; individualized exercise prescription. Eur Heart J. 2013;34:3669–74.

97. Dua JS, Cooper AR, Fox KR, Graham SA. Physical activity levels in adults with congenital heart disease. Eur J Cardiovasc Prev Rehabil. 2007;14:287–93.
98. Müller J, Hess J, Hager A. Daily physical activity in adults with congenital heart disease is positively correlated with exercise capacity but not with quality of life. Clin Res Cardiol. 2012;101:55–61.
99. Sandberg C, Pomeroy J, Thilén U, Gradmark A, Wadell K, Johansson B. Habitual physical activity in adults with congenital heart disease compared with age- and sex-matched controls. Can J Cardiol. 2016;32:547e–553.
100. Tikkanen AU, Opotowsky AR, Bhatt AB, Landzberg MJ, Rhodes J. Physical activity is associated with improved aerobic exercise capacity over time in adults with congenital heart disease. Int J Cardiol. 2013;168:4685–91.
101. Inuzuka R, Diller GP, Borgia F, Benson L, Tay EL, Alonso-Gonzalez R, et al. Comprehensive use of cardiopulmonary exercise testing identifies adults with congenital heart disease at increased mortality risk in the medium term. Circulation. 2012;125:250–9.
102. Swan L, Hillis WS. Exercise prescription in adults with congenital heart disease: a long wayto go. Heart. 2000;83:685–7.
103. Gratz A, Hess J, Hager A. Self-estimated physical functioning poorly predicts actual exercise capacity in adolescents and adults with congenital heart disease. Eur Heart J. 2009;30:497–504.
104. Lunt D, Briffa T, Briffa NK, Ramsay J. Physical activity levels of adolescents with congenital heart disease. Aust J Physiother. 2003;49:43–50.
105. Piepoli MF, Conraads V, Corra U, Dickstein K, Francis DP, Jaarsm T, McMurray J, Pieske B, Piotrowicz E, Schmid JP, Anker SD, Cohen Solal A, Filippatos GS, Hoes AW, Gielen S, Giannuzzi P, Ponikowski PP. Exercise training in heart failure: from theory to practice. A consensus document of the Heart Failure Association and the European Association for Cardiovascular Prevention and Rehabilitation. Eur J Heart Fail. 2011;13:347–57.
106. Therrien J, Fredriksen P, Walker M, Granton J, Reid GJ, Webb G. A pilot study of exercise training in adult patients with repaired tetralogy of Fallot. Can J Cardiol. 2003;19:685–9.
107. Winter MM, van der Bom T, de Vries LC, Balducci A, Bouma BJ, Pieper PG, et al. Exercise training improves exercise capacity in adult patients with a systemic right ventricle: a randomized clinical trial. Eur Heart J. 2012;33:1378–85.
108. Westhoff-Bleck M, Schieffer B, Tegtbur U, Meyer GP, Hoy L, Schaefer A, Tallone EM, Tutarel O, Mertins R, Wilmink LM, Anker SD, Bauersachs J, Roentgen P. Aerobic training in adults after atrial switch procedure for transposition of the great arteries improves exercise capacity without impairing systemic right ventricular function. Int J Cardiol. 2013;170:24–9.
109. Dua JS, Cooper AR, Fox KR, Graham SA. Exercise training in adults with congenital heart disease: feasibility and benefits. Int J Cardiol. 2010;138:196–205.
110. Thaulow E, Fredriksen PM. Exercise and training in adults with congenital heart disease. Int J Cardiol. 2004;97(Suppl 1):35–8.

Case-Based Learning Cardiac Rehabilitation Pacemaker Implantation

14

P. Dendale and I. Frederix

14.1 Pacemaker Implantation

Case (Part 1)

A 55-year-old patient was admitted to the emergency department with increasing dyspnea. He had a history of mitral and aortic valve replacement (metallic prosthesis) for rheumatic stenosis 10 years earlier. Since several months, he noticed swelling of the ankles, a dry cough, and dyspnea on light exercise such as walking. He was treated with anticoagulants. Amiodarone was started 2 years earlier for paroxysmal atrial fibrillation. On admission, he was comfortable at rest, but showed clear swelling of the ankles, diminished lung sounds suggesting pleural fluid, and swelling of the jugular veins and the liver. The blood pressure was 135/85 mmHg and heart rate was regular at 47/min. Valve sounds were normal. An ECG showed slow sinus rhythm and left bundle branch block. Chest X-ray showed a slight enlargement of the heart and pleural fluid bilaterally.

An echocardiogram showed a preserved systolic function (EF of 61 %, biplane Simpson's method) and an important LV hypertrophy (IVS 1.54 cm, PW 1.51 cm, LV mass index 116 g/m², relative wall thickness (RWT) 0.53); the right ventricle was also dilated with a slight increase in pulmonary pressures (TR maxPG 38.25 mmHg) (Fig. 14.1). The mitral and aortic valve prostheses were normal, and the inferior caval vein was dilated.

The diagnosis of heart failure with preserved systolic function was made, and the patient was treated with bumetanide 2 × 1 mg and spironolactone

P. Dendale (✉)
Faculty of Medicine & Life Sciences, Hasselt University, Hasselt, Belgium
Department of Cardiology, Jessa Hospital, Hasselt, Belgium
e-mail: paul.dendale@jessazh.be

I. Frederix
Faculty of Medicine & Life Sciences, Hasselt University, Hasselt, Belgium
Department of Cardiology, Jessa Hospital, Hasselt, Belgium
Faculty of Medicine & Health Sciences, Antwerp University, Antwerp, Belgium

© Springer International Publishing AG 2017
J. Niebauer (ed.), *Cardiac Rehabilitation Manual*,
DOI 10.1007/978-3-319-47738-1_14

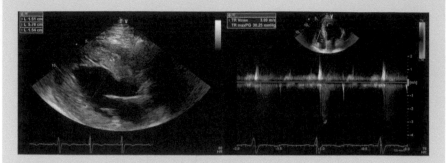

Fig. 14.1 Transthoracic echocardiography. *Left*: parasternal long axis view (1, IVSd; 2, LVEDD; 3, PWd). *Right*: apical four-chamber view

Table 14.1 Maximal cardiopulmonary exercise test results before and after cardiac rehabilitation

	Before rehabilitation	After rehabilitation
Heart rate max	55/min (33 % pred)	59/min (36 % pred)
Load max	80 watt	90 watt
VO2 max	15 ml/kg/min (55 % pred)	16.5 ml/kg/min (61 % pred)
RER max	1.22	1.26
Anaerobic threshold	50 watt	60 watt
VE/VCO2 slope	38	38
Breathing reserve	58 %	60 %

Note: Breathing reserve was calculated as VE max/MVV (MVV = 40 × FEV1). *VE* minute ventilation, *MVV* maximal voluntary ventilation, *FEV1* forced expiratory volume in 1 s. *VO2* oxygen uptake, *RER* respiratory exchange ratio

25 mg and lost more than 6 kg of fluid. He was discharged in NYHA II–III and referred to cardiac rehabilitation.

During the initial visit at the beginning of cardiac rehabilitation, the patient was depressed and anxious, and he worried a lot about his future and the future of his family and his work. He was working full time as a technical engineer before he was admitted for heart failure. His work required moderate physical activity. An exercise test showed a VO2 max of 15 ml/kg/min (55 % pred), with a heart rate staying at around 50–55/min up to maximal exercise. A rehabilitation program was started, consisting of 45-min moderate continuous exercise training sessions between the patient's 1st and 2nd ventilatory threshold for 3 times a week, as well as psychological counselling.

After 3 months of training, the patient remained dyspneic, and his control cardiopulmonary exercise test showed an increase of VO2 max to only 16.5 ml/kg/min (Table 14.1).

Question

What are possible reasons for the lack of influence of rehabilitation on his feeling of dyspnea:

1. Hyperventilation
2. Lack of muscle mass or muscular strength
3. Pulmonary hypertension
4. Chronotropic incompetence

Answer

All four possible explanations may play a role in limiting exercise capacity after rehabilitation in this patient:

- Anxiety and hyperventilation are frequently found in patients with heart failure: a possible clue to this problem is often found when patients do not support the face mask of the ergospirometry. A history of claustrophobia is also often present in these patients. Psychological counselling and breathing control exercises can reduce the anxiety and increase the feeling of control for the patient
- Peripheral muscle atrophy is very common in heart failure, due to disuse, but also to the inflammatory state that often accompanies this pathology. Exercise tolerance and quality of life in heart failure patients are more related to peripheral muscle function than to ejection fraction. Testing and training of the large muscle groups is more and more standard in rehabilitation programs for severe heart failure.
- Respiratory muscle weakness is often present in heart failure and after cardiac surgery. Strength training of the respiratory muscles (inspiratory muscle strength training) was shown to be almost as efficient as endurance training in increasing exercise capacity in severe heart failure.
- The pulmonary artery pressure was slightly elevated at rest, but it is well known that exercise can increase the pulmonary artery pressure importantly in these patients. A sign suggesting that pulmonary hypertension may play a role is the evolution of the VE/VCO2 slope, which in this patient was increased to 38. Exercise echocardiography may allow quantification of the pulmonary artery pressures and confirm exercise-induced pulmonary hypertension, thereby explaining part of the patient's symptoms. Prior research indicates exercise training to be effective in improving pulmonary hypertension patients' exercise capacity, functional class, and quality of life [1]. However, more clinical trials and research are required to assess the effects of different types of exercise programs (including aerobic exercise training, resistance training, inspiratory muscle training, or a combination).
- Chronotropic incompetence, especially in patients with a relatively fixed cardiac output due to the presence of two artificial valves, may also play a role in his dyspnea. In the patient presented in this case, the CPET was maximal during both tests (RER max of 1.22 and 1.26, respectively); however, heart rate max < 85 % pred for age (220 − age = 220–55 = 165; 165 × 85 % = 140) confirms the presence of chronotropic incompetence in the absence of bradycardia-inducing therapy.

Case (Part 2)

A DDDR pacemaker was implanted (indication: persistent symptomatic sinus node, disease type chronotropic incompetence, IIb indication [2]), programmed at a lower rate of 65/min, and a high intensity interval training (HIT) program was prescribed (10-min warm-up, repeating intervals of 4 min at Borg 15 and 3 min at Borg 10, 5-min cool-down), three times a week. Also, the patient was seen individually by the psychologist for breathing control exercises.

After 6 weeks, the patient was scheduled for a follow-up visit with the cardiologist. There he mentioned persistent reduced exercise capacity and dyspnea on exertion NYHA II. Clinical investigation reveals no signs indicative of cardiac decompensation. The patient's blood pressure (123/84 mmHg) and pulse (65/min, regular rhythm) were within normal limits. The results of the performed maximal cardiopulmonary exercise test are shown in Table 14.2.

Table 14.2 Cardiopulmonary exercise test results both before and after pacemaker implantation

	Before PM implantation	After PM implantation
Heart rate max	59/min (36 % pred)	65/min (39 %)
Load max	90 watt	100 watt
VO2 max	16.5 ml/kg/min (61 % pred)	17 ml/kg/min (63 %)
RER max	1.26	1.21
Anaerobic threshold	60 watt	70 watt
VE/VCO2 slope	38	23
Breathing reserve	60 %	65 %

VO2 oxygen uptake, *RER* respiratory exchange ratio
Note: electrocardiographic monitoring during the cardiopulmonary exercise test showed a sustained paced rhythm (65/min), morphologically compatible with monochamber RV apical pacing (left superior axis, rS in V1)

Question

Based on the results of the cardiopulmonary exercise test, what is the most probable cause for the patient's symptoms and rather limited improvement in aerobic capacity?

Answer

The results indicate the cardiopulmonary exercise test to be maximal (RER max 1.21), without ventilatory limitation. The patient's aerobic capacity still remained suboptimal. Electrocardiographic recordings show persistent RV apical pacing at 65/min without clear rate response (although the pacemaker was programmed in DDDR mode). As the pacemaker activity sensor is often more responsive to exercise when the body moves significantly, an exercise test on the treadmill was subsequently performed: in our patient it showed an increase of pacing rate to a maximum of 82/min. Reprogramming of the pacemaker was done by increasing the sensitivity of the activity sensor, and the patient was tested again on the bicycle and the treadmill. Maximal heart rate now rose up to 98/min (59 % pred) on the bicycle and 115/min (70 % pred) on the treadmill. The patient was now able to increase significantly the training load, and a control exercise test showed a significant increase in exercise capacity (VO2 max 23 ml/kg/min, 85 % pred). The patient returned to work after 6 more weeks of rehabilitation.

The rehabilitation program is ideally suited to optimize the settings of the pacemaker. In most cases, at the pacemaker clinic, only the resting values are checked. When the patient is relatively young and physically active, a test during treadmill exercise will nicely demonstrate if a sufficient chronotropic response is present. To know how the sensors react, it is important to know which sensor is used in a particular pacemaker [3–7]. Accelerometers are the most common type of sensor. They will react poorly to an exercise test on the bicycle, and even the treadmill will not always stimulate this sensor optimally. Contemporary pacemakers have a rate response option, based on input signals from multiple sensors (activity sensor/accelerometer, minute ventilation sensor, QT sensor). Repeated pacemaker controls with exercise testing on the treadmill can be necessary to find the optimal settings.

Case (Part 3)

After returning to work, the patient was requested to come regularly to the cardiology department for follow-up (both for his HFpEF and for pacemaker control). The patient however moved and now had very busy professional commitments due to a recent promotion, thereby making it difficult to attend all scheduled appointments. Can we provide the patient with follow-up without necessitating him to come for in-clinic visits?

Follow-up of pacemaker function and of physical activity from a distance can now be done by telemonitoring [8]. Patients with implantable devices such as pacemakers (especially when in combination with heart failure) should be followed up every 3–12 months, which traditionally required in-clinic visits. Latest-generation devices allow data transmission and technical or medical alerts to be sent from the patient's home to the physician (remote monitoring, i.e., telemonitoring). A number of studies have shown its effectiveness in timely detection and management of both clinical and technical events and endorsed its adoption [9, 10]. As a consequence the European Society of Cardiology (ESC) has integrated remote implantable device monitoring in its guidelines (Class IIa indication) [2]. The role of activity monitoring in long-term follow-up or home rehabilitation using these data is still to be investigated.

Conclusion

The rehabilitation of patients presenting with symptoms of heart failure requires a truly multidisciplinary approach: deconditioning, fear of physical activity, post-traumatic stress in patients who were hospitalized with acute pulmonary edema, sleep apnea, weight loss and cachexia, etc., all contribute to the reduction in quality of life in these patients. A cardiac rehabilitation program consisting of patient-tailored exercise prescription (based on primary pathology, present comorbidities, and exercise modifiers), education, and psychological support is needed.

Even though the implantation of a pacemaker is not considered a routine indication for cardiac rehabilitation, this case shows that in active patients, interesting and important information can be gathered during the exercise program. In contrast to the normal pacemaker follow-up, where only resting data are often considered, the rehabilitation program gives the opportunity to fine-tune the pacemaker programming. At the start of a cardiac rehabilitation program, a maximal exercise test on the bicycle and on the treadmill should be performed in pacemaker-dependent patients, to analyze the response of the pacemaker to exercise. The further follow-up of patients with implanted devices is nowadays possible by remote monitoring, not necessitating patients to come for in-clinic visits.

References

1. Babu AS, Padmakumar R, Maiya AG, Mohapatra AK, Kamath RL. Effects of exercise training on exercise capacity in pulmonary arterial hypertension: a systematic review of clinical trials. Heart Lung Circ. 2016;25:333–41.
2. Auricchio A, Baron-Esquivias G, Bordachar P, et al. 2013 ESC guidelines on cardiac pacing and cardiac resynchronization therapy. Eur Heart J. 2013;34:2281–329.
3. Coman J, Freedman R, Koplan BA, Reeves R, Santucci P, Stolen KQ, Kraus SM, Meyer TE. A blended sensor restores chronotropic response more favorably than an accelerometer alone in pacemaker patients: the LIFE study results. Pacing Clin Electrophysiol. 2008;31(11):1433–42.
4. Erol-Yilmaz A, Tukkie R, De Boo J, Schrama T, Wilde A. Direct comparison of a contractility and activity pacemaker sensor during treadmill exercise testing. Pacing Clin Electrophysiol. 2004;27(11):1493–9.
5. Haennel RG, Logan T, Dunne C, Burgess J, Busse E. Effects of sensor selection on exercise stroke volume in pacemaker dependent patients. Pacing Clin Electrophysiol. 1998;21(9):1700–8.
6. Carmouche DG, Bubien RS, Kay GN. The effect of maximum heart rate on oxygen kinetics and exercise performance at low and high workloads. Pacing Clin Electrophysiol. 1998;21(4 Pt 1):679–86.
7. Candinas R, Jakob M, Buckingham TA, Mattmann H, Amann FW. Vibration, acceleration, gravitation, and movement: activity controlled rate adaptive pacing during treadmill exercise testing and daily life activities. Pacing Clin Electrophysiol. 1997;20(7):1777–86.
8. Dario C, Delise P, Gubian L, Saccavini C, Brandolino G, Mancin S. Large controlled observational study on remote monitoring of pacemakers and implantable cardiac defibrillators: a clinical, economic, and organizational evaluation. Interact J Med Res. 2016;5(1):e4.
9. Mabo P, Victor F, Bazin P, Ahres S, Babuty D, Da CA, Binet D, Daubert J. A randomized trial of long-term remote monitoring of pacemaker recipients (the COMPAS trial). Eur Heart J. 2012;33:1105–11.
10. Halimi F, Jacques C, Attuel P, Dessenne X, Amara W. Optimized post-operative surveillance of permanent pacemakers by home monitoring: The OEDIPE trial. Europace. 2008;10:1392–9.

Case-Based Learning: Patient with Peripheral Artery Disease

15

Jean-Paul Schmid

15.1 Clinical Information

A 75-year-old male was addressed to the outpatient cardiac rehabilitation clinic for a supervised exercise training programme and risk factor intervention due to symptoms of intermittent claudication. He is known for bilateral peripheral artery disease (PAD) stage II according to the Fontaine classification (cf. Table 15.1) for 3 years due to a high-grade stenosis of the arteria femoralis superficialis on the left side, treated conservatively until now. Initially, symptoms were present on the left side only, but 1 year ago, they appeared also at the right side, where they actually predominate.

Table 15.1 Classification of peripheral artery disease: Fontaine stages

I	Pathological finding at physical examination; patient without symptoms, also during exercise
II	Claudication intermittents: symptoms during exercise
IIa	Pain-free walking distance, > 200 m
IIb	Pain-free walking distance, < 200 m
III	Pain at rest: mostly during the night, relieve of pain by position change or getting up
IV	Acral lesion, gangrene

What is the evidence regarding a supervised or non-supervised exercise training programme with risk factor intervention in patients with lower extremity PAD?

J.-P. Schmid
Department of Cardiology, Tiefenau Hospital, Bern, Switzerland
e-mail: jean-paul.schmid@spitaltiefenau.ch

© Springer International Publishing AG 2017
J. Niebauer (ed.), *Cardiac Rehabilitation Manual*,
DOI 10.1007/978-3-319-47738-1_15

- A programme of supervised exercise training is recommended as an initial treatment modality for patients with intermittent claudication (Class I, Level of Evidence: A) [1, 2].
- Supervised exercise training should be performed for a minimum of 30–45 min, in sessions performed at least three times per week for a minimum of 12 weeks (Class I, Level of Evidence: A) [3]. The usefulness of unsupervised exercise programmes is not well established as an effective initial treatment modality for patients with intermittent claudication (Class IIb, Level of Evidence: B) [3]; however, non-supervised exercise therapy is indicated when supervised exercise therapy is not feasible or available [1].

Twelve years ago, the patient was also diagnosed a three-vessel coronary artery disease and had to undergo coronary artery bypass surgery with a left internal mammarial artery–left anterior descending artery graft and venous grafts on the right coronary artery, circumflex artery and the first diagonal branch of the left anterior descending artery. Figure 15.1 shows the ECG at rest. The left ventricle at that time showed a concentric hypertrophy with an infero-lateral hypokinesia and a slightly reduced left ventricular systolic function with an ejection fraction of 48 %. Actually, the patient does not complain about cardiac symptoms. An exercise stress test 3 years ago was electrically positive but clinically negative.

As further diagnosis, arthrosis of the left knee with condition after meniscectomy 5 years ago and a condition after hip replacement on the right side due to coxarthrosis 15 years ago are known.

Cardiovascular Risk Factors Arterial hypertension treated for more than 30 years, dyslipidaemia (treated since 12 years), condition after smoking (stopped 12 years ago, 40 pack-years)

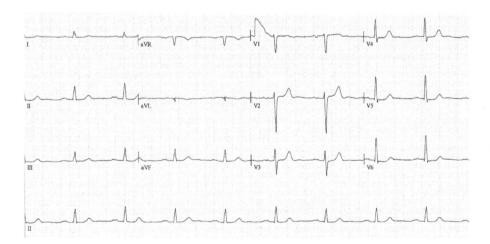

Fig. 15.1 Resting ECG. Sinus rhythm, 60/min

The results of a screening blood sample are as follows: glucose, 5.2 mmol/L (94 mg/dL); total cholesterol, 4.9 mmol/L (190 mg/dL); LDL-C, 3.4 mmol/L (130 mg/dL); HDL-C, 0.9 mmol/L (35 mg/dL); and triglycerides, 1.2 mmol/L (105 mg/dL).

Actual Medication   Aspirin 100 mg/d, lisinopril/hydrochlorothiazide 20/12,5 mg/d, nebivolol 10 mg/d, simvastatin 40 mg/d

> What are the key points of history taking in a patient with PAD?

- Is there any exertional limitation quickly relieved at rest of the lower extremity muscles or any history of walking impairment, i.e. fatigue, aching, numbness or pain?
- Any pain at rest localized to the lower leg or foot and its association with the upright or recumbent positions?
- Primary site(s) of discomfort: buttock, thigh, calf or foot?
- Upper extremity exertional pain, particularly if associated with dizziness or vertigo?
- Any transient or permanent neurological symptoms?
- History of hypertension or renal failure?
- Post-prandial abdominal pain and diarrhoea, particularly if related to eating and associated with weight loss?
- Erectile dysfunction?

15.2   Clinical Assessment

75-year-old patient in good general condition, obese (172 cm, 90 kg, BMI 30.4 kg/m^2). The patient describes classical intermittent claudication with crampy pain of his right calf. The pain-free walking distance in the plain is between 200 and 300 m; in uphill, symptoms occur already after 50–100 m.

Cardiopulmonary auscultation is normal. Blood pressure is 130/75 mmHg on both sides. Heart rate is 60/min., regular. Hip flexion at the right side is limited. No blood flow murmurs are noted over the carotid, subclavian, ilio-femoral or renal arteries. Palpation of the abdominal aorta is normal.

The pulse over the femoral arteries was palpable at both sides, attenuated on the right. Distally, only the posterior tibialis artery on the left side was weakly palpable (c.f. Fig. 15.3). The other examination findings were normal, especially no skin lesions of the legs or feet.

> What are the key points of the clinical assessment of a patient with PAD?

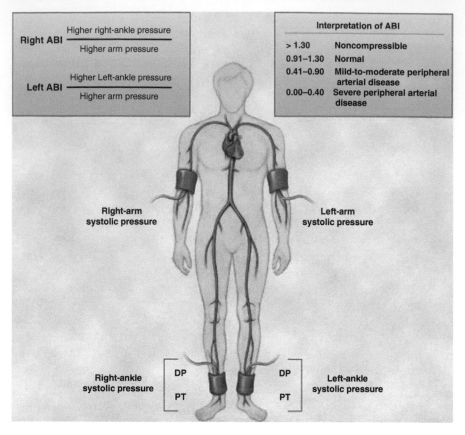

Right ABI = (Higher right-ankle pressure) / (Higher arm pressure)

Left ABI = (Higher Left-ankle pressure) / (Higher arm pressure)

Interpretation of ABI

> 1.30	Noncompressible
0.91–1.30	Normal
0.41–0.90	Mild-to-moderate peripheral arterial disease
0.00–0.40	Severe peripheral arterial disease

Right-arm systolic pressure

Left-arm systolic pressure

Right-ankle systolic pressure — DP, PT

Left-ankle systolic pressure — DP, PT

Fig. 15.2 Measurement of the ankle–brachial index (*ABI*). Systolic blood pressure is measured by Doppler ultrasonography in each arm and in the dorsalis pedis (*DP*) and posterior tibial (*PT*) arteries in each ankle [4]

- Measurement of bilateral arm BP, auscultation and palpation of the cervical and supraclavicular fossae areas, peripheral arteries and abdominal aorta with annotation of any bruits and inspection of the feet for trophic defects.
- Any poorly healing wounds of legs or feet?
- Reduced muscle mass, strength and endurance?
- Ankle–brachial index measurement (cf. Fig. 15.2).
- Functional capacity?

The oscillogram measured at the big toe shows a moderately abnormal graph with a flat peak, an equal upslope and downslope time and a missing dicrotic notch. This finding is confirmed by the ABI which is 0.77 on the right side and 0.92 on the left side (c.f. Fig. 15.3).

How is the ABI correctly measured and which are the pathologic ranges?

ABI Measurement (Fig. 15.2): Systolic blood pressure is measured by Doppler ultrasonography in each arm and in the dorsalis pedis and posterior tibial arteries in each ankle [4]. The higher of the two arm pressures is selected, as is the higher of the two pressures in each ankle. The right and left ankle–brachial index values are determined by dividing the higher ankle pressure in each leg by the higher arm pressure [5]. The ranges of the ankle–brachial index values are shown, with a ratio greater than 1.30 suggesting a non-compressible, calcified vessel. In this condition, the true pressure at that location cannot be obtained, and additional tests are required to diagnose peripheral arterial disease. Patients with claudication typically have ankle–brachial index values ranging from 0.41 to 0.90, and those with critical leg ischaemia have values of 0.40 or less.

Segmental limb plethysmographic waveform analysis is based on evaluation of waveform shape and signal amplitude (Figs. 15.4 and 15.5). Standardized criteria relating waveform changes to anatomic site and hemodynamic severity of disease are used in diagnostic interpretation. Pulse volume recordings are typically performed by injecting a standard volume of air into pneumatic cuffs. The volume of air injected into the cuff is enough to occlude the venous circulation but does not occlude the arterial circulation. Volume changes in the limb segment below the cuff

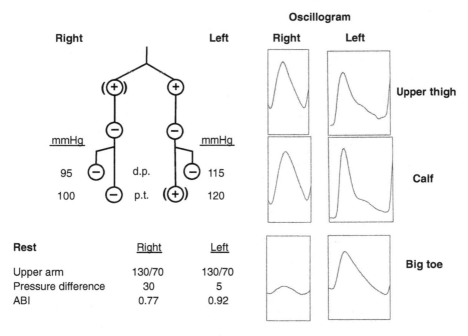

Fig. 15.3 Measurement of the ankle–brachial index and arterial pulse volume plethysmography (oscillogram) of the 75-year-old patient with intermittent claudication, Fontaine stage IIa

Normal
- Sharp upstroke
- Scooped or flat interval between peaks   **Low thigh**
- Possible dicrotic notch

Mildly abnormal
- Sharp upstroke
- No flat period or scooping between peaks   **Ankle**
- No dicrotic notch

Moderately abnormal
- Flat peak
- Equal upslope and downslope time   **Calf**
- No dicrotic notch

Severely abnormal
- Flat peak
- Equal upslope and downslope time   **Calf**
- No dicrotic notch
- Low amplitude

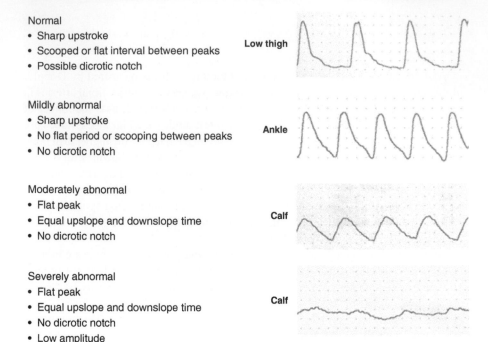

Fig. 15.4 Pulse volume plethysmography: Pulse volume recording contour with increasing vascular disease severity [14]

are translated into a pulsatile pressure, which is detected by a transducer and then displayed by a pressure pulse contour.

A normal pulse volume recording, similar to the arterial waveform, is composed of a systolic upstroke with a sharp systolic peak followed by a downstroke that contains a prominent dicrotic notch. If a haemodynamically significant stenosis is present, dissipation of energy occurs because of arterial narrowing; this is reflected in a change in the pulse volume recording contour, indicating a proximal arterial obstruction. The amount of variation in the pulse volume recording contour is reflective of disease severity, as shown in Fig. 15.4.

15.3 Functional Capacity

For assessment of the functional capacity and possible exercise-induced ischaemia, a symptom-limited exercise stress test on a bicycle (15 W/min. Ramp protocol) was effectuated. The patient performed 102 W, corresponding to 74 % of the predicted value. Blood pressure increased from 130/75 mmHg to 190/80 mmHg, heart rate from 60/min. up to 117/min. (80 % of the predicted). Rate pressure product was 22′230. The reason for test termination was right calf pain. The test was clinically and electrically negative (Fig. 15.6).

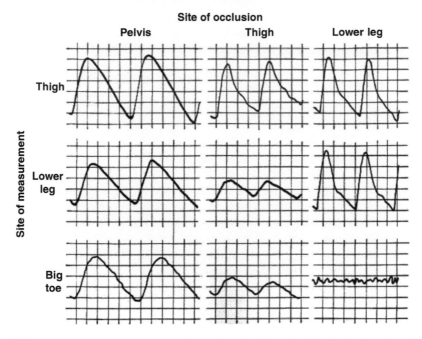

Fig. 15.5 Pulse volume plethysmography: Determination of the site of occlusion by pulse volume plethysmography

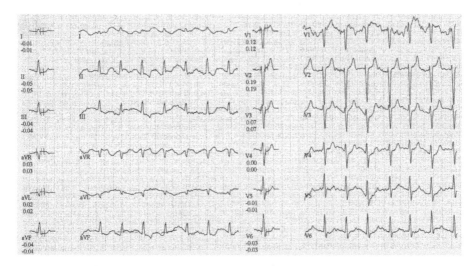

Fig. 15.6 ECG at maximal exercise of a symptom-limited exercise stress test

On a treadmill test with fixed speed (3.2 km/h) and slope (10 %), the pain-free walking distance was 134 m, the maximal walking distance 210 m, limited by claudication of the right calf.

> What is the usefulness of assessment of the functional capacity and exercise testing in PAD patients and which are the appropriate tests?

The roles of exercise testing in PAD patients are the following:

(a) Excluding occult coronary artery disease, monitoring symptoms, ST–T wave changes, arrhythmias, heart rate and blood pressure responses.
(b) Establishing the diagnosis of lower extremity PAD when resting measures of the ABI are normal.
(c) Objectively document the magnitude of symptom limitation in patients with lower extremity PAD and claudication.
(d) Objectively measure the functional improvement obtained in response to claudication interventions.
(e) Differentiate claudication from pseudoclaudication in individuals with exertional leg symptoms.
(f) Provide objective data that can demonstrate the safety of exercise and to individualize exercise prescriptions in patients with claudication before initiation of a formal programme of exercise training.

The recommendations of ACC/AHA practice guidelines for the management of patients with peripheral arterial disease concerning exercise testing are the following:

• Exercise treadmill tests are recommended to provide the most objective evidence of the magnitude of the functional limitation of claudication and to measure the response to therapy (Class I, Level of Evidence: B).
• A standardized exercise protocol (either fixed or graded) with a motorized treadmill should be used to ensure reproducibility of measurements of pain-free walking distance and maximal walking distance (Class I, Level of Evidence: B).
• Exercise treadmill tests with measurement of preexercise and postexercise ABI values are recommended to provide diagnostic data useful in differentiating arterial claudication from nonarterial claudication ("pseudoclaudication") (Class I, Level of Evidence: B).
• Exercise treadmill tests should be performed in individuals with claudication who are to undergo exercise training (lower extremity PAD rehabilitation) so as to determine functional capacity, assess nonvascular exercise limitations and demonstrate the safety of exercise. (Class I, Level of Evidence: B).
• A 6-min walk test may be reasonable to provide an objective assessment of the functional limitation of claudication and response to therapy in elderly

individuals or others not amenable to treadmill testing (Class IIb, Level of Evidence: B).

The patient attended regularly the exercise training programme during 12 weeks, three times a week without complication.

What are the key elements of a therapeutic exercise-training programme for rehabilitation from PAD in patients with claudication [6]?

15.3.1 Warm-up and cool-down

• Periods of 5–10 min each.

15.3.2 Types of Exercise

• Treadmill and track walking are the most effective.
• Resistance training has benefit for patients with other forms of cardiovascular disease, and its use, as tolerated, for general fitness is complementary to walking but not a substitute for it.

15.3.3 Intensity

• The initial workload of the treadmill is set to a speed and grade that elicits claudication symptoms within 3–5 min.
• Patients walk at this workload until claudication of moderate severity occurs and then rest standing or sitting for a brief period to permit symptoms to subside.

15.3.4 Duration

• The exercise–rest–exercise pattern should be repeated throughout the exercise session.
• The initial session will usually include 35 min. of intermittent walking; walking is increased by 5 min each session until 50 min of intermittent walking can be accomplished.

15.3.5 Frequency

• Treadmill or track walking 3–5 times per week.

15.3.6 Role of Direct Supervision

- As the patient's walking ability improves, the exercise workload should be increased by modifying the treadmill grade or speed (or both) to ensure that the stimulus of claudication pain always occurs during the workout.
- As walking ability improves, and a higher HR is reached, there is the possibility that cardiac signs and symptoms may appear. These symptoms should be appropriately diagnosed and treated.

Six weeks after the start, the patient noted the first clinical benefits, and at the end of the programme, he was able to walk 400 to 500 m without rest in the plain. In the standardized treadmill test, pain-free walking distance had increased from 134 to 198 m and the maximal walking distance from 210 to 324 m.

> What range of improvement can be expected from an exercise training?

The positive effects of a formal exercise-training programme for claudication have been demonstrated in many randomized trials [7]. Exercise improves not only maximal treadmill walking distance but also health-related quality of life and community-based functional capacity (i.e. the ability to walk at defined speeds and for defined distances). Girolami et al. [8] reported in a meta-analysis of randomized trials that exercise training increased maximal treadmill walking distance by 179 m (95 % CI 60 to 298). This degree of improvement should translate into longer walking distances on level ground. In another meta-analysis, Gardner et al. [9] showed that exercise training improved pain-free walking time in patients with claudication by an average of 180 % percent and improved maximal walking time by an average of 120 %. A meta-analysis from the Cochrane Collaboration that considered only randomized, controlled trials concluded that exercise improved maximal walking time by an average of 150 % (range, 74–230 %).

The time course of the response to a programme of exercise has not been fully established. Clinical benefits have been observed as early as 4 weeks after the initiation of exercise and may continue to accrue after 6 months of participation [10]. Improvements in walking ability after 6 months of supervised exercise rehabilitation three times per week were sustained when patients continued to participate in an exercise maintenance programme for an additional 12 months [11].

15.4   Risk factor Management

PAD is part of the multisite disease atherosclerosis. An integrated approach to prevention and treatment of atherothrombosis as a whole is therefore highly warranted. After the programme, blood pressure was well controlled with values around 130/80 mmHg, measured regularly at the beginning of each exercise session. To improve lipid control, simvastatin was substituted with rosuvastatin 10 mg and ezetimibe was added. At the end of the programme, total cholesterol was 3.9 mmol/L (150 mg/dL), LDL-C was 1.9 mmol/L (75 mg/dL), HDL-C was 1.1 mmol/L (40 mg/dL) and triglycerides were 1.1 mmol/L (100 mg/dL). The improvement in the walking distance enabled the patient to be much more active in his daily activities, and he is willing to continue his efforts after having resumed the exercise programme.

What are the recommendations concerning risk factor management in PAD patients [1, 3, 12]?

15.4.1 Smoking

- Aggressive smoking cessation efforts constitute one of the most important interventions a physician can make in caring for patients with PAD.
- Individuals with lower extremity PAD who smoke cigarettes or use other forms of tobacco should be advised to stop smoking and should be offered comprehensive smoking cessation interventions, including behaviour modification therapy, nicotine replacement therapy, or bupropion/vareniclin (Class I, Level of Evidence: B) [1, 3].

15.4.2 Physical Activity

- Exercise activities, such as walking, lasting >30 min, ≥3 times/week, until near-maximal pain, are recommended.
- A supervised hospital- or clinic-based exercise training programme, which ensures that patients are receiving a standardised exercise stimulus in a safe environment, is effective and recommended as initial treatment modality for all patients (Class I, Level of Evidence: A).
- Supervised exercise training should be performed for a minimum of 30 to 45 min, in sessions performed at least three times per week for a minimum of 12 weeks (Class I, Level of Evidence: A).
- No data to support the efficacy of the informal "go home and walk" advice and the usefulness of unsupervised ET programmes is uncertain (Class IIb, Level of Evidence: B).

15.4.3 Lipid Control

- The optimization of the lipid profile in PAD patients leads to reductions in mortality and vascular events and may improve symptoms of intermittent claudication and functional capacity.
- All patients with PAD should have their serum LDL cholesterol reduced to <100 mg/dL (2.6 mmol/L, Class I, Level of evidence B). In high-risk patients, LDL should be reduced to < 70 mg/dL (1.8 mmol/L) or ≥50 % LDL cholesterol

reduction when the target level cannot be reached (Class IIa, Level of Evidence: B) [1]. High-risk patients are considered to be individuals with (a) multiple major risk factors (especially diabetes), (b) severe and poorly controlled risk factors (especially continued cigarette smoking) and (c) multiple risk factors of the metabolic syndrome.

- Fibrates may play an important role in patients with low serum HDL (< 40 mg/dL or 1.0 mmol/L) or high serum triglyceride concentrations (>150 mg/dL or 1.7 mmol/L, Class IIa, Level of Evidence: C) [3].

15.4.4 Hypertension

- Individuals with PAD should receive hypertension treatment according to current national guidelines. A blood pressure < 140/90 mmHg or if comorbidities, diabetes or chronic renal disease are present, a target blood pressure < 130/80 mm Hg should be aimed (Class I, Level of Evidence: A) [3].
- Only major reductions in perfusion pressure may worsen claudication.
- ß-Blockers are not contraindicated in patients with PAD and should be considered in the case of concomitant coronary artery disease and/or heart failure [1, 13].

15.4.5 Diabetes

- Proper foot care, including use of appropriate footwear, chiropody/podiatric medicine, daily foot inspection, skin cleansing and use of topical moisturizing creams, should be encouraged, and skin lesions and ulcerations should be addressed urgently in all patients with diabetes and lower extremity PAD (Class I, Level of Evidence: B) [3].
- In patients with PAD and diabetes, the HbA1c level should be kept at ≤6.5 % (Class I, Level of Evidence: C) [1].

References

1. European Stroke Organisation, Tendera M, Aboyans V, Bartelink ML, Baumgartner I, Clement D, Collet JP, Cremonesi A, De Carlo M, Erbel R, Fowkes FG, Heras M, Kownator S, Minar E, Ostergren J, Poldermans D, Riambau V, Roffi M, Rother J, Sievert H, van Sambeek M, Zeller T, Guidelines ESCCfP. ESC Guidelines on the diagnosis and treatment of peripheral artery diseases: Document covering atherosclerotic disease of extracranial carotid and vertebral, mesenteric, renal, upper and lower extremity arteries: the task force on the diagnosis and treatment of peripheral artery diseases of the European Society of Cardiology (ESC). Eur Heart J. 2011;32:2851–906.

2. Bendermacher BL, Willigendael EM, Teijink JA, Prins MH. Supervised exercise therapy versus non-supervised exercise therapy for intermittent claudication. Cochrane Database Syst Rev. 2006;19:CD005263.
3. Anderson JL, Halperin JL, Albert NM, Bozkurt B, Brindis RG, Curtis LH, DeMets D, Guyton RA, Hochman JS, Kovacs RJ, Ohman EM, Pressler SJ, Sellke FW, Shen WK. Management of patients with peripheral artery disease (compilation of 2005 and 2011 ACCF/AHA guideline recommendations): a report of the American College of Cardiology Foundation/American Heart Association Task Force on Practice Guidelines. Circulation. 2013;127:1425–43.
4. Hiatt WR. Medical treatment of peripheral arterial disease and claudication. N Engl J Med. 2001;344:1608–21.
5. Orchard TJ, Strandness Jr DE. Assessment of peripheral vascular disease in diabetes. Report and recommendations of an international workshop sponsored by the American Diabetes Association and the American Heart Association September 18-20, 1992 New Orleans, Louisiana. Circulation. 1993;88:819–28.
6. Stewart KJ, Hiatt WR, Regensteiner JG, Hirsch AT. Exercise training for claudication. N Engl J Med. 2002;347:1941–51.
7. Nehler MR, Hiatt WR. Exercise therapy for claudication. Ann Vasc Surg. 1999;13:109–14.
8. Girolami B, Bernardi E, Prins MH, Ten Cate JW, Hettiarachchi R, Prandoni P, Girolami A, Buller HR. Treatment of intermittent claudication with physical training, smoking cessation, pentoxifylline, or nafronyl: a meta-analysis. Arch Intern Med. 1999;159:337–45.
9. Gardner AW, Poehlman ET. Exercise rehabilitation programs for the treatment of claudication pain A meta-analysis. JAMA. 1995;274:975–80.
10. Gibellini R, Fanello M, Bardile AF, Salerno M, Aloi T. Exercise training in intermittent claudication. Int Angiol. 2000;19:8–13.
11. Gardner AW, Katzel LI, Sorkin JD, Goldberg AP. Effects of long-term exercise rehabilitation on claudication distances in patients with peripheral arterial disease: a randomized controlled trial. J Cardiopulm Rehabil. 2002;22:192–8.
12. Hirsch AT, Haskal ZJ, Hertzer NR, Bakal CW, Creager MA, Halperin JL, Hiratzka LF, Murphy WR, Olin JW, Puschett JB, Rosenfield KA, Sacks D, Stanley JC, Taylor Jr LM, White CJ, White J, White RA, Antman EM, Smith Jr SC, Adams CD, Anderson JL, Faxon DP, Fuster V, Gibbons RJ, Hunt SA, Jacobs AK, Nishimura R, Ornato JP, Page RL, Riegel B. ACC/AHA 2005 practice guidelines for the management of patients with peripheral arterial disease (lower extremity, renal, mesenteric, and abdominal aortic): a collaborative report from the American Association for Vascular Surgery/Society for Vascular Surgery, Society for Cardiovascular Angiography and Interventions, Society for Vascular Medicine and Biology, Society of Interventional Radiology, and the ACC/AHA Task Force on Practice Guidelines (Writing Committee to Develop Guidelines for the Management of Patients With Peripheral Arterial Disease): endorsed by the American Association of Cardiovascular and Pulmonary Rehabilitation; National Heart, Lung, and Blood Institute; Society for Vascular Nursing; TransAtlantic Inter-Society Consensus; and Vascular Disease Foundation. Circulation. 2006;113:e463–654.
13. Radack K, Deck C. Beta-adrenergic blocker therapy does not worsen intermittent claudication in subjects with peripheral arterial disease. A meta-analysis of randomized controlled trials. Arch Intern Med. 1991;151:1769–76.
14. Gerhard-Herman M, Gardin JM, Jaff M, Mohler E, Roman M, Naqvi TZ. Guidelines for non-invasive vascular laboratory testing: a report from the American Society of Echocardiography and the Society for Vascular Medicine and Biology. Vasc Med. 2006;11:183–200.

Index

© Springer International Publishing AG 2017
J. Niebauer (ed.), *Cardiac Rehabilitation Manual*,
DOI 10.1007/978-3-319-47738-1

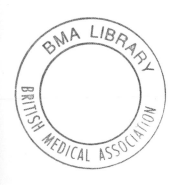